WHAT YOUR
DOCTOR MAY *NOT*
TELL YOU ABOUT
FIBROMYALGIA

WHAT YOUR DOCTOR MAY *NOT* TELL YOU ABOUT

FIBROMYALGIA

The Revolutionary Treatment
That Can Reverse the Disease

4th Edition

R. PAUL ST. AMAND, MD, AND CLAUDIA CRAIG MAREK

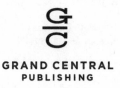

GRAND CENTRAL
PUBLISHING

NEW YORK   BOSTON

Grand Central Publishing
Hachette Book Group
1290 Avenue of the Americas, New York, NY 10104
grandcentralpublishing.com
twitter.com/grandcentralpub

First Edition: May 2019

Grand Central Publishing is a division of Hachette Book Group, Inc. The Grand Central Publishing name and logo is a trademark of Hachette Book Group, Inc.

The publisher is not responsible for websites (or their content) that are not owned by the publisher.

The Hachette Speakers Bureau provides a wide range of authors for speaking events. To find out more, go to www.hachettespeakersbureau.com or call (866) 376-6591.

Library of Congress Cataloging-in-Publication Data

Names: St. Amand, R. Paul, author. | Marek, Claudia, author.
Title: What your doctor may not tell you about fibromyalgia : the revolutionary treatment that can reverse the disease / R. Paul St. Amand, MD, and Claudia Craig Marek.
Description: Fourth edition. | New York : Grand Central Publishing, [2019] | Includes bibliographical references and index.
Identifiers: LCCN 2018044762| ISBN 9781538713259 (trade pbk.) | ISBN 9781538764411 (ebook)
Subjects: LCSH: Fibromyalgia—Popular works. | Fibromyalgia—Treatment—Popular works.
Classification: LCC RC927.3 .S73 2019 | DDC 616.7/42—dc23
LC record available at https://lccn.loc.gov/2018044762

ISBNs: 978-1-5387-1325-9 (trade pbk.), 978-1-5387-6441-1 (ebook)

Printed in the United States of America

LSC-C

10 9 8 7 6 5 4 3 2 1

CONTENTS

PREFACE

So here we are at a fourth edition. Now in my nineties, I should go to pasture, but there aren't many of those available here in Los Angeles. Lacking such havens, I personally have no retirement plans. I'm doing what I was cut out to do and still thrilled at the marvel of getting someone well.

We will offer some changes in this fourth edition. Our treatments of fibromyalgia, hypoglycemia, and the so-called chronic fatigue syndrome are ever evolving—perhaps not by much, but by enough to make them more effective. Former readers will spot ample repetition, since basic facts don't change. Still, new findings will hopefully regain your curiosity and deepen your knowledge. We will update you on this illness cluster and its sick-making fellow travelers that add nuances to this enlarging syndrome. Our research is progressing, albeit slowly, and we aim to tell you about it.

So excusing myself, please allow me redundancy: Our new readers may have just recently filed for metabolic bankruptcy. They know not from whence we came, or how we got here. They should know that serendipity played a large part in the beginning, and it still has a role in our advances. They, too, might be awestruck to learn how luck plays its part along the stumbling path to enlightenment. They should never hold back telling their healers their own astute observations.

I came out from Tufts University Medical School and headed for

Los Angeles. There I was polished up for the profession by my four years of postgraduate training under the tutelage of UCLA. I knew very little about a lot of illnesses because not much was known. However, I well knew how to spot hypochondriasis and anxiety disorder. At least I so labeled myriad patients within just a few early months of creating my practice. They were certainly abundant.

Experience being a versatile teacher, I was busy expanding my skills. An unsuspecting instructor appeared in the patient-person of Mr. G, and he ignited me with a quick post-postgraduate lesson. Please pay reverence to that man who so stirred my imagination; more observant than most, an occult scientist at heart, he did indeed pause to teach. Me, a 1958-neophyte physician, needed that layman to remind him it paid to listen. His observations on dental calculus (tartar) woke a bit of dormant researcher in my character (more on this in chapter 3). I lost sleep because of him. But it was good that he made me call upon my background degree in biochemistry. Better than that: He made me respect observations made by untrained laymen, and that has made all the difference.

In those days we didn't have to go through a gamut of applications, scientific reasoning, and begging for permission to try something new. So I began prescribing gout medicine to a few of my choice and reliably diagnosed hypochondriac patients. The rest is history. This book is about the work that followed and the protocol that evolved.

Controversy continues about that protocol. We've had excellent success using it. Some have tried it and failed. Unfortunately, many of those have not fully vetted its nuances and couldn't possibly succeed. Yet our website and this book provide surefooted steps to clearing fibromyalgia. Patients should certainly be directed to these resources and given a chance to better health. But I'm ahead of myself: New readers will read on and find out what this all means.

Regardless of naysayers, we still offer the only treatment system that will reverse fibromyalgia. All other approaches obtund the brain's perception of symptoms using enervating chemical interventions or unsustainable exercise excesses that do not alter the underlying condition. If there were other equally effective methods, we would happily prescribe and describe them. I'll explain without apology in the text that follows.

Sixty years later we have not yet weathered the storm. Acceptance is reluctant at best, more often none. We describe what we've achieved and what we're doing. I offer my credentials and long experience in practice, research, and teaching as associate professor of medicine in endocrinology at Harbor-UCLA. All that will go for naught until we or someone else produces a diagnostic blood test. We and others are working on just that issue. I'll describe our efforts in these pages.

You will read about my theory, which remains unproven and simplistic. Yet I have good reasons to believe as I do. Throughout these pages, you will find discussions about biochemistry gone faulty. Right or wrong, learn why I think there exist aberrations in phosphate metabolism. As you read, be assured our disease descriptions are exact and that the illness has mostly a genetic basis. I maintain my right to make such statements: I've treated myself, my family, and several thousand fibromyalgics. Collectively, we've been great teachers.

Much is yet to be proven. We're always seeking firmer evidence. We're still seeking facts with the leadership of master researchers at the City of Hope in Duarte, California. We're not stalled out. We simply lack the funds to bring in a quick and definitive close.

As we asserted in past editions:

1. Fibromyalgia is an inherited syndrome.
2. We have an effective treatment that relies on a very old, readily available, over-the-counter, and utterly safe medication, guaifenesin.
3. Body-wide inability to generate sufficient energy adequately explains the full spectrum of the illness.
4. The hypoglycemia syndrome is a frequent co-condition.

We were once in despair realizing that medical practitioners would be reluctant to accept a new entity. Even if they did, it was possible that no biochemical or genetic solution would be found. We've allayed our fears. The diagnosis is now being made on each continent and in most nations. An inherited cause is largely acknowledged. Nature is forcibly giving up her secret concerning the underlying faulty metabolism. That mystery is being probed by many investigators in confirmation that the entity not only exists, but is widely accepted. Surely finalizing results will be forthcoming, however unlikely in my lifetime.

R. Paul St. Amand, MD

ACKNOWLEDGMENTS

I know it's still the politic thing to do, but I wholeheartedly rededicate this book and new edition to my wife, Janell. She tolerates my theft of moments we should have spent together. My coauthor, Claudia, well deserves and gets my warmest accolades for her years of dedication to a disease with which she has lived in the flesh and in our clinic. Our local editor, Mari Florence, was and remains the overseer to keep us straight on point. Our secretary, Gloria Martinez, has lent her expertise to the ever-growing Spanish-language population we serve throughout the Western Hemisphere. We extend our appreciation to support group leaders throughout the world. They, their members, and the rapidly growing list of the internet's social networks well provide the once-lacking missionary zeal that we've sorely needed.

And then the patients—oh my! The patients! They were, are, and will remain my hero-teachers. They've endured some very ignorant gaps in medical care; suffered the vicissitudes of inefficient treatments; observed and pointed out tiny diagnostic nuances; surfaced for us what wasn't obvious; and shared the exhilaration of restored health by gifting us their hugs. In great numbers they've become the knowledgeable support team I've always wanted—the army I yearned for in the first edition. We surely didn't get this far alone. The growing team is huge and unrelenting. Thanks, group. You mustn't stop yet!

R. Paul St. Amand, MD

WHAT YOUR DOCTOR MAY *NOT* TELL YOU ABOUT
FIBROMYALGIA

PART I

THE PLAN FOR CONQUERING FIBROMYALGIA

CHAPTER 1

AN INVITATION TO JOIN US AND FIND YOUR WAY BACK TO HEALTH

Fibromyalgia chipped away at me my whole life, but when I finally had my full crash at forty and was rendered bedbound I decided that I would read every single book in the library because I thought to myself, "Someone, somewhere, knows something." So I ended up with an enormous stack of books by my bed. Luckily *What Your Doctor May* Not *Tell You About Fibromyalgia* was only the second book I picked up. I never read the rest. I started guai within the week, and three years later color and movement have returned to my world, and I am just so thankful.

—*Sophie, Australia*

I t can start off subtly: a bit of muscle pain, along with some generalized aches and stiffness. Then there are periods when concentration is impossible, a day or two of overwhelming fatigue, and maybe a little dizziness, heart palpitations, irritability, and anxieties. Irritable bowel and digestive woes can flare periodically. Symptoms come and go at first, and it's easy to chalk them up to a mild case of the flu that never quite fully develops. You, like most individuals, tend to blame stress or overexertion for these strange little complaints.

Then one day, you realize one part or another of your body always hurts. You're often confused, short of memory, unable to concentrate, and you're always stressed and feeling as if you're at the end of your rope. You wake up tired every morning no matter how much sleep you've had—or you may have difficulty sleeping at all. Your symptoms begin to worsen, and you notice new ones: depression, numbness and tingling of the hands, leg cramps, headaches, abdominal pains, cramps, constipation taking turns with diarrhea, or bladder infections. Now you notice that you can no longer sleep through the night. Sometimes pain keeps you awake; most of the time, though, you don't know what causes the insomnia or what keeps waking you. And what causes your craving for sugar and starch? Why is it that you haven't changed your eating habits, but you still gain weight? You've accumulated enough bad omens that you aren't too surprised when bad days outnumber the good ones. Eventually you just cycle from bad to worse. When you look back, nature gave you ample warnings.

> You feel like you constantly are coming down with the flu. Your body aches and the pain shifts from day to day, and no matter what you do, you simply can't shake it. You try to get more sleep and you try to eat better, but nothing seems to help. Your friends offer advice and try to get you out of the house doing more, and the more you do, the worse you feel. You end up pushing yourself through life until one day, you can no longer push. The pain and fatigue have engulfed you, and you no longer recognize who you have become.
>
> —*Chantal H., Michigan*

You become increasingly immobile, and unconsciously you stop making plans with family and friends because you don't know how you'll feel the next day—or the day after. Go supermarket shopping? You're kidding. That's just one of the many chores you've come to dread. At least you now have the time to review the long list of doctors you've visited. Each time your hopes have been dashed despite the number of tests you've taken and the many tubes of blood you've sacrificed. Sure enough: Results are always normal. Increasingly, doctors are making the diagnosis despite the unrevealing tests and will offer a sequential array of failed drugs. But some will still escort you out of the office and point to the nearest psychiatrist; a few will admit that nothing much will help you but you could do a trial of this or that newest drug. As a result, you may have subsidized your neighborhood health food store or internet vendors by consuming your body weight in various vitamins and supplements. You may have googled your symptoms and found frustrating and contradictory explanations for them. Possibly you have even ordered and tried a "miracle cure" or two. WebMD and Livestrong.com have not had much to offer, but sometimes you still try looking for help on websites.

Your life has entered a downward spiral into more pain, depression, and fatigue. Some of you may be nearing rock bottom. You reproach yourself for everything. Your lament includes a review of all of your inadequacies and poor coping abilities. You put yourself on trial for repeatedly letting down family and friends. You feel as though you've damaged their lives and your own.

Wounded relationships are the most damaging side effect of fibromyalgia. You're not the person your spouse married, and you know it. You fret and sputter about your fragilities, but you can't seem to correct them. You're depressed especially when you look at your children and the parental deprivations they suffer. Suicide may have crossed your mind, but you know that's not the solution. Okay, enough already with the remorse!

It feels like everyone around me is normal and happy and having a good time and I'm so different. I want to have a few normal days.

I don't fit in anywhere because no one understands. People laugh and say, "You look fine," but I'm dying inside and I can't explain it to them. I'm so tired of pretending I'm okay when I want to scream. I have kept a positive attitude for so long but it's exhausting and I just can't do it anymore. I wish I could just go away somewhere and hide.

—*Susie, California*

Fibromyalgia is widespread in all ethnic groups in all parts of the world. In North America, it's generally estimated that about 5 percent of the adult population suffers from it. Since the early cases are not being diagnosed, we feel that over 10 percent of women and 5 or more percent of men are affected. Using our guess, over twenty million Americans suffer from fibromyalgia— about 85 percent women, although men are more likely not to be diagnosed. Fibromyalgia is the most common disorder seen by rheumatologists.[1] It's further thought that chronic fatigue syndrome affects twenty-five million people. I and many other physicians consider the two the same disease. Blending the entities into one would augment the percentage of people with fibromyalgia. We'll develop the thought later on, but we have enough observations to conclude that today's fibromyalgia is the prelude to tomorrow's osteoarthritis, something that affects nearly 40 percent of older people. Adding up combinations of those numbers would lead us to conclude that nearly one third of our population will, even if just mildly, suffer some symptoms of fibromyalgia in their lifetime.

My rheumatologist told me I was too old to have FMS [fibromyalgia syndrome]. At that time I was fifty-four, never mind the fact I had had symptoms most of my life. The disease had become "full blown" when I was about fifty-one...After another year of suffering, I diagnosed myself via the 'net. My DO [doctor of osteopathy] sent me back to the same rheumatologist because he is the only board-certified one in our area. At that time he told me I was too old to have FMS, but even if I did, there was nothing that could be done...I have since been diagnosed with FMS by three other doctors, all of whom have told me the only thing they could do was treat my symptoms. I was as good as I would ever be and would get much worse.

—*Betty, Texas*

In 1843, Dr. Robert Froriep published his observations about the condition we now call fibromyalgia. For centuries, all sorts of muscle pains had been lumped together and called rheumatism. There were no blood tests to separate out things like rheumatoid arthritis, polymyalgia, and lupus. There were no imaging studies to diagnose disk problems in the back and no nerve conduction studies, so doctors relied on physical examination and observations. Froriep described a subset of patients with what he observed as "rheumatism with hard, tender places," which he could feel in many locations on the body. As a result, in nineteenth-century Germany fibromyalgia was called soft tissue arthritis. Unfortunately as time went by the word *hard* (swollen) was forgotten, so the muscle examination was replaced by a search for tender points.

In the early 1900s, Sir William Gowers over in London studied his own lumbago. He observed symptom clusters in his patients, and dubbed the disease *fibrositis* assuming there was some sort of inflammation he could not measure causing the problem. (This name stuck for the next eighty years or so even though it was subsequently revealed that there was none.) Dr. Gowers also observed that his patients were exhausted and that the disease was "so painful it would make a strong man cry out." He tried everything he could think of in an attempt to relieve this pain, including injecting cocaine into the tender points (it didn't work very well). He also gave his patients a newly discovered drug, aspirin, and noted that it didn't work very well, either.[2]

In the 1960s, Canadian doctor Hugh Smythe wrote an article

about fibrositis that was published in a textbook. He is credited with bringing the disease into the modern spotlight. He is also the man who made tenderness a criterion for fibromyalgia; previously, tenderness was not mandatory to make the diagnosis. His colleague Harvey Moldofsky would introduce the concept that nonrestorative sleep was a hallmark (and perhaps causative). This, too, remained a part of the official criteria from then on.

Fibromyalgia, a coined word that suggests "pain in muscles and fibers," has now replaced the previously popular names *fibrositis* and *rheumatism* dating back to the American College of Rheumatology's publication in 1990. On New Year's Day 1993, the World Health Organization (WHO), as part of the Copenhagen Declaration, officially declared fibromyalgia a syndrome (a medical condition made up of a cluster of accepted symptoms) and the most common cause of widespread chronic muscle pain. The WHO incorporated the American College of Rheumatology's 1990 list of the distinguishing features of fibromyalgia as penned by Drs. Muhammad Yunus, Hugh Smythe, Frederick Wolfe, and others.[3] The biggest part of this was the concept of the eighteen most frequent locations of tender points dispersed over the bodies of fibromyalgics, with a symmetrical distribution of nine such on each side, some in all four quadrants. The criterion they created was that at least eleven of these should be sufficiently tender when prodded with a certain amount of pressure. These tender points would become the major diagnostic point until 2010, when the criteria were amended to address the complaint that the other symptoms of fibromyalgia were not included.

But the World Health Organization went a little farther. The Copenhagen Declaration added: "Fibromyalgia is part of a wider syndrome encompassing headaches, irritable bladder, dysmenorrhea, cold sensitivity, Raynaud's phenomenon, restless legs, atypical patterns of numbness and tingling, exercise intolerance, and complaints of weakness." It also recognized that patients are often depressed.

In 2010, new criteria for identifying fibromyalgia would make an appearance. Physicians were instructed to also accept six self-reported symptoms (difficulty sleeping, fatigue, poor cognition, headaches, depression, and abdominal pain) as well as nineteen pain locations, while also recognizing that not all patients experience pain in the same way. "Women are more tender than men; men often don't get diagnosed," explained one of the authors, Robert Bennett. "Even for women a clinician could identify a sufficient number of tender points to make a diagnosis one day but the next clinician could fail to do so. The patient goes from having fibromyalgia to not having fibromyalgia." The tender points were thus abandoned. It had become clear that the number and intensity of symptoms were the identifying characteristics of fibromyalgia.

In 2016, another revision was made in order to clarify generalized pain complaints in patients. Again, no mention is made of the tender points, simply "generalized pain defined as pain in at least four out of five regions" that has been experienced at a similar level for at least three months. Patients must experience widespread pain on an index of less than or equal to 7 and a few other numbers. So perhaps the takeaway lesson is simply that there is not exactly an agreed-upon definition of fibromyalgia. It has been changed by the efforts of patients, examining doctors, and even pharmaceutical companies.

Still, today fibromyalgia is almost universally recognized as a distinct illness and taught in medical schools. Sadly, there remain a few uninformed but increasingly rare doctors who still tell patients that it's just a catchall name for symptoms shared by a bunch of neurotic women. Were that true, I would have long since gone fishing!

Despite all the research and speculation, fibromyalgia remains poorly understood. It's a complex and chronic disease that causes widespread pain and profound fatigue. Its range of symptoms makes simple, everyday tasks daunting or difficult, and often impossible. There are no outward manifestations and no tissue damage, making it one of the so-called invisible illnesses. But it is very real.

> I remember: turning on the bathroom sink and forgetting to turn it off, completely flooding the bathroom; eating half a piece of toast and throwing the other half out because it was too much work to chew it; trying to read the newspaper and reading the same sentence over and over again because I couldn't comprehend it; lying on the couch in a zombie-type state all day long before going to bed; lying on the floor in pain. I remember not getting any diagnosis or any help at all from the medical field and being completely terrified, thinking I was going to die.
>
> —*Cheryl K., Canada*

People who enjoy semantics will argue whether we are dealing with a condition, illness, syndrome, or disease. If you are unwell, you have a condition that causes your illness. *Disease* suggests lack of ease. Symptoms and findings that regularly appear together often enough are regularly grouped in medical terms as syndromes. Use any of those according to your preference or simply acknowledge that you're sick.

Many publications list the symptoms of fibromyalgia, most of them incompletely. Because of this, in some ways, it remains a phantom illness with very few physical findings according to medical literature, though not so to a trained examiner. Though we're closing in, there are no well-accepted validating laboratory, X-ray, or scanning techniques to give physicians an unchallenged diagnostic footing.

A well-conducted medical history, all by itself, will uncover the cyclic and progressive symptoms that point directly to the diagnosis. When coupled with a physical muscle evaluation (looking for those hard, swollen, and often tender areas described earlier), an accurate diagnosis is easy to make. People with fibromyalgia have severe problems in multiple areas that are always different from those without the disease. Diagnosing requires listening on the part of the doctor because patients have so many complaints, but there are differences that make fibromyalgia unique. If you ask people with rheumatoid arthritis where it hurts, they most often report problems in their affected joints. Though fibromyalgia patients can experience this, they also have pain in different, uncharacteristic regions. Fibro patients are particularly tender when examined in specific spots, and present hard areas of contracted tissue in the muscles; neither is seen in rheumatoid arthritis patients. So it's not that hard (actually, it's easy!) to identify fibromyalgia if you stop and listen and then examine the muscles themselves.

The often used physical examination—eliciting tenderness by poking fingers at certain spots—luckily has been officially discontinued as part of the diagnostic criteria. Yet doctors who are not specialists may not know this and persist with this type of exam. Obviously it is far from perfect and totally falls apart in someone with a high pain threshold or someone taking heavy pain medication. Our method of examination involves sliding our hands along body surfaces, looking for any swollen joint, muscle, tendon, or ligament. Though this does not rely on the patient's expression of pain, we continue to do it. We mark the findings on a printed body caricature—a technique we call mapping.

I had watched my mother disintegrate. She died at ninety-four, never knowing what was wrong. No one ever explained why her muscles hurt, why she could not move her bowels naturally, why she had constant headaches, etc. She wanted to die; yet she lived to be just short of ninety-five, suffering terribly. I could not help her. I had no idea what was causing all her symptoms. Then I read Dr. St. Amand's book. By chapter 2, I thought I knew what was wrong. And when Dr. St. Amand diagnosed my daughter, he was also diagnosing the rest of the people in my family that were suffering with FMS.

—*Bonnie J., Florida*

Is there an accurate blood test for fibromyalgia? From reading the internet, you get the impression that one exists and that it is more accurate than the diagnostic criteria above. But is that true?

In December 2012, a study was published in *BMC Clinical Pathology*.[4] The authors measured cytokine levels in the blood of 201 subjects (110 with fibromyalgia). They concluded, "The cytokine responses to mitogenic activators of PBMC isolated from patients with FM were significantly lower than those of healthy individuals, implying that cell-mediated immunity is impaired in FM patients. This novel cytokine assay reveals unique and valuable immunologic traits, which, *when combined with clinical patterns*, can offer a diagnostic methodology in FM" (emphasis added). In other words, even though it's claimed that the blood test will identify fibromyalgia, an exam and medical history have to be used, too. The blood test claims 93 percent sensitivity.

But is it accurate? Cytokine levels are abnormal in many physical and mental conditions. The original study of 110 fibromyalgics compared them solely with the same number of people who had not been diagnosed with the disease. After intense criticism, the authors added tests on twenty-five people with rheumatoid arthritis and twenty-five with lupus. Although they admit that some medications might have colored the results, they did show that the profiles were different to 97 percent specificity.

Another criticism is that the authors provided almost no information about patient selection or other vital data for a comparison trial. The well-accepted CONSORT (Consolidated Standards of Reporting Trials) statement offers guidelines on reporting of data, but these guidelines were not followed. Critics (not just us) have pointed out that as a clinical study, it was very poorly planned and carried out. As a pathology report it might pass muster, but the data did not in any way address the validity and reliability of the test.

In addition, it's been pointed out that the paper was published only after the authors asserted there was no conflict of interest. They did not disclose that they were about to file a patent for a kit that performs the tests outlined in the paper. Since there was (and is) a lot of money at stake for the company and for author Dr. Bruce Gillis, it is certain that the publishers would have appreciated knowing that. This ethical violation would have resulted in most publications withdrawing the paper.

The test currently costs about $950 and is covered by some insurance companies. If your doctor won't order it for you, Dr. Gillis will. You have to take the kit to a lab for blood drawing, which will add to the cost. (The test is now available around the world.)

Most of those who take the test plan to use the result, if positive, to file for some sort of assistance such as disability. However, a positive result on this test is far from a slam-dunk. The test is not able to determine the severity of your disease or how incapacitated you are. You'll still need a doctor's examination, notes, and observations to qualify.

The bottom line is that if you want to find out if you have fibromyalgia, you can do that in less time than it takes for blood to be drawn!

Although fibromyalgia is not a terminal illness, it is a demoralizing and debilitating one. The physical symptoms can be unbearable, and depression and anxiety accompany them. *Psychology Today* estimates that suicide rates are ten times higher in patients with chronic pain conditions. This is not acceptable—not when something can be done. Our purpose in writing this book as a new edition is to continue clarifying the only treatment that works. We will also tell you about our exciting new findings, along with those of our research colleagues.

Although few patients can tolerate even a token amount, many physicians simply advise exercise. That suggestion usually comes with the offer of a series of chemical Band-Aids in an attempt to mask the expanding list of symptoms. Medical professionals unwittingly promote eventual disability when they prescribe ever-stronger medications that, sooner or later, further deplete energy and deepen the mental haze. They have nothing else to offer and justifiably defend the practice because they can't sit idly by and watch people suffer. But many of those people end up disabled due to the side effects of their medications.

Long-term disability insurance companies are enjoined in battle with sufferers, but they're hardly disinterested parties. It's to their advantage if they can get a fibromyalgic diagnosed as a psychiatric case via the common co-complaints of depression and anxiety. They do have growing difficulty in finding a compliant psychiatrist or other professional who will ignore fibromyalgia. Yet because the vast majority of insurance policies do not cover mental disability, the companies keep trying.

Since there's a great deal of money at stake, certain ploys are regularly used. They hire physicians (often retired from practice in a different field) who call and talk with the patient's doctor, then quote him or her only in part. What they end up reporting is twisted in favor of the employer. Insurers give patients a dictum—"Your disability will end on [date]"—and enforce it no matter what the personal physician writes. In other words, "We won't pay you anymore." The implication is, "Go get a lawyer if you want to fight." Insurance companies defend themselves by pointing out that fibromyalgia cases have reached epidemic proportions and are assaulting their bottom line. US Social Security, state disability, and workers' compensation are also reacting to the financial reality of the situation. More than 35 percent of American fibromyalgia patients have received some form of disability or injury compensation, and that does not include lost income from employers and lost wages to employees and other forms of assistance. We are the first to agree that the country can ill afford to swell these ranks. Even when compensation has been granted, we want to get patients motivated to heal and reenter the workforce. Yet neither can we turn our backs on very real suffering. We see only one solution to this dilemma: Get to the sick ones much sooner, and get them well.

The basic problem for patients and physicians is that there is no consensus regarding the causes of fibromyalgia. Considerable amounts of time and money have been spent searching for one, yet few experts agree on anything. The purpose of this book is to present mutual findings: our patients' and our own.

The vast majority of physicians are skillfully trained, well intentioned, and dedicated to their oath-driven principle of trying to help patients. Fibromyalgia is such a system-wide illness—with so many seemingly unconnected, rapidly shifting complaints—that doctors are understandably confused. Add to that the professional frustration they experience when they're stymied at every turn no matter what they prescribe. They eventually respond by referring patients to another doctor who should know more than they do about some "new" symptom. In the process, patients receive a fast-track medical education as they go from specialist to specialist.

It's also no wonder that most of our colleagues consider treating fibromyalgia hopeless. All they can do is relieve symptoms as best they can, often by prescribing the latest drug promoted by a drug company—if a patient's insurance company will cover it. With no known cause to treat, it makes total sense to attack individual symptoms with whatever may ameliorate them. Polypharmacy soon emerges, making use of NSAIDs (nonsteroidal anti-inflammatory drugs), various analgesics, antidepressants, sedatives, tranquilizers, stimulants, and ultimately narcotics. The process is unstoppable. Patients get sicker and are forced by the side effects of their medications into a far worse state than before treatment. For many, the picture is truly bleak.

What do you do when fibro is causing your whole life to come apart? Your money situation has gone from bad to worse because you can't work and you can't think well enough to budget. You forget to make a deposit or your lights get turned off because you forgot to pay. Your husband wants to know when you'll get better because he feels lonely when all you can do is drag yourself through the day let alone make passionate love all night. Your kids are having trouble in school and you can't help them because you can't think. Neither can you skate with your daughter or play basketball with your sons. You look at your laundry piled up and you can't imagine sorting it let alone carrying it over to the laundry room. I can't think, can't talk, and can't feel. I feel dead.

—*Debbie, California*

Over the years, we've used different drugs to treat fibromyalgia. In the past, we mainly prescribed gout medications that were thoroughly effective. Unfortunately, each had certain side effects that left a small group of patients in a treatment limbo. In 1992, our search led us to try guaifenesin, a widely available medication. It is well tolerated and has no known side effects. It's available over the counter without a prescription in both long- and short-acting formulations, often in combinations that we'll cover later on. Prices vary among these preparations, and despite the fact that the cost has gone up in recent years the drug is still relatively inexpensive. It is likely that the drug will be coming down in cost as the patents on Mucinex expire.

We use guaifenesin as the mainstay of our treatment protocol. It actually addresses the basic disturbance caused by our defective genes. It does not work by masking symptoms the way pain and brain-altering medications do. This book is the culmination of six decades of research and hands-on examinations. We've treated thousands of patients who have traveled from all over the world seeking relief from this enervating disease. With our approach, all the symptoms including pain reverse, and will completely disappear in most patients if joints have not been damaged. Most individuals resume normal lives with minimal residual problems. Recovery is not immediate: We have to find the effective dosage of guaifenesin and try to clear out what it took years to accumulate. There are other crucial factors in our treatment that we will explain.

In order for guaifenesin to work, it must have unrestricted access to receptors in the kidneys. These are like little docking stations where the medication must park and unload its contents before it will be effective for fibromyalgia. Unfortunately, a common chemical can enter these stations preferentially. Many ingredients in the products we use every day—pain medications, muscle rubs, vitamins and herbal supplements, skin care products, toothpastes, and sunscreens—contain the chemical known as salicylate. You'll find that we stress, again and again throughout this book, that in order for our protocol to succeed, patients must strictly avoid all sources of salicylate.

Approximately 30 percent of female fibromyalgics also have hypoglycemia, or bouts of low blood sugar, with symptoms that greatly overlap those of fibromyalgia. For complete success, both conditions must be addressed simultaneously. If hypoglycemia is overlooked and patients fail to make required dietary adjustments, fatigue, cognitive, and intestinal symptoms will persist even though fibromyalgia overlaps will reverse on guaifenesin.

As we will expand on in this book, our protocol must be followed very carefully if patients are to achieve the positive results we describe. We've heard too often from patients and physicians alike who missed the mandatory step of cleaning out all sources of salicylates, "I tried Dr. St. Amand's treatment and it doesn't work."

We will share our knowledge of fibromyalgia throughout this book. We know firsthand the nature of the disease: the cognitive distress, the unrelenting exhaustion, and the pains that cumulatively induce deep depression, and finally even suicidal thoughts. We know how hard it is to be understood in a healthy world, where perfectly healthy people are all around you, when friends and even family say (dare we repeat?), "You don't look sick!" We've poured our hopes into yours in the succeeding chapters. We'll try to explain simply and discuss clearly all of the important lessons you must learn if you plan success. We'll stress what you must change, because most of you need more than just a pill to get fully reenergized and relatively pain-free. Patients of any age can follow our protocol, designed to reverse fibromyalgia in far less time than it took to develop the illness. Despite damage in later years from osteoarthritis that guaifenesin cannot reverse, clear thinking and full energy can be restored.

We readily admit that the guaifenesin protocol is not entirely accepted in mainstream medicine. We have not provided the coveted double-blind study, but we now have published papers in medical journals for those willing to decipher their contents. Word of our protocol is spreading thanks to grassroots support from our healed patients, and given that there are few alternatives, many practitioners are open to ways to help. As a result, many physicians and other practitioners are using the protocol or at least directing patients to our books and website. In addition to face-to-face, hands-on training with doctors who've come to us, Claudia and I have spoken at medical meetings, mixed patient–doctor groups, and guaifenesin support groups worldwide; we've even participated in occasional television and radio interviews to deliver our simple message. During these events, we regularly extend invitations to join us in fighting the battle. In short, we've been preaching to anyone who'll listen for many years now. Whether through this book or in person, we keep repeating, "Guaifenesin works, but you must follow the protocol as written."

I have never contacted an organization or a website for any reason so I'm not sure what I'm doing. I just hope you receive this. I do not know what else to do. I'm divorced, single mother of two daughters, sixteen and ten. I've been through some extremely stressful years while trying to work, raise my girls, and go to numerous doctors, some of which claim they specialize in fibromyalgia. I don't know what to say next except I'm hoping you can help me. I'm forty-two years old, and for the past few years, I feel like I'm seventy-two. I'm always exhausted, experiencing pain, irritable, dizzy, issues with my bowels, skin problems... I've always lived my life feeling that no matter what was handed to me, my glass was always half full, but now it feels like my glass is empty. I want my life back. I want to be the person I was in the past.

—*Lisa, Maryland*

By now we are sure you know that you must take charge of your own illness. Physicians will never spend the time (which they do not have) to look for salicylates in products other than prescription drugs. They're not going to shop at cosmetics counters using magnifying glasses to scan labels. No one will hover nearby to slap your hand when you reach for a piece of pie if you're hypoglycemic. But look at it this way: Not reading labels or cheating on the diet will obviously harm you, but it will also discourage your doctor, who's observing you and hoping for your success if only to acquire a method for treating other patients. Even practitioners who've feigned disinterest and only allowed that guaifenesin can't hurt you will become attentive as you begin to feel better. They will see the change in you, and they won't be able to deny that what you are doing is working, at least for you. Since you're reading this book, you must still be motivated to try again despite all of your previous setbacks. That speaks volumes. For each one who picks up this book, we know that there are some who'll put it down because it "looks too hard," and "I'm too sick to try this."

Eleven years ago this evening I took a deep breath and swallowed my first half-pill of guaifenesin. I had been following all the standard treatments—antidepressant for pain and sleep, pain meds for pain, sleeping pills for sleep, following a very rigid schedule of waking and sleeping and activity every day, avoiding stress whenever possible, and meditating for half an hour morning and evening. But I got sicker and sicker anyway. At night, I would hear somebody scream in my sleep, and wake up to realize it had been me, crying out in pain when I changed position. I was sure within six months I would lose my job and never be able to work again. I was planning to commit suicide before I became totally incapacitated. But I had decided that first I would give the guaifenesin protocol a try.

—*Anne Louise, Minnesota*

We invite all fibromyalgia sufferers (and their loved ones) to embark on the journey to improved health. Let us be your tour directors. We're passionate about providing you with the information you need. We've both done it, paid our dues, guided thousands through the same process over the years, and we are eager to share what we know. Realize up front that this trip is not for the faint of heart. For most of you, the road back to good health will seem long, with days of discomfort living in a cognitive wasteland. In the beginning, this may be more intense than what you have suffered to date. But the destination is worth the effort: There is nothing worse than continuing the semi-life you have now. This treatment is designed to flush the body of the metabolic debris that's clogging up your energy-producing factories, the tiny mitochondria buried deep inside all your cells. While that's happening, your emotional and physical pain will most likely increase. But with time, you'll notice symptoms easing and you'll soon find that you have some good hours, eventually better ones, and ultimately great days. You'll actually bounce back after an illness, injury, or hard work, just as you once did. You'll regain the ability to participate in activities with the energy and enthusiasm that have eluded you for years. By following our treatment regimen to the letter, along with your doctor's advice, this is all within your reach. We want you to resume living your life to the fullest. The best definition of *happiness* we've ever heard is: "Happiness is freedom from pain."

CHAPTER 2

THE FIBROMYALGIA SYNDROME

An Overview of Symptoms and Causes

> Fibromyalgia is real, fibromyalgia hurts, and fibromyalgia intrudes into lives and relationships in a real way. The two basic challenges that face a newly diagnosed patient are the following: learning about your illness so that you understand it and then explaining it to everyone else in your life so that they do as well.
>
> —*Claudia Marek,* Fibromyalgia Is Real

What is fibromyalgia? The medical community and patients are still looking for a simple way to answer that question. My coauthor, Claudia, asked her son, Malcolm Potter, that very question when he was about ten years old. His response was, "It feels like all my muscles want to throw up!" That intuitive response still seems as descriptive as anything else that's been offered. Another one is "the irritable everything syndrome," coined by Dr. Hugh Smythe of Toronto, Ontario. From ten-year-old boy to prominent researcher—two phrases that pretty well cover it, wouldn't you say?

Fibromyalgia is different from other illnesses. If we were to describe thyroid diseases, diabetes, or rheumatoid arthritis, for example, we could easily recite their distinguishing characteristics. Most conditions have a single set of lab tests to help confirm the diagnosis. Often, one major organ or gland is the culprit. That's not so with fibromyalgia, because it doesn't pick on just a single type of cell or limited body part. Instead, it shows up with myriad seemingly unrelated symptoms in endless combinations. At first glance, the only thing these complaints seem to have in common is that they coexist in a single human being. Fibromyalgia symptoms don't neatly fit into diagnostic categories. Perversely, they spill profusely over the borders that define any particular medical specialty. You just can't quite tuck it in. It remains elusive, treacherous, troublesome to pin down, and taxing to treat.

Though there is no set pattern, fibromyalgia assaults enough systems to raise a warning flag to the alert physician. It certainly requires more time to handle than the few minutes allotted per patient by insurance companies—which leaves both doctor and patient frustrated. Often physicians in family practice, internal medicine, and rheumatology, who more routinely perform complete patient evaluations, are more adept at identifying the many outlying symptoms.

A cluster of dominant symptoms often drives patients to seek help from whatever specialist they deem best suited to handle them. Specialists, by definition, work in somewhat limited spheres. That narrow focus may not allow a panoramic view where all the symptoms are displayed. Thinking within their particular fields, they find it difficult to expand perspectives to include minutiae into an all-encompassing diagnosis. So they end up treating just a few symptoms as if those represent the entire disease. Therefore, irritable bowel syndrome, interstitial cystitis, vulvar pain syndrome, chronic fatigue syndrome, chronic candidiasis, and myofascial pain syndrome are handled as separate entities though they represent facets of fibromyalgia. Even if a patient experiences improvement from local interventions, the remainder of symptoms continue unabated and progress with time.

FREQUENCY OF SYMPTOMS BY PERCENTAGE OF OCCURRENCE									
Symptom	%	Symptom	%	Symptom	%	Symptom	%	Symptom	%
Fatigue	98	Sweating	66	Eye Irritation	72	Gas/Bloating	76	Itching	77
Irritability	89	Palpitations	47	Nasal Congestion	79	Constipation	69	Rashes	64
Nervousness	76	Frontal Headaches	72	Abnormal Tastes	65	Diarrhea	63	Sensitivities	49
Depression	89	Occipital Headaches	58	a) Bad	55	Dysuria	32	a) Chemical *Rash from contact*	7
Insomnia	90	General Headaches	26	b) Metallic	49	Pungent Urine	46	b) Light	21
Impaired Concentration	86	Dizziness	81	Ringing Ears/Tinnitus *(fleeting)*	65	Bladder Infections *more than 3 lifetime*	68	c) Odor	34
Impaired Memory	89	a) Vertigo	38	Numbness	83	Vulvodynia	43	d) Sounds	13
Anxiety	75	b) Imbalance *(fleeting)*	74	Restless Legs	62	Weight Gain *20 or more lbs.*	57	e) Allergies	26
Sugar Craving	73	c) Faintness	21	Leg Cramps	71	Brittle Nails	75	Growing Pains *Before age 14*	63
Salt Craving	39	Blurred Vision	66	Nausea	62	Bruising *Non-injured*	75	Pain	99

BASED ON 4,000 CONSECUTIVE PATIENTS

In my early years in practice, patients with numerous complaints visited me. Each had many doctors and had taken many medications. They still weren't well, but were certainly more frustrated. Their family doctors had examined and tested them, often in memorable detail. The inevitable conclusion was: "Everything's normal; it's just your nerves." Family and friends eventually echoed those words and accepted the fact that their loved one was just a neurotic who was cracking up under stress. I equally fell into that trap because I was taught that methodology and had seen no evidence to contradict it.

What we were all missing was the connecting thread among patients. Glaringly obvious was the fact that there was a similarity in all the accounts. Sure, many patients found it difficult to pinpoint exactly when their symptoms had begun. Most had great trouble discerning the order in which they appeared. They wilted under questioning as if they were being cross-examined and a wrong answer would result in condemnation. Listening to the cascade—migraines, fatigue, depression, muscle aches, dizziness, nasal congestion, gas, diarrhea, breaking nails, numbness, bladder infections—shouldn't someone have caught on sooner? A whole group of patients were repeating the same things!

> Some mornings I would wake up and feel so lethargic it was all I could do to make it to work. For several years, I'd attributed my muscle pain to the few fender-benders that I'd been in. I'd thought the migraine headaches were hereditary. And I would tell myself I'd caught a "bug" when the dizziness and fatigue became a problem. The strange thing was the symptoms seemed to get worse as time went on, not better, despite the treatment I'd received from traditional MDs, chiropractors, holistic practitioners, acupuncturists, masseuses, and herbalists.
>
> About a year ago, I was so frustrated I rattled off all my recurring symptoms to my [previous] doctor and demanded, "I've been here before with these problems. What's wrong with me?" To which she replied, with annoying frankness, "I don't know."
>
> —Michelle, California

As with other illnesses, the severity and impact of fibromyalgia differ greatly from patient to patient. Some are able to lead relatively normal lives. Often they live with a number of irritating symptoms for years when almost suddenly a full-blown, unrelenting disease hits. Others become considerably debilitated early on, even homebound. There are those who feel well until traumatized by an accident, surgery, extensive dental work, infection, or emotional stress. They single out those events as triggers that precipitate their illnesses. In most cases, when taking a more detailed history, we can elucidate many, much earlier complaints. But for the vast number of people, symptoms sneak up insidiously, wax and wane, gradually intensify, and eventually never go away.

In addition to the physical complaints, the vast majority of patients also have difficulties with memory and concentration—cognitive difficulties that have been nicknamed fibrofog. This embarrassing entanglement often takes a heavier toll on patients than do the aches and pains. It raises fear of serious brain deterioration, and begs reassurances that it isn't the appearance of premature Alzheimer's. You can appreciate the alarm invoked by the neurological involvement upon reading the following description.

> I sit at a computer at work with a headset on, answering calls from people about computers of all types...I have to solve their problems, at the same time "teach" them. Many times I have found myself not knowing whom I am talking to (man or woman?) and what we were talking about. It is like just waking up from a dream. So I have to keep notes of what I'm doing on my calls, or just plain ask the person to repeat what they just said. This will eventually cost me my job...I don't know what my future holds. I've gotten in my car and forgotten how to turn the lights on, or where the windshield wipers are. Sometimes I can laugh about it, later. But it's getting more frequent and I'm not laughing anymore.
>
> —*Cyndi S., Arkansas*

At the beginning of my medical career, I knew of no disease that could encompass the multiple and weird symptoms expressed by this group. The sheer number of people reciting the same litany of complaints made it ever more likely there was some undocumented disease. The depth of cycling and rapid shifting from good to bad days didn't quite fit into the description of neurosis. I also noticed that sick days were not always related to tensions and stresses at home or work. Neurotics are neurotic and don't usually experience great days out of nowhere. The fact that my patients were inexplicably better at times despite living under identical conditions made me more attentive to the repetitious nature of their symptoms.

There was no doubt that these patients were emotionally upset, frequently at the end of their rope, and often on the defensive. They complained of varying degrees of pain and at least some stiffness, affecting many parts of their body. That seemed pretty tangible and at least represented specific locales for me to start probing. I kept trying to find some palpable abnormalities in the designated painful areas. Eventually I did feel them: very detectable swellings, scattered pattern-like, everywhere. I soon made the connection that worse-pain days meant worse-everywhere complaints. It wasn't long before I realized that the entire symptom cascade was interrelated somehow. It became obvious that pain hurts whether it stems from an emotionally floundering brain or from a gut in spasm, a burning and irritated bladder, or a headache. It was indeed one great big mess! I was literally feeling my way and reinforcing my ever-growing conviction that everything was linked and had to have a single cause. What on earth could it be?

THE SYMPTOMS OF FIBROMYALGIA

By and large, fibromyalgia symptoms can be grouped into the following categories: central nervous system, eye-ear-nose-and-throat, musculoskeletal, dermal, gastrointestinal, and genitourinary. There are a few other, isolated problems that don't fit easily into any classification other than miscellaneous. We'll look at all of those affected areas and present you with a tableau of fibromyalgia. Each of these biological systems earns a chapter later in this book. We'll separate them just to make the full ramifications of the disease more comprehensible. But please remember, they are all very much connected, all stem from the same cause, and all are equally reversed by one medication, guaifenesin.

- **Cerebral**—Fatigue, irritability, nervousness, depression, apathy, listlessness, impaired memory and concentration (fibrofog), anxieties and suicidal thoughts, insomnia, frequent waking, and nonrestorative sleep.

- **Musculoskeletal**—Pain and generalized morning stiffness in the involved muscles, tendons, ligaments, and fascia that may arise from such structures surrounding the neck, shoulders, upper and lower back, hips, knees, inner and outer elbows, wrists, fingers, toes, and chest as well as from injured or old operative sites. Pain can assume any form and intensity, such as throbbing, burning, stabbing, stinging, grabbing, or any combination of these. Joints may be swollen, red, and hot, or just painful as in the temporomandibular joint (TMJ). Numbness of the extremities or face and tingling anywhere arise from contracted structures pressing on nearby nerves. Facial and head pains spring from the neck or skull bone connections (sutures). Tiny parts of muscles often twitch, and restless leg syndrome makes it impossible to find a comfortable position. Sensations of electrical impulses in muscles and a feeling of generalized weakness along with leg and foot cramps complete the list.

- **Dermal**—Undue sweating; various rashes may appear with or without itching: hives, red blotches, acne, tiny red or clear bumps, blisters, eczema (seborrheic or neurodermatitis), and rosacea. Nails are often brittle, and chip or easily peel. Hair is of poor quality and either breaks or falls out prematurely, sometimes in bunches. Strange sensations are common, including cold and hot patches (especially of the palms, soles, and thighs), crawling, electric vibrations, prickling, hypersensitivity to touch, and flushing that is sometimes accompanied by an unpleasant pungent and irritating sweat.

- **Gastrointestinal**—Symptoms that are labeled as separate entities such as irritable bowel syndrome, leaky gut, or spastic colon. Transient nausea, cramping or stabbing gas pain, bloating, constipation alternating with diarrhea, mucus in stools, and sometimes stomach hyperacidity with burning reflux.

- **Genitourinary**—Pungent urine, frequent urination, bladder spasms with very low (suprapubic) abdominal aching, burning urination (dysuria) with or without repeated bladder infections or so-called interstitial cystitis. Suspected vaginal yeast infections without the usual cottage cheese discharge are mimicked by vulvodynia (vulvar pain syndrome), which includes vulvitis (painful, irritated, burning, and sometimes raw vaginal lips), vestibulitis (same symptoms deeper into the opening), vaginal spasms or cramps, burning mucous discharge, increased menstrual-uterine cramps, and painful intercourse (dyspareunia).

- **Head-eye-ear-nose-and-throat**—Headaches that may be labeled migraines if they are of sufficient intensity. Other, less forceful ones could be restricted to the back of the neck and head only (occipital); front only (frontal), often erroneously blamed on the sinuses; one-sided only (unilateral); or generalized (entire head); dizziness, vertigo (spinning), or imbalance; dry eyes as well as itching and burning with or without a sticky or gritty discharge (sand) first thing in the morning; blurred vision; excessive nasal mucous congestion and postnasal drip; painful, burning, or cut tongue; abnormal tastes (bad or metallic), scalded mouth; brief ringing (tinnitus) or lower-pitched sounds in the ears; ear and eyeball aching and tenderness; sensitivity to light, sounds, and odors. New late-in-life-onset asthma and hay fever are sometimes caused by fibromyalgia.

- **Miscellaneous**—Weight gain; low-grade fever with night sweats; lowered immunity to infections; morning eyelid and hand swelling from water retention that slowly gravitates to the lower extremities and by evening stretches tissues, impinges on myriad surface nerves, and causes restless leg syndrome.

TENDER POINTS

> It took years to happen. It was not until I turned sixty-three that I became totally aware of the fact that my body was breaking down. Before that I had plenty of indications that my health was disintegrating; eighteen years of chiropractic adjustments, visits to many nutritionists, and a kitchen cabinet filled with at least twenty different homeopathic remedies purchased from people who charged me for their alternative practices. I tried that route because my mom, who had similar symptoms, had had no success with regular doctors. Researching FMS took me to Devin Starlanyl's book *Fibromyalgia and Chronic Myofascial Pain*. I was relaxing on the beach, reading her book, and saw a diagram of the tender points. I found all eighteen on me. And then I knew what I had.
>
> —Bonnie J., Florida

In the 1840s, "painful hard places" was used to describe some people with rheumatism. These sensitive spots are now referred to as tender or trigger points. The latter designation is used for the so-called myofascial pain syndrome. These sensitive spots have been mapped, poked, prodded, biopsied, injected, and scanned. They're frequently assessed using a contraption called a dolorimeter, a spring-loaded device that measures the pressure load when a patient cries out or flinches.

When questioned, most patients confirm tender areas throughout their bodies. Most are located on muscles, tendons, and ligaments. Pain complaints move around a lot, but tender sites don't vary all that much. In reality, the most painful spots of the day take precedence and drown out the others. Swelling changes with fluid content, and pain is determined by how much pressure squeezes neighboring nerves. That's why small swellings can sometimes hurt much more than the bigger ones.

We always found the old tender-point concept unduly limiting. Pain sensitivity is largely inherited and varies in a spectrum of tolerance. Of interest, though, is the amount of involvement in the tissues. So, after taking a patient's history, we begin our search for any involved areas in a process we call mapping. This manual examination turns up many large and small spastic zones, sometimes involving an entire muscle bundle. These areas are distinctly swollen, but not always tender, so we simply call them the lumps and bumps of fibromyalgia. We record each of these, noting its location and size on a sketch of the body. (See chapter 7 for a description of our technique and a blank body map.) Some patients can barely be touched; others can be prodded with little concern. Our examination doesn't rely on what a person feels: They've already told us about their pain distribution. We are purely objective and record only what we can feel without added input from the patient.

WHAT CAUSES FIBROMYALGIA?

Given the broad spectrum of bodily functions and tissues affected by fibromyalgia, it's only natural to wonder: What kind of pathology would affect so many, diverse systems of the body? Can brittle nails and migraines really be connected? Why haven't we found abnormalities in the customary diagnostic tests? Such issues have perplexed physicians and patients alike. Those of us who've studied fibromyalgia for years still don't agree on the answers, but luckily the enigma is breaking up, as you will learn.

There are controversies in the medical community about the nature of fibromyalgia. I've seriously studied the proposed concepts, and I disagree with them. I've long ago joined in and expounded my own theory. Luckily, I have a lot of data: firsthand experience and much gleaned from basic science, as well as published results from our own research. The current treatments being offered don't hold up well and mainly mask the developing disease. Before delving into details, here is my authentication. I've gathered first-hand evidence from examining more than ten thousand patients and from their follow-up visits. I add to those numbers daily, and I've examined every single one of them personally. For the past fifteen or twenty years, I have only treated fibromyalgia. Therefore, I hardly feel pompous saying "in my experience." What we're about to share makes the most sense coming from the perspective of physiology, biochemistry, and clinical medicine. We continue expanding on a concept that fits, because we have a treatment that works.

Here we ask you to bear in mind that a theory is nothing more than a set of assumptions based on many accumulated facts. Encountering a theory, immediately recognize that it undoubtedly contains errors and oversights. This edition of the book will tell you how we are improving it by actively delving deeper into the biochemical and genetic factors we've always thought were at the root of fibromyalgia. We're completely satisfied that the illness responds well to guaifenesin and other medications we've used in the past. Our published research papers give a glimpse into the effects of how these medications work. The truth is revealing itself at last. Please remain patient with us. Our theories are undergoing rigorous testing, and so far so good!

We wish we could choose a more descriptive name for the disease that would fit all of its symptoms. *Fibromyalgia* is a Latin term meaning "pain in muscles and fibers," but that's clearly inadequate to define the rest of the illness. *Chronic fatigue syndrome*, the second most commonly used moniker, focuses mainly on brain exhaustion and malfunction. For most patients, both labels apply at various times during their illness but can't be easily combined into one classification. At times, the symptoms of one condition are prevalent and tilt the scale to one or the other diagnosis. However, it just takes a careful history and appropriate examination to make it very clear that we're dealing with one and the same condition. It's merely a matter of tissue sensitivity, disease intensity, and individual pain threshold.

For these reasons, fibromyalgia badly needs a new name—not that this is likely to happen. We proposed *dysenergism syndrome* (faulty energy) in our first edition. Since then, a learned Greek colleague invoked his native language to suggest *energopenia*, meaning "dearth of energy." That would cover it well, but it's not being accepted. Indeed, our treatment restores vitality by lifting the biochemical blockade we're about to describe. Once this is done, the symptoms of the illness recede. I use myself as an example. At age ninety-plus, I'm still able to do some things I couldn't do in my thirties. As much as we'd love to change the name, at this time we'll go along with common usage and stick with *fibromyalgia*, but bear in mind the term may reflect nothing of your most distressing symptoms.

THE MALFUNCTION JUNCTION OF FIBROMYALGIA: A BIOCHEMICAL THEORY

What in the world could be the metabolic difficulty that springs up to cause such a body-wide failure? The stack of symptoms we've listed above strongly *confirms* that many bodily functions have gone on strike, and *all* at the same time. You and your doctors may have been just looking at the surface effects of fibromyalgia. There certainly has to be some type of deeper, more fundamental breakdown. Aches and pains arise from spasms; the brain is obviously too tired to remain functionally alert. But why do the bladder, skin, intestinal tract, eyes, nose, throat, and more all join in? There must be some altered chemistry behind all this—a truly basic connection.

There is a saying in medicine that either too much or too little of a given element will interfere with function. Not surprisingly, cells best work within a very narrow range for each of their chemical constituents. Logically, to preserve itself, the body spreads surplus concentrations among a variety of cells. However, there is a critical level that, when exceeded, induces malfunction—in fibromyalgia, an energy deficit. We believe that this illness is caused by an excess of a specific biochemical substance that enters individual and intercommunicating cells. This process begins at birth and accrues until the body's safety membranes are overstretched and become porous. The time from birth until the symptoms appear varies with the individual's genetic traits. We think there's an inherited malfunction in specific areas of the kidneys that allows accumulation and excesses of normal body components that, in normal people, are kept under control by excretion. We strongly suspect inorganic phosphate.

Every bodily function needs energy—not only in moving, running, exercising, and speaking, but also to simply grow hair, breathe, digest food, fight illness, and, especially, maintain brain function. Eighty to 90 percent of our food is converted to fuel. All cells produce a currency of energy known as adenosine triphosphate (ATP). The chores we've just listed and whatever else a body does all depend on this vital compound. That's true for all living things: plants, bacteria, and animals large or small. This process involves extremely complicated biochemical mechanisms.

To understand how fibromyalgic cells mess up, we need to study how energy is produced. In proper function, the concentration of every substance essential to energy formation is meticulously maintained. Tiny power stations called mitochondria, where raw materials are processed, are where our story properly begins. Those structures are present in all cells of the body, and especially loaded in brain and muscle cells. They are complex little factories that convert 80 percent or more of our foods into adenosine triphosphate—three phosphates (tri-) hooked onto a single parent molecule named adenosine. When a cell is called upon to perform some function, it rips one high-energy phosphate off adenosine, and expends it as fuel to energize the chosen activity. This chemical expenditure provides most of the energy required by living tissue. Almost magically, electrons are released in these chemical outbursts and are somehow directed to the right place to do the right job at precisely the right time. Think of ATP as a fuel analogous to the gasoline in your car's tank that's ever ready for burning. It's also like plugging in an electric cord: The energy's been there all the while, just waiting for a signal to connect. The body also releases electrons that flow through cells, charge up various enzymes, and run electrical currents in tissue "appliances." In healthy bodies, cells seem to have an almost unlimited supply of ATP. In fact, within thousandths of a second, cells can resurrect new high-energy phosphates from a series of reservoirs to replenish ATP.

So how does an energy deficit occur in fibromyalgia? We know that this is the problem. It had been suggested much earlier, but a study reported in 1989 actually measured ATP levels in tissues of fibromyalgics.[1] Two Swedish researchers, Drs. Bengtsson and Henriksson, found a 20 percent reduction in muscle biopsies taken from such sites. They sampled bits from the swollen and tender bumps in the trapezius muscle located at the top of the shoulder. Adjacent, normal tissue was also biopsied and studied but showed no similar ATP deficits. A few years later, low ATP levels were found in red blood cells of affected individuals. These studies, along with the more technical magnetic resonance spectroscopy that can probe inside living cells, support our theory of inadequate energy as the cause of fibromyalgia.

We like having our theory validated, but the question still arises: Why this depletion? What has interfered so stressfully to suck out ATP? The body is superbly geared to prevent such an occurrence, since major losses would mean cellular death. Obviously, that doesn't happen in fibromyalgia, since no damage occurs. So something must be lacking or have entered the cells, accumulating sufficiently to gunk up and slow or idle its generators.

It's well known in physiology and biochemistry that phosphate excesses in the inner core of mitochondria, the matrix, slow down these power stations. Eventually, this not only eats up surplus ATP but slows basic production as well. Blocking ATP generation means there won't be enough high-energy phosphates available for the cell to do any real work beyond simply surviving. Cells with the highest activity are the first hit and worst affected by this shortage. The more cells that are pressed into service, the more intensely they are affected. So it's no small wonder that brain and muscle are the heaviest hit! Optimal function is permitted only when energy is sufficiently replenished. Is any of this news to a fibromyalgic?

But phosphate is not the only problem. It can't pile up indiscriminately inside cells without causing permanent damage. Because each phosphate ion carries two negative charges, electrical equilibrium can only be sustained by a counterbalancing (buffering) with an element that sports two positive charges. Enter calcium, the preferred companion for phosphate. Whenever and wherever phosphate goes, so does calcium.

Calcium normally sits quietly inside storage bins, known as the endoplasmic reticulum, and mitochondria, or lurks just outside the cell's wall. When a stimulus arrives, the command is given to the endoplasmic reticulum to release stored calcium into the fluid chamber of the cell, the cytosol. The amount released is just enough to perform the desired task, no more and no less. If more is needed to amplify the signal, liberal amounts can be imported from the readily available external pool. Focus on the fact that calcium is the final battery terminal—the ultimate messenger that commands any cell to "Get going and do what you're told!" (See figures 2.1 and 2.2.)

Calcium won't end its demands for performance as long as it sits in the cell's liquid interior, the cytosol (known as the sarcoplasm in muscles). So the poor cell must strive to keep working as instructed until it's relieved of duty. To interrupt go-ahead signals, calcium must be either pumped back into storage within the endoplasmic reticulum, or totally pushed out from the cell. (Enzyme pumps exist that are used just for this purpose.) As you've learned, any function performed by the body uses up ATP for energy; the pumps need the same motivation. Some 40 percent of cell energy is expended simply to move calcium into and

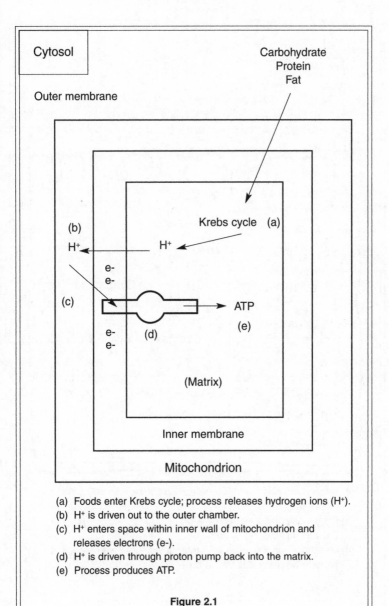

(a) Foods enter Krebs cycle; process releases hydrogen ions (H+).
(b) H+ is driven out to the outer chamber.
(c) H+ enters space within inner wall of mitochondrion and
    releases electrons (e-).
(d) H+ is driven through proton pump back into the matrix.
(e) Process produces ATP.

Figure 2.1

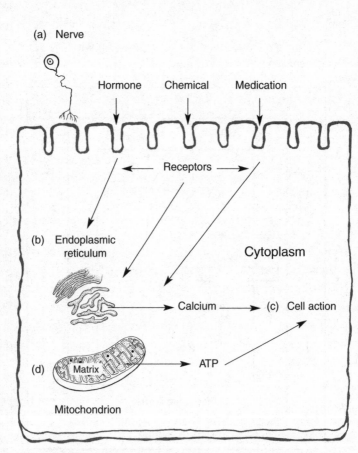

(a) Nerve, hormone, chemical, or medication signals endoplasmic reticulum (ER).
(b) ER releases calcium into cytosol.
(c) Calcium initiates cell action.
(d) Mitochondrion produces ATP that provides cell with energy to perform whatever it is told to do.

Figure 2.2

out of internal storage or to extrude it from the cell. Depleted ATP in fibromyalgia permits calcium to sit far too long where it's no longer needed. Simply put, there's not enough energy to fully staff the pumps and bail out calcium where it's no longer wanted. As a result, affected tissues are under stress and continue to over-work day and night to the point of exhaustion.

As we've stated, the numerous lumps and bumps we palpate are found predominantly in muscles, tendons, ligaments, and on the outside of a few joints. These areas are in a contracted state—they're working twenty-four hours a day. Only calcium out of its proper storage confinement and sitting in the cytosol (sarcoplasm) of a cell can force that overworked condition.

It's not difficult to accept this premise, since patient distress points directly to the core of the basic abnormality. There isn't anything else we can surmise that would cause such steadily con-tracted tissues. There is an overwhelming tension state as a result of this condition. Readers with fibromyalgia know without being told how many seemingly unrelated parts of the body are affected. "My whole body is tired, it aches, my bladder is irritated, my gut doesn't work, my brain is addled, and even my fingernails keep breaking." The extent of these common complaints should alert my profession to the fact that the malady is a fundamental assault at the very heart of life. The widespread metabolic mayhem can all be explained by inadequate sources of ATP.

We tend to focus on the brain deficits and musculoskeletal pains of fibromyalgia and ignore the fact that they, too, are symp-toms of a larger problem. Multiple studies have revealed problems all over the body in the tissues that produce various molecules, hormones, and neurotransmitters. In other words, journals have reported on abnormalities including low levels of growth hor-mone, insulin-like growth factor, serotonin, certain amino acids, and free urinary cortisol. These and numerous other results have still failed to produce a single accurate diagnostic test for fibromy-algia despite the dedicated efforts of many researchers.

Energy deprivation is certainly at the root of this illness. No matter what findings pop up in the future, the shortage of ATP will continue to explain the disturbance. Many capable MD and PhD investigators are looking for a culprit, and findings are finally emerging—things new to this edition. Any new theory would need to propose a similarly debilitating disturbance, serious enough to destroy what was once a well-functioning body. But only restoration of normal ATP production can give back to patients their mental and physical energies.

In genetics, the term *polymorphisms* refers to multiple variations in a single gene. We're now certain that there is more than just one of these variations scattered in various chromosomes in fibromyalgia. We defended this position early on because we had treated several patients under the age of five, but also many individuals who displayed neither the symptoms nor characteristic findings until later in life—even one who began at the age of seventy-four. That last observation suggested the presence of one or more less destructive genes. The addition of kinder (recessive) genes to less gentle (dominant) ones permits all sorts of combinations (permutations), which in turn determine how intensely and when the illness is first expressed. If both parents have such defects, their mutual children will, too.

In our first edition, I erroneously predicted that the X chromosome would be the likely site for the major genetic defect. When we wrote a book about childhood fibromyalgia, Claudia realized that prior to puberty we had equal numbers of boys and girls (ninety-three to ninety-four, respectively). So why is it that, postpubertally, women make up 85 percent of the fibromyalgia population? It dawned on us that bones and muscles require huge amounts of phosphate to sustain rapid growth. That timing put to rest the myth of "growing pains." They occur mostly in the preteen years of relatively slow growth and usually disappear during the spurt that signals puberty. Testosterone-fed male tissues beef up and sustain lifelong phosphate requirements. Such buffering offers men partial protection from fibromyalgia, but does not eliminate them as genetic carriers.

The human genome has now been mapped, and though there are yet slots to fill in, we and others have identified some mutations. So many people have fibromyalgia that geneticists might at first consider the variations as normal subtypes. We and our patients remain involved in an ongoing study with a premier research institute in Southern California, the City of Hope. I personally suspect that our adverse traits encode defective enzymes that are normally dedicated to precision control of phosphate or other ions. They would be less responsive and would neglect the retention or elimination of phosphate that should accommodate to bodily needs. Initially, the defects would still allow the body to tuck retained excesses into receptive sinkholes, particularly in bones. The daily retention would be minute, but we believe that "tuckability" is eventually exceeded. Other cells must take up the slack even though they get sick doing it.

Had enough of the technical explanations? It's time to discuss our treatment for reversing fibromyalgia.

CHAPTER 3

GUAIFENESIN

How and Why It Works

> I will consider changing my medications, my physical ther-
> apies, and even my exercise routine, but I will not consider
> going without guaifenesin, nor will I take anything that
> might block its effect. It's too important to my well-being.
> —*Devin Starlanyl, author of* The Fibromyalgia Advocate

As often happens in medicine, I stumbled upon the treatment for fibromyalgia quite by accident. I was young and naive, and I was lucky. It all began with a patient's chance observation.

In 1959, long before our illness had been defined or officially named, a patient came to see me on a revisit. He suffered from gout and for two years had taken the only drug available at that time, probenecid (Benemid). He was feeling fine but unexpect-edly said, "Hey, Doc, does this drug take tartar off your teeth?" He then scraped off bits and pieces of tartar (clinically referred to as dental calculus) and flicked them onto my office floor. Though I was not particularly pleased with his newly discovered skill, I responded the way a poised physician should. I harrumphed appropriately and said, "I don't think so." Yet my curiosity was piqued, and I began to reflect on this finding, asking myself what this flaking might indicate.

My knowledge of dentistry was limited so I consulted a textbook that had a page or two devoted to dental calculus. I learned that the mineral backbone of tartar was 75 percent calcium phosphate in a chemical structure called apatite. Tartar develops from saliva, which in turn derives from the serum of blood. Water, all varieties of minerals, proteins, abundant calcium, and phosphate are secreted from blood plasma into the salivary glands. These glands modify and manufacture their own proteins, such as mucus and digestive enzymes. They then mulch and concentrate such things with the above elements to make saliva. My search taught me that salivary phosphate concentrations were four times that normally found in blood. The level of salivary calcium, on the other hand, is just about equal to what's inside the bloodstream. Chemically speaking, this makes for a very unstable solution. We multiply the calcium level by that of phosphate and produce a number called the solubility constant. Sufficient instability caused by too much or too little of either element allows crystals to form deep under the gums and on the teeth; that's the material we call tartar. Though dental calculus can wreak havoc on the gums, teeth, and oral hygiene, that was all the information I could find.

Not everyone creates dental calculus, and those who do produce the stuff at variable rates. My quest was to learn what was metabolically different about tartar formers. I began by looking more closely at people with gout, since it was a gout medication that let my patient chip tartar off his teeth.

I'd been interested in gout and suspected that there was more to the illness than merely joint pains and swelling. I reread the original description written by Thomas Sydenham in 1683. He described gout as a disease with joint pain and one manifested by "great mental torpor," "suffusion of the sinuses," generalized flu-like aching, and malaise or fatigue, along with many other complaints, all in the dramatic language of his day. In other words, there were system-wide effects that were often overshadowed by the pain and throbbing of the joints.

Gout—A metabolic disease unrelated to fibromyalgia. Diagnosis is helped if a high plasma uric acid level is discovered. Aspiration of a gouty joint will show needle-like uric acid crystals. Gout is treated with two types of medications: uricosuric drugs such as sulfinpyrazone and probenecid, which cause the kidneys to excrete excess uric acid; and—more commonly used nowadays—allopurinol or febuxostat, which inhibit the formation of uric acid. Gout has many symptoms, but the most diagnostic is a red, hot, or swollen joint usually located from the knee down. It is inherited, and ten times more common in men than in women, and then only after menopause.

Uric acid—A waste product from the breakdown of nucleic acids in body cells; it is also produced in the digestion of some foods. Most uric acid passes by way of the kidneys into the urine and is excreted, although some is passed through the digestive tract. When the kidneys do not excrete uric acid properly, high levels can build up in the body. This can lead to gout or, to a lesser extent, kidney stones.

Gout is usually inherited, and we know the cause. In susceptible individuals, accumulations of uric acid crystallize and form deposits in certain joints. Sydenham's description of systemic symptoms preceding a joint attack made me wonder if there might be a gouty syndrome. If so, people would have all of the preliminary symptoms of gout without an acute arthritic attack. The condition would appear in cycles owing to minideposits in certain tissues such as the brain and the gastrointestinal tract.

Muscles would be slightly affected and joints spared altogether until very much later in the disease. An elevated plasma uric acid level would be the only way of alerting a physician about such a syndrome, which would predate the typical red, hot, swollen joints seen later on.

I soon found a few patients whom I thought might have these earliest gout symptoms: cyclic bouts of fatigue, irritability, nervousness, depression, insomnia, anxieties, loss of memory and concentration. They also described generalized, flu-like aching and stiffness (mainly in muscles), headaches, dizziness, numbness and tingling of the extremities, and leg cramps as their most prominent complaints. Indigestion with a sour stomach, gas, and flatulence completed the picture. Blood tests revealed higher-than-normal levels of uric acid (urate). When I treated these patients with gout medication, their uric acid dropped to normal. I was exhilarated by the fact that their symptoms also disappeared. Oddly enough, although patients quickly felt better, they still relapsed off and on: They suffered less often and intensely during each subsequent attack by staying on the medication. I'd always known that lowering the blood uric acid actually precipitated acute attacks of gout. As uric acid crystals are pulled from joints, they create pain just as they did going in. My gouty-syndrome patients indeed suffered reversal symptoms similar to those they experienced before treatment. It was exactly the same as Sydenham had described—except, I must stress, that there was no joint involvement. This was surely gout at its inception, before it could be diagnosed by the telltale dramatic symptoms.

Flushed as I was with success, my confidence in my new "gout syndrome pre-gout" was soon shaken. Here came another group of patients who had all of the symptoms suggesting my new condition. Yet no matter how many times I tested, they never showed elevated uric acid. Their aches and pains emanated from the entire musculoskeletal system and only mildly in joints. They had tenderness and swelling in tendons, ligaments, and especially muscles, structures that are only very rarely affected by gout. I decided to try gout medication on their symptoms anyway. To my surprise, they began recycling their symptoms in the same way that high-uric-acid group had. They improved in the same way: Gradually, cyclically, and progressively, they accumulated more good than bad days; ultimately, some went on to complete clearing and remained well if they stayed on the medication. In short, results were identical in all three groups: those with the classic symptoms of gout (red, hot, and swollen joints); those without joint symptoms—the gouty syndrome; and now this no-uric-acid condition. The same drug was effective for all three, but what in the world was the cause of this third thing? I suspected that they were clearing something different out of affected tissues since it couldn't be uric acid.

I began to concentrate on what was different about the group who didn't have elevated uric acid. They suffered from multiple aches and pains, but their fatigue was more overwhelming and constant. Women greatly outnumbered men, whereas gout predominantly affected men. (Gout in women is almost nonexistent before menopause.) It was unlikely there was a connection with gout or the uric acid group despite the similarity in their symptoms, and despite the fact that probenecid was working to reverse both conditions. My sleeping brain must have been mulling this over, and I woke up one night with the thought: Could there be an entirely new disease that acts like the gouty syndrome and is somehow connected to my patient's tartar?

I found it difficult to stop thinking about this idea. There existed no name to describe this entity. *Fibrositis* had fallen into disuse, and *fibromyalgia* wasn't yet born. I had been guilty of dismissing patients with these odd complaints, considering them hypochondriacs. I'd been taught about these psychological misfits, the anxiety neurotics. In school, we were drilled to look for unbalanced hormones, unhappy marriages, empty-nest syndrome, inadequate upbringing, or just plain social maladjustment. When I lingered to elicit all the symptoms, I became fascinated by how similar their stories were. If psychosomatic, how could all these women invent closely identical complaints?

They didn't know each other; they represented every ethnic group; they came from all over the world and from widely disparate socioeconomic demographics. Yet their recitation of symptoms seemed choreographed! Some were stoic, some slightly militant, but most just psychologically whipped. Their lips twitched and they sometimes sobbed a bit when one by one I extracted their unpredictable complaints. They usually recalled good and bad days in the earlier phases of their disease. Most remembered what happiness was before they succumbed, despite having the same marriages, children, stress, and anticipated fun times. I knew it was ludicrous to continue in my belief that all of this was due to their nerves, no matter what psychiatry books iterated. I was soon convinced there existed a prevalent, unidentified, unexplored, but very real disease.

When I initially used the first gout medication, probenecid, I had variable success. The first two patients began the cyclic reversal I had learned to expect in the gouty syndrome. My enthusiasm was soon dashed when I failed with the next three patients. After some initial teeth gnashing (mine), something told me to try a higher dosage. I did, and the rewards were swift: All three patients began the hoped-for reverse cycling. It now seemed even more likely that there actually was a tartar, or apatite crystal, syndrome—as I first named it. It was, however, clear that uric acid played no part in the condition, since I could never detect abnormal levels in any of these people.

As I paid close attention, I found progressively more patients who fit the mold. So many, in fact, that I soon knew I was look-ing at a very common and major illness. Moreover, it was a debilitating disease that inexorably and ultimately destroyed quality of life. Vast numbers of these patients soon swelled my practice; I learned a great deal from them. I quickly realized the illness was familial. The oldest related their horror stories with a longer litany of complaints, but even the youngest of them had a list.

I was routinely touched by the years patients had suffered. Nuances in their stories made each one different, but left no doubt they were ill with the same sickness. It would have helped to have an electronic tablet to record the number of prior physician visits, tests, surgeries, and oddball diagnoses. Probably you readers can add to that list: "It's a bad menopause," "you're depressed," "inner ear disorder," "defect in your neurotransmitters," "rheumatoid arthritis," "migraine syndrome," "early lupus," or "multiple sclerosis."

For too many in those days, it was only a matter of time before most were told: "It's all in your head; you need a psychiatrist." Some had seriously considered suicide, so compromised was the quality of their lives. They were frustrated and guilt-ridden about not being able to care for their families. They fiercely resented being different from other people. When I told them they suffered from an honest-to-goodness illness, I had to hand many of them the Kleenex box.

One day in August my body just said, "That's enough," and I hardly got out of bed for six months. With a teen, a tween, and a first grader, that was very rough. The years of migraines, body aches, shooting pains, sharp pains, numbness, restless legs, bladder issues, intolerance to so much, the feeling of throbbing, overwhelming heaviness that was nonstop...The list was embarrassing every time I went to a new doctor or tried a new approach. If it wasn't for a stranger who pushed me in the direction of Dr. St. Amand, I would have never gotten my life back, and who knows how long I could have kept living. I was on fifteen prescription pills a day for all of my symptoms and the doctors told me that sometimes this "just happens." I began to believe what everyone else said, this *was* all in my head, *maybe* I just need to accept all the pills and the cane to help me walk and the missing out on virtually everything in life. Because of the guaifenesin protocol, I was able to kick that bad attitude and brainwashing to the curb and fight back to not only getting off *all* my prescriptions, but also ditching the cane and eventually getting back to work again.

—*Gennessee A., California*

New uricosuric medications appeared in subsequent years: Anturane, Flexin, and Robinul. Each acted at a well-defined kidney level to increase uric acid excretion and was effective for gout. Strikingly, each also worked for our gouty syndrome and for fibromyalgia. But remember, fibromyalgia is not connected to uric acid. Several articles and books have said that I believe uric acid is involved in the disease. I have consistently denied that I ever believed such a thing. There are similarities, but something other than uric acid is being extruded. Whatever genetic defect manifests at that location, it is mitigated by guaifenesin as well as by all the uricosuric drugs we have tried.

With treatment, other patients began flicking tartar. That wasn't much help to us since too many healthy people can do the same. Nevertheless, those early observations had put me on the right track. The successes forced me to suspect that the body was improperly handling either calcium or phosphate. Patients commonly described chipping and peeling of their fingernails in cycles. Nail minerals are predominantly calcium and phosphate—the same as tartar. I theorized that nails were also cycling and depositing similar excesses at their roots. Compare this to the concentric rings of trees created as they grow. As with fibromyalgia, trees make defective layers during adverse cycles.

Calcium was not the problem. Our gout medicines worked on

the negatively charged urate part of uric acid (sodium urate). Calcium, unlike urate, is an ion with positive charges. If I could eliminate calcium as the culprit, logically I would suspect its companion in tartar, phosphate. There were ample biochemical reasons that pointed to phosphate. Like urate, it carries negatively charged ions. Calcium tablets sometimes helped patients feel slightly better. Calcium bound chemically to phosphate in the intestine, decreased its absorption, and helped eliminate it into the stools. Kidney reabsorption or excretion of phosphate into the urine is handled in about the same area as uric acid. Calcium was a clue, but not effective enough alone to reverse fibromyalgia.

Although the uricosuric drugs I was using to treat fibromyalgia were successful, they had side effects. Sulfinpyrazone could raise stomach acidity enough to cause ulcers. Probenecid is a sulfa drug, and if allergy develops, the resulting hives can last for weeks. Robinul causes dry mouth or eyes (dangerous in glaucoma), nausea, and abdominal pain, and increases fatigue or a spacey feeling; it may also cause major urinary retention in men with an enlarged prostate.

So due to these limitations, I was always on the lookout for a more effective, better-tolerated medication. In 1991, more than thirty years after I began my initial research, I got lucky. My nurse's ten-year-old son, Malcolm Potter, had been on our treatment for fibromyalgia since the age of seven. As he grew, he needed somewhat larger amounts of his medication, sulfinpyrazone (Anturane), to continue his reversal. As mentioned above, this drug causes hyperacidity and gastric upsets in 8 percent of patients. As my young patient grew taller, we raised his dosage and as a result, his stomach began to hurt. I didn't want to try the other medications since I worried about their particular side effects. This was a kid who would need some drug for the rest of his life, so I intensified my search for a safer substitute.

Luckily for Malcolm, it wasn't long before I recalled a little clipping about another drug that could ever so slightly lower uric acid. I was able to confirm this in a newer edition of the *Physicians' Desk Reference*. The effect of this medication on uric acid is far too weak to successfully treat gout.[1] But you'll recall that anything I'd used so far with that effect had also worked for fibromyalgia. A bit later, I came upon a corroborating article in an old copy of the *Journal of Rheumatology*.[2]

The FDA-approved use of guaifenesin is for producing and loosening mucus in various respiratory infections. Thus, it's found in many cold preparations. It originated somewhere around 1530 as a boiled tree bark distillation called guaiacum and, believe it or not, was widely used for rheumatism.[3] It was even used to treat gout. In 1928, a medical paper extolled its virtues for treating growing pains in children. It also relieved symptoms we would now recognize as fibromyalgia. Guaiacum was later purified to guaiacolate, and made its first appearance in cough mixtures some eighty years ago. It was eventually synthesized and about forty years ago was pressed into tablets and named guaifenesin. Its original use isn't completely ignored, however. In the *"Physicians' Desk Reference" for Herbal Medicines*, *Guaiacum officinale* remains a liquid medication indicated for rheumatism.[4]

The standard guaifenesin dosage for creating looser phlegm in bronchitis, asthma, hay fever, and nasal and sinus congestion is 1,200 mg in the morning and in the evening (2,400 mg per day). For many years, guaifenesin was a prescription drug. Now the drug is sold over the counter and in differing strengths, making it widely accessible. It's available in 600 and 1,200 mg extended-release strengths, as well as combined short- and long-acting 600 or 1,200 mg tablets. There are also immediate-release (or short-acting) guaifenesin preparations in various strengths, but most commonly 200 or 400 mg tablets. Since 2004, the brand name is Mucinex (a bilayered long and short combination), but there are now various generic forms. Guaifenesin is quite well absorbed from the intestinal tract at rates that differ among preparations.

Guaifenesin (gwy-FEN-e-sin) is an expectorant that thins mucus and helps to loosen phlegm. Guaifenesin is quickly absorbed from the gastrointestinal tract, and is rapidly metabolized and excreted into the urine. Guaifenesin is also known to lower uric acid levels. No serious side effects have been reported.[5]

—*Physicians' Desk Reference*

To learn more about guaifenesin, go to such sources as www.drugs .com or bring it up in your computer through your search engines. Your pharmacist could copy a printout for you. But the newer *Physicians' Desk Reference* reference book no longer describes it, because it's sold over the counter.

But let's return now to my willing test subject, Malcolm, who had been off his original medicine for some time because of his irritated stomach. I surmised that I'd see some kind of reversal symptoms within a few days if guaifenesin was effective. Luckily for all of us, Malcolm, on the second morning after beginning guaifenesin, stumbled out of his bedroom moaning, "Mom, I can't walk—even the bottoms of my feet hurt!" So pervasive were his stiffness and aching that we knew we'd struck therapeutic gold! Indeed, we had stumbled upon the safest and most potent weapon against this disease. Since guaifenesin has no significant side effects, his symptom onslaught could only mean that we were purging his fibromyalgia. Unconvincingly for him during his full-blown torture, he was to lead us all back onto a safer road to recovery!

HOW DOES GUAIFENESIN WORK ON FIBROMYALGIA?

Do you remember our discussion in chapter 1 about the lumps and bumps of fibromyalgia? We find them on every single patient with the disease. We transpose each onto a body caricature, or map, for future tracking. These swollen places are for the most part tender. They're located in tendons and ligaments, but mostly in muscles. Ninety to 95 percent of the swelling is simply water that has collected under considerable pressure. We suspect this fluid has been lured into cells because of the forced entry of a slight excess of phosphate and calcium. Overconcentration of these two elements could seriously threaten survival of the affected cells, making dilution mandatory. That's accomplished by sucking in salt (sodium chloride) accompanied by water. Proper dilution is achieved; cells are saved from destruction, but some malfunction results. A lump appears that can be easily felt when we examine a patient. The worst part of this process is that swelling presses on nerves, and they transmit messages of discomfort to the brain. Only when each element is tucked into relatively safe storage areas is some of the water allowed to leave. That actually reduces the size of the bump and somewhat eases pain.

Why did his getting worse tell us that Malcolm was actually improving? The answer is reversal pain, the opposite of what happens when the disease develops. The body can't pull concentrates out into more diluted areas, because this would defy some chemistry and the body's dictum of equilibrium. When reversal begins, water has to reenter the affected cells wherever clearing is about to start. That extra fluid again causes swelling and pressure on nerves to signal pain messages. When guaifenesin initiates purging, the newly retained fluid reverses direction and is expelled from cells, taking the excess ions of phosphate, calcium, and sodium along with it. The expanded cells shrink down a bit and lessen pressure on nerves and some of the miseries of fibromyalgia.

When cells do their cleaning, they sweep phosphate and its fellow travelers back out into the bloodstream. Varying with the amount of waterborne material being extracted, the blood undergoes a miniflooding with the same debris it just tried to hide.

This time, the phosphate flows into the kidneys for excretion. But the kidneys can't immediately process all of that sudden inflow. You'll recall our theory that fibromyalgia occurs because the kidneys are sluggish when it comes to expelling phosphate. Since the urine is the only elimination route, the waste backs up, waiting its turn for elimination. The blood is impatient and, meeting renal resistance, responds by stashing minideposits into temporary staging areas all over the body. Muscles absorb up a fair share, which causes generalized, flu-like aching. The brain also cooperates and stores enough debris to intensify fatigue, cognitive impairment, irritability, depression, anxiety, and insomnia. It's as if the disease were heading entirely in the wrong direction. In fact, it seems worse than ever, since purging is moving detritus out of cells at least six times faster than it had been allowed to enter. The difference this time, however, is that the kidneys are now working in the right direction, thanks to guaifenesin. They're now at full capacity trying to eliminate the unacceptable excesses. As you'd expect, symptoms of fibromyalgia worsen until the kidneys catch up.

What pours out under treatment are the accumulated chemical energy blockers that induced fibromyalgia. Guaifenesin will pull out some excess phosphate in small batches with help from the kidneys. During this purging, along with the above symptoms, patients also describe unpleasant tastes, scalded mouth, bad breath, and burning perspiration and urine as the body dumps the acidic phosphate into all bodily fluids. Even tears and vaginal secretions may sting. During this leaching-out period, people often notice small amounts of particulate matter or bubbles in the urine. Each cycle ends when that's all that can be done metabolically for the time being.

Between reversal cycles, relative rest periods follow. They could last for just a few hours, sometimes days, or even weeks. During more peaceful periods, it's still likely that some reversing is going on at a subliminal level. What patients experience varies greatly, since so much depends on individual pain thresholds and ability to cope. Only one thing is sure: It soon becomes clear that the next attack is under way. Over time, these symptom onslaughts diminish in intensity and frequency. The severity of symptoms lessens, and patients gradually get closer to restoring their health. Reversal symptoms, however intense, should reassure the patient that guaifenesin is working, because the drug has no known side effects. These attacks and serial body map improvements tell us that restoration is in process.

My daughter was diagnosed with FMS after two years of searching for what was wrong. That year she missed over seventy days of school. Then I found the information about guaifenesin. I took it to my doctor, who had heard of it and didn't know if it would work. Together we followed the directions.

Now, for the first time in over five years, my daughter was able to go on a vacation and not be afraid of the pain. She was able to go to school without fear and went outside and played with her girlfriends! When school started this year, teacher after teacher stopped her and asked her what had changed over the summer; she looked so good and different! She is thirteen years old and in junior high...to be pain free and to be able to go out on the soccer field with her friends without the fear of the pain has been amazing.

—*Irene, California*

We commented earlier that we have used five totally different medications that worked to clear fibromyalgia. These had nothing in common except that they act at the same site in the kidney. It is well documented that each urges the kidneys to excrete a lot or a bit more uric acid. Yet because it is easily measured, we know uric acid is not the culprit in fibromyalgia. Years ago, while searching for a clue as to what else these drugs might expel, I had measured the urinary output of phosphate, calcium, and urate before and during treatment with probenecid. Later we performed the same experiment on patients using guaifenesin and got virtually the same results. We found a 60 percent increase in phosphate excretion and a lesser (30 percent) unloading of oxalate and calcium. But where the gout medications significantly increased uric acid excretion, only a minimal discharge occurred with guaifenesin. This finding cemented our belief that phosphate is the culprit in fibromyalgia.

How does guaifenesin purge phosphate from the body? It's somewhat like opening a spigot that lets the kidneys drain out the problem. Think of your home water system. You open the tap, and water flows out of the faucet from the pipes that connect to the main line, which pulls from a larger source. Ultimately, the reservoir to which your pipes are connected gets lowered by the amount you've used at home, no matter the distance between the two locations.

We can use this analogy to explain our version of fibromyalgia. Those of us with defective genes have perfectly normal kidney function. The problem arises because this inherited defect produces some slightly crippled proteins called enzymes. In non-affected people, these allow well-controlled opening of the spigot whenever the bloodstream offers up waste for renal filtering. Our theory suggests that affected kidneys badly direct the fate of inorganic phosphate (symbol: P_i). Our genetic malfunction doesn't let the tap open fully; phosphate still leaks out, but sluggishly. There may be considerable daily variability, but that back-damming effect will eventually accrue P_i and redistribute it throughout the body. Different tissue susceptibilities determine which ones will best scoop up this excess phosphate.

The process works roughly like this. Metabolic by-products are transported via the bloodstream to the kidneys for filtering.

Flushing through these structures are surplus minerals, chemicals, and water in concentrations almost identical to those of the blood—with some notable exceptions such as inorganic phosphate (P_i). Huge amounts of that are absorbed from our foodstuffs and mainly used to make cellular energy, and for this reason the body requires a huge amount. But as with most other body ingredients, there are always leftovers. A lot are recycled, but some get extruded from cells and pushed into the bloodstream. That excess baggage is what's sent downstream to the kidneys for possible elimination. There the no-longer-needed substances and water are extracted to form urine. This major interface of blood and kidney occurs at places called glomeruli.

Our kidneys are the command centers when it comes to designing urine. At some point, cells lining the walls of the renal tubules make decisions. They solicit nerve or hormonal advice before releasing filtered products such as phosphate into the bladder. At the same time, impulses can arrive from multiple sources urgently requesting extra P_i. Tubules are capable of reabsorbing whatever may be needed. Cells lining the millions of kidney tubules face the developing urine stream on one side, and the blood capillaries on the opposite end. That's where choices are made concerning many urine-borne substances, including P_i. Tubules can open side gates to retrieve P_i and allow it through to the blood side for reuse. Depending on the incoming signals, they can also keep them closed, deny access, and direct partial or total excretion. You can see in figure 3.1 how this works.

Phosphate thus has two ways to go. Both are through the bloodstream's capillary walls. The first system shoves it directly into the fluid that's about to become urine. The second extracts it from the blood straight into the tubule-lining cells from one side and ejects through the other side into the urine. While this sounds like an unnecessarily duplicated effort, these two venues are under different yet synchronized control. Phosphate

Kidney Phosphate Control

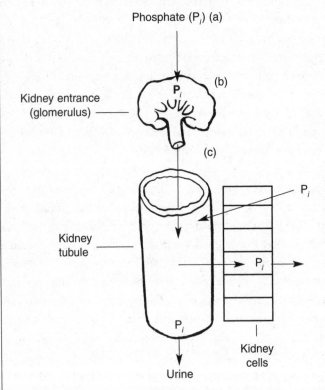

(a) Blood brings inorganic phosphate P_i to the kidney.
(b) P_i is filtered through the glomerulus and is delivered to the tubule.
(c) P_i can also be delivered directly through the blood and through the kidney cells into the tubule.
(d) P_i can go two ways from the tubule:
      1. Out into the urine.
      2. Reabsorbed from the tubule into the kidney cell and back into the bloodstream.

This is how kidney cells "decide" to keep or eliminate phosphates according to what the body needs.

Figure 3.1

concentrations are sensed; nerve and hormonal suggestions are respected to please the body's requirements. It sounds simple, but these activities count on enzymes responding correctly to the body's needs. In fibromyalgia, it is probable that one or more of the involved enzymes are genetically defective or malformed. This would fit with our theory: Fibromyalgics just can't get rid of enough phosphate.

Now we can choreograph the whole scene. Cells work so we can live, but require a huge amount of energy in the process. Most of our food is expended to create ATP in the many mitochondria that sit inside each cell. Once formed, this adenosine triphosphate can flip off attached, energized phosphates one at a time and make metabolic things happen. It's highly energy-expensive to keep body parts functioning. Normal wear and tear of cells adds more waste phosphate to the dietary surpluses not earmarked for immediate use. All of that is dispatched to the kidneys for the sorting out, as we've just discussed.

The body won't tolerate P_i accumulation in the blood, because it's a reciprocal to calcium. This means that when phosphate rises, calcium must fall. There are four parathyroid glands in the neck that are constantly policing such an imbalance. They pour out hormones that protect calcium levels. Phosphate can't escape in the urine, and it isn't even allowed to linger in the bloodstream. So what is the solution to that? In some predetermined pecking order, certain tissues must accept some phosphate to help clear the blood. This process drives inorganic phosphate back into cells willing to accept the responsibility. Muscles and sinews are the most obvious targets, as the body always seeks to spare vital organs. At some point, P_i excesses slow down the mitochondrial generators, and energy production starts lagging. It's chemically necessary that water enter affected cells to keep incoming phosphate and its fellow traveler, calcium, in proper concentration. Sodium and chloride surf along to permit such mandatory dilutions. Those cellular visitors cause swelling and produce the lumps and bumps of fibromyalgia. In turn, that squeezes nerves and sends distress signals to the brain. There the problem is interpreted to express the symptoms of fibromyalgia: pain, burning, crawling, tingling, and numbness. The brain itself isn't immune to the process, so add fatigue and cognitive impairment. We've sketched this sequence in figure 3.2.

Earlier we explained how excess phosphate interrupts energy (ATP) production in mitochondria and causes the symptoms of fibromyalgia. We solve the problem by helping the kidneys back into efficiency. Purge excess phosphate and, no surprise, watch the body's cells eagerly produce all of the ATP we need. Calcium that's been tied up by P_i is also siphoned out of overladen stores. Rid of misplaced calcium, cells get out of overdrive and can relax. Such restoration predictably reenergizes our systems to their full capacity. We believe guaifenesin to be the best and safest agent to prod reluctant enzyme spigots to open wide and let us get on with the business of robust living. (See figure 3.3.)

A very difficult aspect of treatment is what patients must go through during reversal. This is especially tough as too many have already been disappointed by promises of cures that never materialized. They enter the initial recycling phases desperate for a glimmer of hope flashed by getting a few decent hours. We tell our patients that these will be their assurance of success ahead. Once the body provides a few better hours or days, it's signaling that it can do so on a permanent basis. Only when people feel the first pain-free moments will they begin to trust the benefits of guaifenesin and believe what we have told them. It takes guts and perseverance to keep faith when confronted by sometimes intense early reversal symptoms. Later cleansing cycles are also tough, but by then patients have had a taste of recovery: a series of good days with diminished pain and fatigue. That makes coping a lot easier. Even so, each early reversing cycle evokes former concerns.

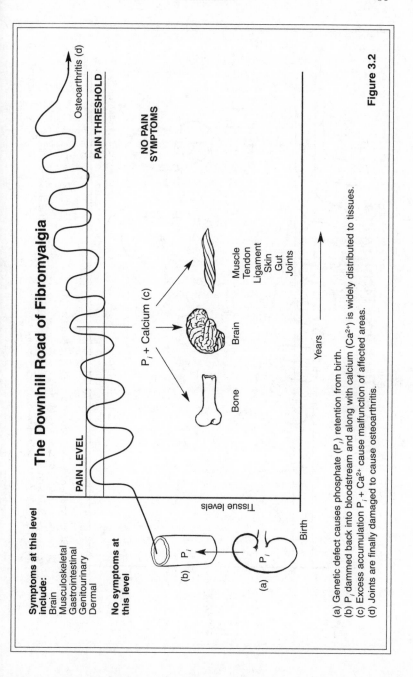

The Downhill Road of Fibromyalgia

Symptoms at this level include:
Brain
Musculoskeletal
Gastrointestinal
Genitourinary
Dermal

No symptoms at this level

PAIN LEVEL

PAIN THRESHOLD

NO PAIN SYMPTOMS

Osteoarthritis (d)

Tissue levels

Birth

Years

P_i + Calcium (c)

Bone

Brain

Muscle
Tendon
Ligament
Skin
Gut
Joints

(a)

(b) P_i

P_i

(a) Genetic defect causes phosphate (P_i) retention from birth.
(b) P_i dammed back into bloodstream and along with calcium (Ca^{2+}) is widely distributed to tissues.
(c) Excess accumulation P_i + Ca^{2+} cause malfunction of affected areas.
(d) Joints are finally damaged to cause osteoarthritis.

Figure 3.2

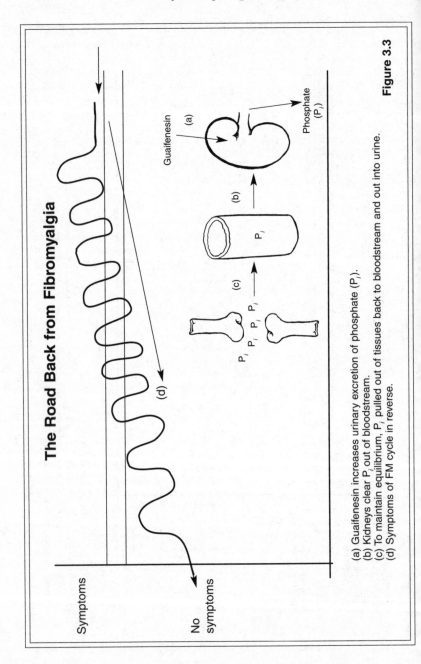

The Road Back from Fibromyalgia

(a) Guaifenesin increases urinary excretion of phosphate (P_i).
(b) Kidneys clear P_i out of bloodstream.
(c) To maintain equilibrium, P_i pulled out of tissues back to bloodstream and out into urine.
(d) Symptoms of FM cycle in reverse.

Figure 3.3

The pain in my shoulders and calves was so intense. It was worse in the mornings and made getting out of bed very difficult. My morning routine included slathering on lots of analgesic cream before I could even think of heading to work. I hoped that my students wouldn't say that their twenty-four-year-old teacher smelled funny. After two months on the protocol, that intense pain subsided greatly and soon enough I didn't need the analgesic cream! Some days I just got up and went to work—without a thought about the pain I was missing.

—*Andrea F., California*

I was diagnosed in 1987, when it was called fibrositis, while in physical therapy school. I was lucky to be where I was because my diagnosis was quick but I was in no way prepared for the destruction this new entity would have on my life. From the day of my diagnosis until the present, I have studied and searched for anything that would help me have a more functional life. It has been hit or miss at best, from consuming shark cartilage to applying magnets to my body. There have been chunks of time taken away from me where the only thing I wanted to do was stay in bed. I have been limited as a mother of two boys and as a wife and at times felt totally inadequate at both.

Two years ago I found Dr. St. Amand's book and began the protocol. A year ago I went on the liberal diet. I began running, although I was told a long time ago that was a big no-no. I just turned forty-five and I have gone from fibromyalgia to 5K. In the last year, I have completed five 5Ks and just came in first in my age group, winning a medal. I am still on my medication but feel nothing can stop me now. I am more active and have more energy. Enjoying life is now my priority, not my fibromyalgia. In my wildest dreams, I would have never guessed I would be where I am now.

—*Cheri M., California*

A common reaction from patients is to suspect that their bodies are different from those of other fibromyalgics. They have trouble overriding the fear that arises from previous disappointments. As treatment progresses, confidence mounts, and relatively soon they become old pros at the ins and outs of their disease. They know good days will return in greater numbers, attacks will be milder, more bearable, and leave progressively fewer areas to purge. Though the initial reversal cycles might have attacked ten or twenty places at one time, later reversals work on only one or two sites simultaneously. This alone greatly diminishes the severity of subsequent attacks. Purging phases get progressively farther apart, making setbacks minor in comparison with the past.

Every patient asks: "How long will it take for me to clear?" There's no easy answer. It depends on several things: the duration of the illness, genetic makeup, and the dosage of guaifenesin required for response. The fastest-responding patients receive low doses (300 mg twice a day), but clear with intense and almost constant attacks. Slower patients need larger dosages and have reversal rates spread over a spectrum of possibilities. We rely on a well-tested rule that the slowest people clean out one year of fibromyalgic debris every two months. The clock doesn't start ticking, however, until they've found the proper dosage and become totally salicylate-free. Yes, it's gradual for some, and unbelievably fast for those lucky ones. Slow responders can go faster under a doctor's guidance by raising the dosage using either longer- or faster-acting guaifenesin. Just don't lose heart.

I think I am reaching a turning point now where the good days are as frequent as the bad days. I told my husband last week I don't feel like I need to have a parade thrown in honor of a good day anymore. I just enjoy it (at first I felt like he should drop everything and celebrate it with me). You know that Celebrex commercial on TV, "I don't want to run a marathon, I just want to give Timmy a bath"? Well, I appreciate the simplest things these days—feeling good enough to scoop dog poop in the backyard, or hang clothes out on the line, or mop the floor.

I've lost fifteen pounds, am able to get around better even on my worst days, and occasionally feel up to a walk in the park across the street. I make a point of building extra steps into my housework, and extra trips up and down the stairs, especially on good days.

—*Marti T., Ohio*

Another patient, who went through years of hardship with fibromyalgia and had difficult cycling during treatment, recounts her experience:

I want to brag about my second thirty-mile bike ride. I am very proud of myself. I want you to know how far I've come. I am forty-eight years old and suffered all my life with progressively more and more pain and depression. I have been on most of the powerful painkillers and antidepressants over the years. I closed my business and quit working in 1994. My mind was worthless, the fatigue and pain made getting out of bed impossible on most days, and I had horrid insomnia for years. The symptoms would come and go, and most of the time I "looked normal," although I put on a lot of weight. Life has always been a fight against body and mind pain. In February of 1997 I was hit hard. My entire body swelled, my skin burned all over, my mouth burned badly, and I salivated constantly. My stomach contorted. My mind went crazy. Most of my muscles were in spasm. I couldn't move without sweating profusely.

—*G. M., California*

FREQUENTLY ASKED QUESTIONS

Before we leave the subject of guaifenesin and end this chapter, let's deal with some of the questions most commonly asked.

Does guaifenesin have side effects?
Other than infrequent and transient nausea in the early treatment stages, guaifenesin has no known side effects.

Which guaifenesin should I use?
Any pure (or plain) guaifenesin free of added medications such as pseudoephedrine or dextromethorphan will do just fine as long as it is a longer-acting or extended-release compound. We do advise patients not to use pills that contain blue dye due to its ability to inhibit energy production at the cellular level, which is exactly what is *not* needed in fibromyalgia.

Can I get guaifenesin over the counter?
Currently, all single-ingredient guaifenesin is sold over the counter.

Can I just treat myself?
We don't particularly recommend self-treatment unless you have a doctor to supervise you. There are many symptoms in fibromyalgia that could easily mask some other condition. Although you should always have those excluded before you begin, it's important to remain vigilant because you can develop another condition. You always need to have a medical doctor who can help you if you have worries about certain symptoms and perform exams and blood tests periodically.

Do I need to drink lots of water with my guaifenesin?
That's not necessary. Pushing fluids *is* urged if you're taking guaifenesin for lung or sinus problems. Extra fluid helps loosen mucus, which is not necessary when using the drug for fibromyalgia.

Should I continue my other medications when I start guaifenesin?
Guaifenesin mixes safely with anything (except salicylates). Your doctor will undoubtedly want you to continue other medications, and many cannot be stopped abruptly. Since you will need to observe your cycles, you do not want to introduce new variables by changing around your medications. But you must stop all aspirin: Avoid Soma Compound (replace with plain Soma), Fiorinal (replace with Fioricet), Empirin, and Percodan (replace with Percocet). We'll tell you more about such things as Pepto-Bismol, Excedrin, muscle rubs, and other products in chapter 4. Don't discontinue or change dosages of prescription medications without consulting your physician.

Some people refer to the guaifenesin protocol as detoxification. Is that correct?
There are no toxins in fibromyalgia. Whatever causes FMS is not foreign to the body, because the body mounts no inflammatory response or antibody attack. We think fibromyalgia is caused by customarily friendly phosphate—there's just too much of it in the wrong places. Since there are no toxins, guaifenesin does not "detox."

Is guaifenesin safe to take if I get pregnant?
Guaifenesin has actually been used to help women get pregnant. It was thought to be helpful solely for its ability to liquefy the mucous plug that normally sits at the opening of the uterus. Later findings identified spermatocidal qualities of this mucus in some women, a defect that is corrected using guaifenesin. Thus, it is safe to take guaifenesin until you know you are pregnant. We suggest each woman discuss this issue with her own doctor. We advise our pregnant patients to stop all medications before attempting to become pregnant. With the permission of your obstetrician, you may resume treatment after the sixth month of pregnancy, since the baby is fully formed by then. This way, fibromyalgic

women can avoid the sudden burst of symptoms that often follows delivery.

Am I at greater risk of osteoporosis when taking guaifenesin?

The calcium excreted by guaifenesin is limited to the inappropriate surplus temporarily locked within your cells. So you don't have to worry about causing osteoporosis. Remember, the medication has been used for more than four hundred years in some form or other. Problems would have shown up by now.

Can guaifenesin cause kidney stones?

No, there are no connections between kidney stones and guaifenesin or fibromyalgia. Most stones are calcium oxalate, some sodium urate, and others complexes of calcium-clutching phosphates and carbonates. We repeat, guaifenesin has been used for years and never implicated with kidney stones. One tiny study found a possible connection, but as confirmed by the authors, subjects were not taking pure guaifenesin. They were abusing combinations of guaifenesin and pseudoephedrine. (The latter is the drug used in the unlawful manufacture of methamphetamine.) Pseudoephedrine was the likely suspect, not guaifenesin.

Is it okay to drink colas while taking guaifenesin?

We have not had to restrict colas though they do contain phosphoric acid. Phosphate is what we're trying to purge from the body, but guaifenesin overcomes that added load rather easily.

If I have asthma, can I take guaifenesin?

Guaifenesin is frequently used for asthma. It's actually marketed as being "mucolytic." That helps cells produce lighter mucus, making it less tenacious and easier to raise. Anyone with added medical conditions should always ask their physician for permission to add any medication.

*   *   *

Are you ready to move on and learn about the protocol? The next few chapters will describe lots of things that will help you understand and successfully treat fibromyalgia.

> Finding your dose is a serious business. The fastest way to reverse your fibro is to take the time to start the journey right. Take a breath. Slow down. Follow the steps in the book. There are no shortcuts.
>
> —*Sophie, Australia*

CHAPTER 4

THE FLY IN THE OINTMENT

Aspirin and Other Salicylates

You can easily manage to get by without salicylates. In the beginning, if you are unsure and too confused to understand, just use fewer products. It's funny that we do without so many things when we are sick, but then want to argue about giving up mint toothpaste. There's no point in reading the book and getting guaifenesin and hoping that you'll get better if you don't do your homework about salicylates. There are many resources to help you and now there are even companies that make special products.

—*Gloria M., California*

Critics say our protocol is difficult (or impossible) because it's just too complicated to avoid salicylate by its many names. We've written this chapter to prove that it's not, especially when compared with living with fibromyalgia. It takes time to learn how to avoid salicylates but it is worth the effort, and certainly in time becomes second nature. Thousands of patients have learned to do it. This book will guide you, and this chapter will help you better understand why it is so important. Figuring it out might be a bit stressful at first, but it's a lot better than being sick every day of your life. Next to that, reading labels whenever you buy something new seems barely an inconvenience. We think you'll agree when you have your first good day.

A BRIEF HISTORY OF SALICYLATES

All five of the medications we've used over the years to treat fibromyalgia have one other thing in common. In each case, the compound salicylate (salicylic acid) blocks their chemical activity at the precise kidney location where we need help.

We must stress that there are no known drug interactions between guaifenesin and any medication. Mixing guaifenesin with salicylates will not make you ill. Guaifenesin will still help liquefy your mucus, and make a cough more productive, but the action we need to treat fibromyalgia will be totally neutered—or blocked. There won't be any outward manifestation of this blocking effect; that's both good and bad news. You won't feel sick if you make a mistake, but it also means that you won't be able to tell by how you feel that your medication isn't effective. In time, of course, you'll suspect the blocking when you start to feel ill more of the time. That's why it's so absolutely necessary to read and review this chapter until you understand what's written here. Unless you successfully avoid salicylates, no amount of guaifenesin can do *anything* to heal you.

Salicylates have been used medicinally since as early as 1500 BC, when ancient Egyptians recorded a pain-relieving recipe using dried myrtle leaves. In the fifth century BC, Hippocrates, affectionately known as the father of medicine, promoted juice extracts from the bark of willow trees for treating aches and pains. Diverse cultures, such as the Native Americans, made the same discovery and used barks and meadow grasses to prepare topical or internal preparations for the same purposes. During the late Middle Ages, a willow bark concoction to alleviate pain and fevers was so popular in Europe it had to be outlawed when trees were being cut down faster than they could be replanted—almost destroying the wicker industry. That law was repealed in 1806 because the alternative drug, quinine from Peru, couldn't reach Europe during Napoleon's blockade.

Whenever plants are found useful in treating disease, a search begins to find the active chemical that's responsible. Then it can be extracted, purified, and made into doses that are uniform in potency. In 1823, the chemical salicin was successfully extracted from the bark of a willow and named for the tree's Latin moniker: *Salix*. Later it was extracted from meadowsweet and many other plants. *Salicin* is still the name used to identify the naturally occurring compound.

Once the chemical was identified, a race was on to synthesize the molecule—that is, to make it from scratch in a laboratory. No longer would entire trees be sacrificed just to extract a few milligrams of drug. It was hoped that this process would be less laborious and expensive than the extraction, and of course that it would result in a successful capitalistic venture. In 1853, this was accomplished, but soon abandoned because the substance proved too acidic for humans to tolerate. For the next fifty years, chemists established the chemical structure and came up with more efficient ways to produce it.

Finally a German chemist, Felix Hoffman, decided to search for a stomach-friendly, less-toxic salicylate in order to alleviate his father's arthritic pains. He was successful and convinced his employer, Bayer, to market it. In 1899, aspirin was born in the form of a prescription powder. A tablet soon followed, and in 1915, it was made available without prescription as a condition of the Treaty of Versailles, which ended World War I. Bayer lost its trademark to the name Aspirin in the US in 1918; today that is used as a generic name in many countries, such as the United Kingdom, Australia, and New Zealand. In Canada, Aspirin with a capital letter is still trademarked, but if it is shown with a lowercase *a* it is a generic. That's why you'll often see *aspirin* and *acetylsalicylic acid* used interchangeably on labels. Avoid them both, obviously.

Aspirin's full effects on the body are still being explored. Its pain-relieving aspects are enhanced by reducing the internal production of prostaglandins and clipping their role in inducing inflammation and nerve sensitivity to pain. Aspirin also lessens the adhesive tendencies of blood platelets and so cuts the risk of a repeat heart attack and certain types of strokes in men and older women. It has actions that might help lessen the risk of colon cancer and possibly cataracts. It costs very little because it's so inexpensively produced. It has wide application as the concentrate salicylic acid used to remove warts and corns; more dilute in cosmetic creams and lotions for treating acne and dandruff; and in chemical skin peels made with weaker concentrations to achieve a mild exfoliation. It's used primarily as a sunscreen in the US even though it does not provide protection against the rays that cause skin cancers.

HOW SALICYLATES BLOCK GUAIFENESIN

Why do salicylates cause such problems for our protocol? The answer isn't very complicated. There is a particular area in the kidneys where guaifenesin must be allowed access to work unimpeded. Unfortunately, it's precisely the same location where salicylates attach to targeted cells: in the renal tubules. These cells have surface areas that house thousands of receptors. It's easy to visualize the process if you think of each receptor as a custom-made garage designed for use only by certain specially shaped cars. Each garage will allow parking only for cars that fit perfectly.

In the human body, every receptor on every cell is precision-made to accommodate only a specific hormone or chemical. For any medication to succeed, it must find and neatly fit into that receptor, which is always a space designed for a natural molecule.

This is what the science of pharmacology is all about. Drugs are manufactured to occupy an existing receptor that will either trigger or block an action.

Unfortunately, guaifenesin and salicylates compete for the same receptors, but salicylates are a better fit and so get preferential parking. Even small amounts of salicylate can occupy all the available sites, leaving none for guaifenesin. In a manner of speaking, once the parking garage is full, it shuts down. As an aside, even with abundant circulating salicylates, guaifenesin still successfully liquefies mucus because it continues to fit into the altogether different receptors in tissues other than the renal tubules. But its benefit for fibromyalgia is nonexistent when salicylates are present.

We've worked since the beginning with this problem we call blocking. We didn't discover it. We already knew patients would have to avoid aspirin. Salicylate's blockade of uricosuric compounds is well documented in medical literature, and the older gout medications all carry a printed warning on the bottle. We had learned by using those medications that their ability to reverse fibromyalgia was blocked in the same way. We knew that guaifenesin wouldn't work to reverse fibromyalgia when taken with aspirin. But we had a lot to learn about other forms of salicylate and what potent effects they had.

There are many studies that have demonstrated the ability of skin to absorb salicylates. Skin biopsies have shown that salicylate topically applied directly at the top of one shoulder muscle (trapezius) was found within one half hour in almost equal concentration in the opposite side. Clearly it was absorbed into the bloodstream and transported effectively throughout the body. It's well known that topical creams applied for muscle pain easily penetrate into underlying tissues and provide relief. But initially we had no idea how quickly and thoroughly they did so or how well the salicylates were moved throughout the body. Once we began observing patients with worsening symptoms and mappings while using muscle rubs such as Salonpas and Asper-creme (methyl salicylate), we were alerted to this issue.

These days we're accustomed to topically applied medications, none of which existed when we first began using guaifenesin. Nicotine patches, migraine sprays, hormone gels and patches, pain patches, and so on are in common use. We know that drug delivery through the skin has advantages. It makes for lower dosages as well as direct delivery into the bloodstream, bypassing the intestinal tract and avoiding degradation by digestive juices.

There are still skeptical physicians who consider it impossible when we expound on how small amounts of salicylate can block guaifenesin. To this we simply say that we know it's true: We've created thousands of maps on our patients that graphically illustrate what we have found. Ignore any and all voices to the contrary; salicylates block with devastating efficiency.

Sensitivity to blockage is genetically determined, but since none of us knows the level of our personal susceptibility, each of us should meticulously abide by the protocol as written. To our readers, we plead—do your job and give guaifenesin a fair chance. If you don't do the protocol properly, you'll never know whether or not guaifenesin would have worked for you. Don't miss your chance to get well.

AVOIDING SALICYLATES

Even before medical school, I had a love affair with medicine. Yet I have to admit that over the years, that affection has been strained by the torment of ferreting out the source of salicylate that's blocking a particular patient. It's certainly been a learning curve! We counsel patients on how to check all their products. It's not as simple as not using aspirin or Pepto-Bismol. Even our best efforts have not prevented errors by intelligent and diligent people.

My first visit with a new patient begins predictably. I take a medical history and complete my examination, which produces a body map displaying the patient's lesions. After that, I make a sketch as I unfold a story—our version of fibromyalgia. I run through the details of how I began to treat it, thanks to an observant man who flicked tartar off his teeth. I move through the metabolism of calcium and phosphate, as I believe it relates to fibromyalgia. I dwell a bit longer on the cyclic but progressive nature of the illness and what we are learning from our current research. Next I spend considerable time explaining the role of guaifenesin in correcting our faulty chemistry, offsetting our genetic problem. Patients grimace a bit when I get to my description of the reversal process as I explain that they will see great swings in symptoms. I describe how they'll cycle quickly or gradually from worse-than-ever to better-than-in-a-long-time. Patients handle this information quite well—so far, so good.

I always brace myself when I move into the next part of my explanation. Now I must address the issue of the salicylates they'll have to avoid in topical products and the herbal medications they must discontinue. We've actually had a few patients dump both guaifenesin and us rather than give up a cherished item. One actress came out and said that the protocol was "too hard" and then simply failed to appear for her next appointment. Believe it or not, we've also heard: "I'd rather have fibromyalgia than give up the products I need to use!" It can be equally difficult to convince patients to part with their Juice Plus+, liver cleansers, or herbal laxatives. At this point, we remind patients that were those things effective, they would have saved themselves the expense and time involved in visiting our office. Of course, there are also those who immediately say they'd give up anything at all to feel better!

Over the years I've tried so many things, avoiding chemicals and certain foods. I've done elimination diets and stopped using gluten. None of them made my condition better. Now I have to check products for salicylates and I don't see a problem with reading more labels. And I know I have to do it right but I'm up for a challenge. I just want to get well.

—*Alecia, Oregon*

SYNTHETIC SALICYLATES

We'll start the discussion with the easiest group of salicylates to identify: the synthetic or pure chemical form. Since salicylate or salicylic acid is exactly what you can't use, obviously that's the first thing you should look for on product labels. Simply put: If you see the words *salicylate* or *salicylic acid* on the label of any product you take as a medication or use on your skin—you must discontinue that product in order for your guaifenesin to be effective.

The most common salicylate is good old aspirin or acetylsalicylic acid. It may appear on labels by either name or by the abbreviation *ASA* (a common designation, especially in Canada). Many pain medications contain aspirin, especially those for headaches. Examples include Anacin, Excedrin, and Fiorinal. Their aspirin-free counterparts (Excedrin Tension Headache and Fioricet) pose no problem. Anything marked aspirin-free is okay to use.

It's slightly more difficult to spot the compound when it's blended into a long chemical name. Examples include Pepto-Bismol (bismuth subsalicylate), or Trilisate (choline magnesium trisalicylate). As you can see, all you need is the chemical (or generic name) to check a medication either prescription or over the counter (for example, sodium salicylate, magnesium salicylate, salicylic acid, salicylsalicylic acid). Notice how easily you can spot *sal* buried within those names? When you see it, dump the product.

You'll also find synthetic salicylates in topical products that employ an acid to work. That's why acne soaps, dandruff shampoos, chemical peels, and callus-removing products may contain salicylic acid. It's also used to treat psoriasis and seborrheic dermatitis of the face and scalp, and to remove dead skin. Plantar and common warts are treated with varying strengths of salicylic acid. Peels, scrubs, dandruff shampoos, and the like should not be used if they contain salicylic acid, but any other acid (lactic, glycolic) would be no problem. The only acid that blocks guaifenesin is salicylic acid.

Overzealous patients sometimes confuse silicate or sulfate and think they're potential blockers. Not so. We repeat: The three telltale letters are *s-a-l* when it comes to the synthetic chemical salicylates.

There are several other chemicals that are also salicylates. These are derivatives of camphor and menthol and can be easily spotted because they contain the syllables *camph* or *menth*. No matter how long a chemical name—even if it has twenty-five letters—if it doesn't contain those syllables—*sal, camph,* or *menth*—you can use it. *Meth*—as in *methyl paraben*—is safe. Without the *n*, it is safe to use. But products like Carmex or Icy Hot will block.

As mentioned earlier in this chapter, sunscreens often contain a salicylate. But none of the sunscreen ingredients you need to avoid are the ones that protect against skin cancer or photoaging. It's true that effective sunscreens are more expensive than those that don't actually protect you from anything other than sunburn, but it's important to use them. Look at it this way: You'll save on wrinkle creams later! The ingredients to avoid in your sunscreen are spelled a little differently: octisalate, homosalate, mexoryl, and meradimate. Let me stress that these are ingredients, so you will need to check *any* product that contains a sunscreen or SPF. If your ChapStick has an SPF, if your day cream contains an SPF, if your foundation contains an SPF, you must check the active (sunscreen) ingredients to make sure you do not see those listed above. Any other sunscreen—zinc oxide, titanium dioxide, avobenzone—is fine. Remember that when you are checking a topical product like a sunscreen, you'll also have to check the inactive ingredients armed with all the information in this chapter.

So far we've covered synthetic salicylates (the manufactured chemical will be listed as salicylate, salicylic acid, or—in medications—compounds that contain either of those words); chemicals with the syllable *sal*, *camph*, or *menth*; and products with the sunscreen octisalate, homosalate, mexoryl, or meradimate.

NATURAL SALICYLATES

All plants make salicylates.[1] The publication of the article proving this, in 1984, was a defining moment for the guaifenesin protocol, as well as a missing piece of the puzzle. What had been hazy and not quite appreciated was suddenly clear. Just as the realization many years before that there was a condition called hypoglycemia had hit me like a ton of bricks, this headline was staggering. It took a few more years, some refinements, and some missteps, but an important piece of information had suddenly dropped into our laps, and we knew it the minute we read the article in the journal *Science*.

It required no great leap of faith to realize that if taking aspirin—or acetylsalicylic acid—would block guaifenesin, then so would taking white willow bark, which harbors the natural salicylate, salicin. Once past the mouth, these chemicals—because they are identical—fit the same receptors and have the same diverse effects on the body. Only the source is different. So then, if all plants make salicylates, then all herbal medications contain them. And because herbal medications are concentrates, they contain substantial amounts of salicylate. Medicinal herbs, like all medications, are designed to deliver the active chemical(s) into the bloodstream in sufficient quantities to alter some kind of body function. They are designed to override the body's own natural defense system.

In the early days of the protocol, herbal medications were not as commonly used. The supplement market was almost nonexistent except for a few multivitamins. Self-respecting patients back then didn't take alfalfa, borage seed oil, wild Mexican yam, or bioflavonoids. But as time passed, everything old was becoming new again. People who wouldn't dream of taking eight aspirin a day would take white willow bark with a passion, commenting that it was natural and could not hurt them. Women who wouldn't take horse estrogens or synthetic (another nasty word) hormones saw no problem with taking black cohosh or yam, which contain other forms of steroids. Exotic juice extracts like goji and acai and seemingly strange herbal names like *dong quai* have suddenly appeared on the shelf in every market. Asking what was natural about taking grape seed or seaweed extracts in concentrations that didn't exist in nature was suddenly very politically incorrect. And, of course, the herbal pain preparations helpful for fibromyalgia quite simply work because they contain the highest levels of natural salicylate.

NATURAL SALICYLATES AS MEDICATIONS

Gather up all your dietary supplements, no matter the form—single-ingredient formulations as well as those with added vitamins or minerals; powders along with pills, capsules, drops, et cetera. If the information panel on the back says "Supplement" or offers "Supplemental Facts," you must check the ingredients list closely: This is a *medication*, meaning that it's concentrated enough to change the chemistry of your body. The concentration is what makes it medicinal. If the label instead offers "Nutrition Facts"—which you'll see on things like protein powders, drinks, and the like—this is a food. It isn't concentrated, in other words, and you don't need to check it out.

Look for the words *oil*, *gel*, or *extract* with a plant name. In nature, only plants make salicylates, so you can use anything you can identify as not being a plant. Simply put: If an ingredient doesn't have the name of a plant, you can take it. For example: Calcium, magnesium, and zinc aren't plants, so no problem. Glucosamine, 5-HTP, malic acid, fish oil...again, not plants, so they can't block guaifenesin. On the other hand, turmeric, *Ginkgo biloba*, green tea extract, valerian, evening primrose oil, flaxseed oil, and wild yam are plants or come from plants, and so they do block guaifenesin. Also check for bioflavonoids (quercetin, hesperiden, or rutin), which are concentrated plant pigments and will block guaifenesin. (Don't forget to recheck labels when replacing a product to make sure there have been no ingredient changes.) It's simple: If it has the name of a plant or contains bioflavonoids, don't use it.

Make sure you check the labels on all your vitamins—look for plant names such as *rose hips* or *ginseng*, and for bioflavonoids. Vitamin C or multivitamins that contain vitamin C often have bioflavonoids added to them.

Ingredients such as lutein or lycopene that are not the names of plants are okay. Your product label may helpfully tell you the plant from which they are derived (marigold, tomatoes), but they are single chemicals extracted and purified in a factory and are not blockers. Unless the chemical extracted from a plant contains the syllables *sal*, *camph*, or *menth*, it is not a blocker. Whole plants can be easily identified as oils, gels, or extracts.

Hormones are fine; hormones are not plants. But don't take a whole plant (such as saw palmetto or yam extract) to get the hormone. Instead, use the purified form.

In short: You must not take plants as medications with guaifenesin. If the ingredients list of the supplement you want to take contains the name of a plant with a strength (measure of potency), then you cannot take it or it will block you.

NATURAL SALICYLATES IN TOPICAL PRODUCTS

The next step is to check your topical products. Gather up everything you use on your skin: shampoo, conditioner, bubble bath, body lotions, deodorants, lip balms, face cleansers, bar soap, eye makeup removers, nail polish remover, massage oils, cuticle creams, makeup, and so on. You're going to have to check the ingredients in all of these. Any product for which you do not have the full list of ingredients should be set aside. This includes products without labels (or without the packaging that had the ingredients printed on it), as well as any product that lists only active ingredients. Later in this chapter, we'll explain how to research these products. Don't be distracted by the pictures on the front of any product. Many have lovely drawings of flowers but don't contain any actual plants. The only way you can check a product is by looking at the list of ingredients. A product that reads "Vanilla Hand Soap" on the front may not contain vanilla. Go directly to the ingredients list.

Once you've made sure that the syllables *sal*, *camph*, or *menth* aren't listed, do a quick scan of the ingredients. (If the product you are checking has an SPF, you must look for octisalate, homosalate, mexoryl, or meradimate. These ingredients are found *only* in sunscreens, so if the product you are checking doesn't have an SPF, you can skip this step.) If you don't see the name of a plant, the product is okay since only plants make natural salicylates. So, for example, plain Vaseline (petroleum jelly) is fine to use. So is single-ingredient baby oil—mineral oil cannot be a blocker.

Once you've completed the above step, it's time to concentrate on the products left in your pile. Now look for oils, gels, or extracts with a plant name. Remember that natural salicylates are found only in plants, but not in animal or mineral products. Thus, mineral oil, vitamin E, emu oil, and lanolin are all safe to use. You are looking for plant names coupled with the indication that the ingredient is a whole plant—oil, gel, or extract.

Check everything. All topical products including lipsticks, mouthwashes, suppositories, chewing gums, cortisone creams, nasal sprays, breath mints, toothpastes, razors, as well as shaving creams have the potential to block guaifenesin. Some of these products contain camphor, menthol, or castor oils. Others add mint—spearmint, peppermint, or wintergreen oil—which easily provides enough salicylate to block guaifenesin. Razors may have strips coated with aloe adjacent to the cutting edge. The salicylates in the aloe slide into the tiny cuts you can make when you shave your legs, underarms, or face and readily block guaifenesin. Don't forget that you must check any product that contains a sunscreen (SPF) for octisalate, homosalate, mexoryl, or meradimate.

Plant ingredients in most products are not difficult to identify. Witch hazel, lavender, arnica, rosemary, ginseng, chamomile, and aloe vera are some of the well-known ones. Seeing the word *bark*, *stem*, *leaf*, *root*, or *flower* in the ingredients list is a tip-off that you're dealing with a member of the plant kingdom. If you see the word *oil*, *gel* or *extract* and it's coupled with a word you can't identify, you'll need to find out if it's a member of the plant kingdom. Unfortunately, there are some plant names that are more difficult to find in standard reference books. Since the basic ingredients in all cosmetics are similar, manufacturers search for unique-sounding additives that will set their product apart on labels and in advertisements. The more expensive the product, the more common exotic ingredients are. Rain forests and tropical islands are being raided for cajeput, quillaja, bibia, padauk, and other native plants. Fortunately, these exotic but obscure substances are easy to check, too. The simplest way to identify them is with the aid of an online search engine such as Google, Bing, or Yahoo.

If your reference tells you the ingredient coupled with *oil*, *gel*, or *extract* is a plant, then you can't use that product. You don't need to google it or look it up on Wikipedia; all you need to know is if the funny name on the product label is actually a plant. Not all of them are. You don't need to locate the molecular structure or learn where the plant grows in its native form. If it's a plant name coupled with *oil*, *gel*, or *extract*—don't put it on your skin.

> Things have become so much easier now with so many ways to order products online. You don't have to stand in stores anymore with a magnifying glass to try to read tiny print on the back of boxes. Most places have free delivery and easy return policies.
>
> When I first started out, I just didn't use very many things because it was too hard. I could understand how people felt they couldn't do the protocol because they were too exhausted to shop and try to figure things out at the same time. But now there's no excuse—it's much easier to start the protocol now.
>
> —*Meghan P., California*

All plants make salicylates. However, not all parts of all plants contain the chemical. There is no way to know this except by careful research. In the plant kingdom, there is only one category of plant that doesn't contain salicylates and that is grains (the actual grain, not the plant it grows on). Thus wheat germ oil is salicylate-free, but wheatgrass extract is not. So on the protocol, you can use topical products that contain grain oils, gels, or extracts. This includes oatmeal products as long as they contain no other plants such as chamomile or lavender.

Dental Products

What sits in your mouth is really topically applied. Nicorette gum, sublingual nitroglycerin, and orally disintegrating migraine tablets are examples of medications that can be quickly absorbed into the bloodstream. Guaifenesin can be blocked by oral hygiene products that contain salicylates. Some contain salicylate by name (the first ingredient in Listerine is methyl salicylate), but most commonly the blocker is some form of mint. All mint is methyl salicylate, whether it's synthetic or extracted from the natural plant. If you smell or taste mint in a product, it will block your guaifenesin. (It will also block if it's there but you can't taste it.)

Most mouthwashes and toothpastes celebrate mint (*Fresh mint! Mint blast! Cool mint!*) or menthol—the more powerful, the better. In the United States, no law says the individual ingredients of toothpastes, including flavors, need to be listed. Labels generally only tell whether the product contains fluoride. Even when the inactive ingredients are listed, those in the flavor are lumped together simply as "flavor"; mint oil, salicylic acid, and methyl salicylate are not listed separately. Wintergreen is 98 percent methyl salicylate, but there is no way to tell this from packaging or ingredients lists. You just have to know to avoid all forms of mint.

Our advice is that it's best to stick with dental products that we know won't block guaifenesin. The Cleure brand of dental products, designed by Flora Stay, DDS, are all salicylate-free. Tom's of Maine voluntarily reveals all their ingredients, including flavor components, so you can check these by reading labels. Alternatively, simply dip your toothbrush in baking soda. You can also sprinkle it with hydrogen peroxide or use a peroxide gel such as Arm & Hammer that contains no flavor. Any dental product that is unflavored is a good solution to the mint problem.

Don't ignore dental floss, breath strips or sprays, cough drops, lozenges, gum, or hard candies. Fruit and cinnamon flavors are fine, but be aware of mint that is hard to taste because of other strong flavors. Dr. Flora Stay has a number of products and suggestions on her website (www.cleure.com). There you'll find such products as salicylate-free tooth whiteners, fluoride gel, and mouthwashes, and a question–and–answer board for personal assistance.

Products Without Listed Ingredients

When you gather up your products to check, you'll find some without listed ingredients. This can be because they were on the packaging you threw away or because the list was on the display at the store. Luckily it's not too difficult in most cases to retrieve them.

If you're checking a medication such as, say, Midol or Pepcid, you can simply put it in a search engine on your computer. This will give you the information you need. Midol's own website contains the information: "None of the products in the Midol family are formulated with aspirin. Midol Complete, Midol (caffeine free), and Midol Long Lasting Relief all contain acetaminophen. Menstridol contains naproxen sodium." A similar search for Pepcid reveals that its chemical name is famotidine—also not a problem with guaifenesin.

Many websites list the ingredients for products they sell. CVS, Walgreens, Target, Walmart, Amazon, Ulta, and Sephora are examples. Companies have their own websites, and some such as Lancôme, L'Oréal, Neutrogena, Olay, and NYX list ingredients for each product. Even when websites don't list ingredients, there's always a CONTACT US button you can use to submit a query. Always ask for the list of ingredients; don't allow them to check for you. Trust only your own eyes! If a company won't give you the ingredients, don't use the product. You'll find some companies more difficult to deal with than others, but since there are so many options it's easy to find what you need with cooperative manufacturers.

Dietary Salicylates

The only foods you need to avoid when taking guaifenesin are those in the mint family. Even those with higher salicylate content, such as berries, fruits, colored vegetables, cooking herbs, and spices, won't block if eaten in normal quantities. Salicylates in foods are diluted and partially destroyed by digestive processes. They're further neutralized metabolically when the liver degrades some of their effects by tagging them with glycine.

Salicylate levels can be measured in the blood and in the urine. The average daily intake from foods is in the range of 10 to 20 mg. Experiments with various diets have supported the conventional wisdom that foods add insignificant amounts into the urine and therefore, presumably, into the bloodstream.[2]

You don't have to avoid small amounts of herbs used to flavor a recipe. But we do need to mention one of the often overlooked blockers—tea. Tea is made from the leaves of the camellia plant, which are high in salicylate. Do not drink green, black, or white tea or any beverage that contains them. Coffee and cocoa drinks won't block, nor would beverages made from grains. Sodas—even root beer—won't block.

WHAT AREN'T NATURAL SALICYLATES

Just because a plant name appears in the list of ingredients in a product other than oral supplements doesn't mean it can keep your guaifenesin from working. All through this chapter, we've been stressing that in your topical products you must avoid oils, gels, or extracts with a plant name. So what about a plant name that's not an oil, gel, or extract?

The answer is simple. We've already explained how single chemicals are acceptable as long as you avoid salicylate, camphor, and menthol. The source of a chemical doesn't matter. If a label reads "sodium laurel sulfate," you don't need to google it to see where it comes from. It is a chemical, and the origin doesn't matter. Salicylates will block no matter the source. If a chemical isn't a salicylate, it will not, even if it is manufactured from a plant.

When you look at a chemical name, sometimes it's easy to spot the raw material from which it was made. Poly cottonseedate, palm glyercides, coconut sterols or fatty acids, and jojoba wax are examples. Some of them offer no clue to their origin: Squalene, beta-carotene, sodium laurel sulfate, and alpha hydroxy acids are some of those. But that's more than you need to know. You don't need to do genealogy on chemicals. Don't use Wikipedia or WikiProject Chemicals because those will confuse you, we promise. Just look at the chemical in question: Does it contain the syllable *sal*, *camph*, or *menth*? If not, you can use it. How can you tell if it's a chemical? If it's not a plant, a mineral, or an animal oil, gel, or extract, it is a chemical. Even if the raw material was a plant, the ingredient you are looking at was made in a chemical factory and isn't a whole plant anymore. So don't worry about gums, waxes, starches, glycerides, monoglycerides, or any word that isn't *oil*, *gel*, or *extract*.

A NOTE ABOUT BUTTERS

True butters from plant sources will not block guaifenesin. These are pure isolated fats and are solid at room temperature. For example, shea butter is a triglyceride (fat) derived mainly from stearic acid and oleic acid. So how can you tell what is a true butter? All butters must be made from fats. Those that come from nuts or seeds that are fatty are true butters. Some are easy to spot, like mango seed butter. But if you see an ingredient such as aloe butter, you should be suspicious since aloe does not contain fat. Here's what I learned when I googled it:

*"Remove the pan of melted **butter** from the heat. Add 8 oz. of **aloe** vera gel, stirring as you go."*

So aloe butter is not a true butter, it is aloe gel (a gel with a plant name) added to something else. Another reason to *always* do your research.

Salicylates and Cosmetics

This protocol is not a quick fix. It's a long-term thing. And you get well one day at a time. And if you make a mistake, you get back on track and keep going. It's kind of like trying to lose a lot of weight or dealing with an alcohol problem. You have to learn to be patient with yourself. I have never been a patient person. I think I have developed more patience on this protocol because I needed to. I was too sick to do anything else. If you spend all your time worrying that it might not work for you, you are wasting your healing energy. Your body is stressed to the limit with being sick. Using your energy to worry means that your energy can't be used in healing. So...follow the directions to the letter. Titrate your dose exactly as it says to. Use as few products as you can in the beginning and make sure they're all salicylate free. Be kind to yourself. Be patient. Try to take one day at a time, one hour at a time.

—*Cris R., Michigan*

We hear a lot of complaints from patients taking guaifenesin who lament the loss of their "natural" products. How can they possibly give up items like jojoba oil face masks, almond oil skin creams, or cleansers with aloe, witch hazel, arnica, or mint? Many have simply been brainwashed by advertising campaigns that have convinced them that if it's from a plant, it's "natural," and so it's safer and better. There's just no evidence that this is the case.

Minerals come from Mother Earth and are natural. Animal oils such as emu, lanolin, or cashmere oils have shown beneficial effects on our own animal skin. And the fact is, many people have started to be leery of ingredients, no matter what the source, with unknown actions on the body. For example, those with a family history of breast cancer often decide to use mineral salt deodorants to avoid aluminum. The bottom line is that plants contain many compounds, some good and some not so good for you.

It's important to know that the FDA doesn't regulate cosmetic claims or ingredients, including the use of words such as *pure* and *natural*. *Natural* on a label can designate something partly human-made combined with a natural ingredient. It could just as surely indicate an ingredient synthetically extracted from plants using some very potent chemicals through a wholly unnatural process. Many "all-natural" toothpastes contain sodium laurel sulfate—a chemical implicated in canker sores. What is natural about sodium laurel sulfate when it comes from a chemical factory?

It's also important to remember that when plant extracts are used, preservatives must be added to maintain freshness. These chemicals are often potent allergens and topical irritants. Skin creams containing cucumber extract have a shelf life of several years. How long can a cucumber last in its natural state, even in the refrigerator? Many dermatologists share this information with patients and suggest that those with allergies and sensitivities use simple fragrance-free products with as few ingredients as possible.

There aren't very many actual moisturizers and humectants—ingredients that seal moisture into the skin. The workhorse ingredients in most products boil down to a very few chemicals whose names you'll see repeated over and over again on labels. Basic soothing ingredients are such things as mineral oil, glycerine, cyclomethicone, dimethicone, and petrolatum. All are laboratory-made and are mainstays in almost every skin cream no matter what else has been added. The most effective moisture-holding agents are glycerine, ceramide, lecithin, hyaluronic acid, sodium hyaluronate, sodium PCA, collagen, elastin, amino acids, cholesterol, glucose, sucrose, fructose, glycogen, and phospholipids—and none is the name of a plant. There are only three ingredients that protect the skin from photoaging and skin cancer: avobenzone, titanium dioxide, and zinc oxide.

Cosmetics companies shovel plant material into ordinary moisturizers and makeup to make them seem more exotic and to command higher prices. While some plant ingredients do the job asked of them, none are essential to maintain or protect skin. In fact, it's not unusual for us to hear patients say that the quality of their skin improved when they stopped using so many products. Patients with skin allergies can attest that using products with fewer ingredients seems to be easier on the body.

We can all agree that not every plant is beneficial or particularly desirable. Tobacco comes from a plant; poison ivy, poison oak, hemlock, oleander, and toadstools are all well-known, potentially lethal toxins. Many people have plant allergies and will develop dermatitis from products containing them.

Paula Begoun first published *Don't Go to the Cosmetics Counter Without Me* in 1991. She also maintains an informative website that reviews products and includes ingredients in most cases: beautypedia.com. She analyzes literally thousands of products from companies such as Almay, Avon, The Body Shop, Charles of the Ritz, Dior, Estée Lauder, Maybelline, Revlon, Vaseline Intensive Care, and Wet N Wild. She reminds us that results are what matter; gouging prices and exotic ingredients don't guarantee a better outcome. Her book provides an overview and evaluates many ingredients in cosmetics, both natural and synthetic, for their efficacy. Her readers get an inside look at how cosmetics are created, manufactured, and marketed. That's interesting and helpful for everyone, not just patients taking guaifenesin. There is no question that we should all be concerned, because ingredients in topical products don't require evaluation for safety by the FDA.

The guaifenesin protocol has benefited hugely from the expertise of Flora Stay, DDS. Her company, Cleure, has products for dental needs, skin care, hair, and cosmetics—all of which will always be salicylate-free. Cleure toothpaste and other offerings benefit from her experience and knowledge as a teaching and practicing dentist who has searched for effective, safe ingredients. Her website, www.cleure.com, contains information about her products and fibromyalgia. She is the author of *The Fibromyalgia Dental Handbook*, published in 2005. In her topical products she relies on vitamin E and pure, true butters; she does not use parabens. Her products are all gluten-free as well.

Ruthie Molloy of Illuminaré Cosmetics was inspired by her sister's battle with fibromyalgia. She has a liquid mineral makeup line that can be purchased through her website (www.illuminarecos metics.com) and other beauty sites.

We should mention one other resource before we leave the subject: Marina del Rey Pharmacy (www.fibropharmacy.com) sells products that have been carefully screened for salicylates. If you're ordering from more than one company, you can save shipping costs as well as be provided with helpful, understanding service. We know of many who have called in, too sick to think, and just asked them to send them one of everything essential: deodorant, toothpaste, mouthwash, and soap. Later, when they recovered enough strength to go out, they added lipstick, eye pencil, and sunscreens and travel sizes of their favorite new products!

I have been in pain since the birth of my oldest daughter. This has been a really long time to be in pain. I thought I had some form of arthritis that no one could find. Eventually, I was in so much agony I had to quit my job because I could no longer potty train the two-year-olds in my preschool class. I could not pick them up without almost crying.

I had a friend who told me I might have fibromyalgia. I made an appointment with Dr. St. Amand. I read his book, *What Your Doctor May* Not *Tell You about Fibromyalgia*, twice in two weeks. At the time, I was on six different pain meds throughout the day. I am not saying it was an easy thing to do. I got worse before I got better. I also am on a hypoglycemic diet. Now I walk every day, sometimes even hitting the ten-thousand-step mark on my knockoff Fitbit. It is a process and I am better.

—*Elaine B., California*

BUYER BEWARE

You will find, if you do any searches on the internet, a lot of resources on salicylate-free products: YouTube videos, support groups, Pinterest and Facebook pages. You'll likely come across the German support group's salicylate-search dictionary—which, if you read this chapter, is entirely unnecessary and makes checking products more laborious. You'll find a number of websites that claim to be affiliated with Dr. St. Amand, but only our website at www.fibromyalgiatreatment.com actually is. We urge you to use caution when availing yourself of these resources and, if you have questions, refer back to this book, our Facebook page, or our website and the support group there. You can only count on those resources to support the protocol as written by Dr. St. Amand. Remember that if and when changes or additions are made to our work, they will be posted on our website.

FREQUENTLY ASKED QUESTIONS ABOUT SALICYLATES

Which dishwashing liquids are salicylate-free?
Dish soaps are usually okay to use. It's hard to find ones that contain actual whole plants. Exceptions might be found at places such as health food stores.

I have eliminated all salicylates from my topically applied products and still don't notice any effect from the guaifenesin. What should I do now?
Recheck everything, even your chewing gum and breath mints for mint, peppermint, spearmint, or wintergreen. Search your vitamins and supplements for bioflavonoids, rose hips, or other plants. If you find nothing, double your dose of guaifenesin. Within a week, you should feel distinctly worse. If you don't, you are most likely blocking. Ask for help from the online support

group at www.fibromyalgiatreatment.com. If you find nothing, your dosage may need further adjustment.

Should I avoid laundry detergents with phosphates?

You do not need to avoid phosphates in anything. Extra phosphates are not a problem. It's impossible to eliminate them from your life, and your body needs a huge amount to form energy. Laundry detergents don't come in direct contact with the skin since they're rinsed out of your clothes before they're worn. So the answer is no.

I'm a gardener. Is there anything I should be careful about?

Yes, you should be very careful doing certain gardening chores. Plant juices and oils are readily absorbed through the skin. You should wear gloves if you will make contact with them. The thin gloves worn by surgeons are ideal for delicate tasks, while thicker, waterproof gloves should be worn for heavier work. Leather gloves if used for long tasks can become progressively saturated with salicylates that eventually soak through. There are many new gardening gloves that are not unwieldy and actually support your hands while you garden. Check your local gardening store or online.

What about smoking cigarettes?

With everything we know today, it's obvious that you shouldn't smoke, even if you don't have fibromyalgia. You should know that more than one study has shown that smokers have more pain and circulatory problems, which is obviously something you do not want to contend with.

However, the topic of this chapter is salicylates. We don't really know the full impact of smoking, but some observant patients noticed a distinctly faster reversal at the same guaifenesin dosage only when they quit smoking. We do know from experiments that tobacco plant leaves contain methyl salicylate. They're treated, and dried, but that would not destroy that chemical. Does the burning or filter change that, and if so, by how much? Obviously, menthol filters create a separate distinct problem.

There's a strong possibility that smoking could make guaifenesin partially or totally ineffective. It might merely depend on the crop's potency, but we tell patients to be as pure as possible and avoid any substance they can't safely validate, and this includes smoking.

Take the easy way in the protocol. By this I mean, don't play around with your dosage, don't use products with salicylates, and try to think positively about the future. Don't let vanity keep you from giving up certain products that interfere with your guaifenesin. If makeup is absolutely necessary in your life, use only what is approved. BE DILIGENT! I can't say this enough. Ultimately you are the one who is going to put yourself into remission. All the information you need is on the website and in the book. You have to have a mind-set that you want to be well. I am extremely SERIOUS. YOU CAN DO IT. You Have to do it if you want a good life. It will take time. Just because we live in an instant satisfaction society doesn't mean you can rush your remission by changing the rules. GO FOR IT with all your moxie. Step up to the plate and declare yourself a person who is going to conquer fibromyalgia.

—*Nora D., Georgia*

CHAPTER 5

PATIENT VINDICATION

I'm now seventy years old and doing great. The fibro pain has been gone for so long but I haven't forgotten how hard it was. If you will do the protocol exactly as Dr. St. Amand teaches, you will be like me...PAIN FREE, FUNCTION-ING, ENJOYING LIFE, and hopefully helping guide other fibro patients through the protocol. I now ride my adult tricycle and wear my goofy hat to keep the sun off my face. I'm known in my town as "The Fibromyalgia Lady" and, after all these years, still get calls from desperate men and women who have been diagnosed. I always guide them to "the book."

—*Nora D., Georgia*

This chapter is one compelling reason for writing this new edition of our book. It presents another opportunity to thank our many patients, not only those who volunteer for our multiplying studies, but others who've done what they can in support. They have had to steel themselves against derogatory remarks, and have encouraged us while we were guiding them and others we will never meet back to health. Scientific reports continue to bolster our theory. We can now address some of the alleged weaknesses of our almost sixty-year-old theory and provide you with some solidly vindicating findings.

Our theory of fibromyalgia and our protocol have been frequent sources of derision, especially by rheumatologists, and we know it. Their initial responses were blatant and attacking. The tone was usually contemptuous with the attached questions: "Where's the proof? Where's the double-blind study?" Yet we have results. We understand that they are retrospective and so despite the volume of records we have meticulously kept we know they are of less scientific value than a controlled double-blind study would be. But they are not meaningless, and even our strongest critics have grudgingly conceded when approached that we do "help some patients."

Attacks continue on our theory, no matter how many thousands of patients have provided supportive data—though it is considered anecdotal because it is not rigorously collected. Of course, the lack of objective tests for fibromyalgia makes it difficult to do more. If we had blood markers to follow, we could more easily demonstrate in a way we could not influence that patients were improving. As it stands, medicine ignores "anecdotal" evidence no matter the volume of words and voices raised in support.

We, too, decry unsubstantiated claims. Yet it is undeniable that we and other physicians in the trenches have learned a lot from actually treating patients and observing what works. It is by listening to patients that our entire treatment protocol was developed and honed over the years. At the same time, we gleaned much scientific data from a variety of journals in the past sixty-some years, and we continue searching for clues. This two-pronged information collection has solidified our thinking.

Sometimes something new does exist under the sun. In 2005, we were given a boost when the *Lancet*, a prestigious British journal (equal to our *New England Journal of Medicine*), published a letter to the editor. The July 9–15, 2005, issue had this quote emblazoned on its cover: "If everything has to be double-blinded, randomized, and evidence-based, where does that leave new ideas?"

That was a spear-like thrust into the realm of medical academia. It fed our resolve and gave us further impetus to keep seeking unassailable, technical defenses for our simple method of treatment. What follows should nudge some skeptics to think again, because it's difficult to refute the evidence.

Our one attempt at a double-blind study failed in 1995 in that both patients and controls improved overall during the year they were followed. To refresh your memory, *double-blind* means that patient-subjects don't know if they're on a real medication under testing or on a placebo (or fake). The *double* refers to the fact that neither do the research physicians conducting the study. Records are kept secret and identified in computer logs using classified numbers. Only when the project is completed are the codes broken and the results statistically analyzed to determine the efficacy of active treatment over placebo.

This study failed largely because of our ignorance regarding salicylates. At the time, all the researchers (ourselves included) were unaware of the impact of topical salicylates. The speed with which the skin and inner membranes assimilate this compound still amazes us. Procedural errors were also made when it came to excluding hypoglycemic individuals, which skewed the wellness questionnaires. The design of the study did not allow for raising doses as it progressed, something we do daily in clinical practice when a patient is not responding. We also have to mention the size of the study: only twenty patients in each group (placebo and guaifenesin) when it began, fewer when it ended, some having dropped out near the beginning because they felt so much worse. We reproach ourselves for these errors, which undoubtedly caused the study's results to be what they were, but we did not know what we did not know and since then have been unable to find a research center and funding to do another.

It is our belief that no successful double-blind study will be forthcoming. Guaifenesin is now readily available over the counter. However willing to help, fibromyalgics would hardly continue in a study for a year or two if they could not see improvement. Remember that only half the patients in a double-blind are given an active medication; the other half receive a placebo, or sugar pill. The placebo group would continue to suffer for a year or more, the time that would be required to harvest interpretable effects. Because our protocol is so well known, it would be obvious to participants once they are told to give up salicylates what drug they are testing.

We recognized the likelihood that our double-blind study was destined to be the last for us immediately after the results were made public. We knew the next step was genetic and biochemical research to expose the disturbed, but currently occult physiology that renders a person fibromyalgic. We're quite excited to introduce you to what our ongoing research is unveiling. Now, how about a little *evidence-based, new-idea* science that needs no double-blinding?

Claudia and I have participated as researchers with the world-renowned Beckman Research Institute at City of Hope. Their scientists have melded some of our observations with invigorating data. We've been on an emotional high ever since their teams began searching for genetic mutations and defective biochemistry in our patients. Their dual disciplines blend perfectly to blaze a well-marked trail that will make it easier for others to follow. The team has produced four published papers.

The first study was under the direction of John E. Shively, PhD. He tested blood from ninety-two of our fibromyalgic patients, sixty-nine family members, and seventy-seven controls (nonfibromyalgics). His team measured twenty-five cytokines or chemokines. Those are tiny proteins generated in many tissues throughout the body. They serve multiple functions and, in combination with other compounds, greatly affect metabolism, induce immune reactions, and may protect—or perversely attack—the body.

Our highly technical paper was published on June 5, 2008, in the *Journal of Experimental Biology and Medicine.* Twenty-three cytokine/chemokines were elevated in our patient subjects. (Another abnormal one has surfaced since the paper was published.) Of these, four main cytokines stand out. Those of you without knowledge in chemistry and immunology may struggle a bit, but you may still enjoy reading the paper.

Many of the disturbed cytokines and chemokines we found are highly inflammatory, yet there is no inflammation in tissues affected by fibromyalgia. That's probably the explanation for why standard blood tests are consistently normal in patients. We interpret the findings to show that a mulch of those little errant proteins, in combination, neutralize one another. That is likely why multiple biopsies from swollen places in fibromyalgia have shown no inflammatory cells. Our coauthors did not address this issue or our interpretation in the published paper, but we've certainly discussed it.

Please pay attention to the sheer number of the abnormal proteins we found. If your head doesn't swim just a little, let's make that happen. The preceding paragraph is an indictment of all those who told you, "It's all in your head." Your blood does reflect the bad stuff going on in your body. We're not sure how those many cytokines interplay with thousands of other compounds surging through your genetically unique self. They can wreak havoc as they interface with hormones and other chemical messengers. Intriguingly, each of them has a function, at times favorable, but likewise destructive when in the wrong company. It seems that combinations are what count in fibromyalgia.

Now for the clincher: On guaifenesin, ten of the elevated chemo/cytokines dropped lower, some to normal. Five stayed about the same. Eight went up even higher as patients were improving on our protocol. Savor this for a moment. Not only has this one paper shown distinct defects in fibromyalgic chemistry, but it also shows the favorable changes from using guaifenesin. We can now safely dismiss the common criticism that "it's good only for mucus."

But we're not done yet. We've also been working with the

genetics department at the same institution. Our first paper on the genetics of fibromyalgia was published in the online journal *PloS One* in December 2009.[1] One common and three rare mutations were found in 15 percent of one hundred patients ("probands") and two hundred of their parents (three hundred total people). That combination of test subjects and parents provides "trios" to produce reliable genetic screening. Since that publication, another gene has surfaced that affects another 15 percent of our patients: A total of 40 percent of our fibromyalgics have shown mutations.

Is it getting obvious? Since several genes are involved in fibromyalgia, by pure chance, many patients will have various combinations, some dominant, some recessive. Elevated cytokines might waylay messengers sent out to do the bidding of those genes. Then add such factors as injury, surgery, infections, indolence, obesity, or other illnesses into the mix. Complicated? You bet it is. We're even skipping over the involvement of strange little proteins known as micro- and silencing RNAs. Those of you with this disease have always known there wouldn't be a simple answer.

Studies are ongoing as we write. Enough new gene aberrations should exist among them to expand on the earlier findings. The more we can locate, the more likely we'll develop a simple, diagnostic blood test unique to fibromyalgia that would even be able to track improvement. We're certainly getting closer.

Let's simplify what we've just written. Think of a guitar player when trying to understand genes (DNA), message carriers (RNA), chemokines, and hormones. The player sets the music in his brain, then sends out nerve messages to the fingers. A gene is like a finger plucking a string. RNAs are like emanations caused by vibrations that spread tones throughout the room. However, obstructive barriers exist everywhere: walls, curtains, open windows, and breezes. Sound waves get deflected, muffled, or echoed depending on where the listener is seated. The sound obstructors are like micro- and silencing RNAs and their companion chemo/cytokines. They're directed to certain positions along the way or to the keenest acoustic site. They can muffle, stifle, and alter the melodic message by insert-ing a flat or a sharp. That changes what is picked up by those within hearing distance. The brain knows that its musical score will be mitigated and differently interpreted by each member of the tissue audience. The renovated sound mix is usually harmonious, but not when disease moves barrier-proteins around and adversely impacts the original composition. That's where we aim our treatment: We alter the cytokines, chemokines, hormones, and nerve impulses to better synchronize their effects with their target organs.

CHAPTER 6

HYPOGLYCEMIA, FIBROGLYCEMIA, AND CARBOHYDRATE INTOLERANCE

The doctor determined that I was hypoglycemic...and he also explained that hypoglycemia and fibromyalgia often go hand in hand. There was a name for what I had, an actual medical term! And there were also websites with information I could read. I was less than thrilled when he told me about the diet I would be on...Sugar was a no-no, as was caffeine...I gulped as he rattled off the list of the carbohydrates I should avoid, including the "Big Five" that figured heavily in my diet: pasta (my Italian heart literally broke in two), rice, potatoes, bananas, and corn...The doctor handed me a list of the permissible and said "Good luck."

This diagnosis meant that a morning might come when I could open my eyes and actually feel good to be alive, without fear of pain. Now four months later, I am pleased to say that I've experienced many such mornings...I have more energy, I sleep better, and I'm in a better mood. Friends, family members, and coworkers all say they've seen a change in me...Six months ago I would not have thought such a change was possible. But thanks to my own stubbornness...and the dedication of my current doctor, I have finally found relief. I guess what my doctor and I have in common is that we refused to give up the search for answers and we chose to ignore people who said there were none. For us both, perseverance has definitely paid off.

—*Michelle Fisher, California*

Hypoglycemia is a frequent unwelcome companion to fibromyalgia, and a contributing factor to your lack of energy. As boring as it may be, let's say it again. Determining whether or not you have this additional misery is an important step. The symptoms of these two conditions interweave, and this overlap makes working with them a little more challenging. You can certainly reverse your fibromyalgia while ignoring your blood sugar problems—but don't expect a full energy boost if you do.

In 1964, I was treating a podiatrist who suffered from fibromyalgia. Luckily for me, she had many scientific interests and studied a great deal. At one of her checkups, she brought me a pamphlet describing a host of symptoms that it attributed to low blood sugar. As an endocrinologist, I was certainly familiar with severe hypoglycemia, the kind that made patients implode with severe systemic symptoms, even passing out. Most of these were diabetics who were injecting themselves with the hormone insulin. There aren't many other conditions that can induce such a dramatic scenario. Once anyone witnesses those wild displays, it is difficult to mistake the diagnosis.

Hypoglycemia—From the Greek, meaning "low [*hypo*] sugar [*glyc*] in the blood [*emia*]." The accepted medical criterion for this condition is a blood sugar reading falling below 50 milligrams per deciliter (mg/dl).

As I read through the gauntlet of listed symptoms, I realized that if the information was even 50 percent accurate, I had been missing the chance to help a lot of sick people. The brochure listed fatigue, irritability, nervousness, depression, insomnia, sweats, headaches, impaired memory and concentration, anxieties, dizziness, blurred vision, leg cramps, sugar craving, flushing, nausea, gas, bloating, and constipation alternating with diarrhea as the most common symptoms. We soon realized those were the chronic effects, which we now segregate from the more dramatic ones we recognize as the acute symptoms of hypoglycemia. The latter occur suddenly: shaking tremors, clamminess or sweating, palpitations, faintness or syncope, confusion, and panic attacks. Of course, these are the easiest ones to spot because they are so dramatic and sudden.

Using gout medications the preceding five years, I had been generally successful in resolving fibromyalgia in the majority of patients. But there was a subset of people who weren't doing as well. Though they complained less about former pains, and though I noted improvement by palpating regression of lumps and bumps, they were not getting any perfectly normal days. Something was different about these patients, who were better on paper but still not feeling well.

Reading the brochure, it became clear to me what the problem was. With a few pertinent additional facts, the picture was now complete. Enter hypoglycemia. As I gained experience, it became progressively easier for me to separate the two and attack them simultaneously. As I learned more about the more subtle symptoms and less dramatic cases, I came to realize the volume of afflicted patients.

Luckily, the treatment for hypoglycemia was already well known. No medication is necessary or even useful. It simply requires eating the proper diet. This diet consists of simply not eating certain foods. No weighing, measuring, or special recipes are involved.

I had just begun to hope that I would finally be able to live without the pain from fibromyalgia. The guaifenesin treatment from Dr. St. Amand gave back my energy and mobility. It was all the more difficult, then, to be disabled by headaches. I was aware that my health was not good, so I ate a vegetarian diet and followed the food pyramid recommendations closely; I ate a diet rich in carbohydrates and low in fat, and the worse I felt, the more carefully I followed these recommendations. Despite this, I was always hungry and faint, and my headaches were steadily worsening.

Claudia showed me the diet recommended for hypoglycemia and offered me the hope that by following this regimen I could control my headaches. I would have tried anything; I had nothing to lose. In fact, I had a lot to lose: pain, fatigue, and even excess weight. From one day to the next my headaches all but vanished; during the first few weeks my migraines diminished to one or two a week and I had no other headaches, either mild or severe. The improvement was so immediate and so unmistakable that I had no difficulty whatsoever following the diet, even though it was just before Christmas and I was surrounded by sweets.

—*Cynthia C., Michigan*

As my education and experience progressed, I became familiar with patients who had hypoglycemia as a stand-alone illness as well as those who suffered from simultaneous fibromyalgia. At the time, I was a spokesman for the Los Angeles County Medical Association. NBC News wanted to present a segment on hypoglycemia, which was at that time the new fad. Because I was an endocrinologist, I was interviewed and asked to join a discussion about the condition on camera with various UC professors.

The story aired on three consecutive evenings as five-minute, serialized segments during the prime-time newscast. Owing to overwhelming viewer response, the program was shown a few more times in the following months. The Los Angeles County Medical Association, UCLA, and Harbor General Hospital were bombarded with phone calls. Since I was the only physician in the segment who was in private practice, all the inquiries were funneled to my office. We were inundated with calls from people with hypoglycemia, as well as the as-yet-unnamed fibromyalgia. Combinations of those two were no longer puzzling to me, but the spectrum of symptoms made patients with other conditions quizzical, and they, too, sought help. Many of those were justified in their suspicions. My patient base grew rapidly to include people not only from our area, but also from other parts of California, soon the entire country, and eventually all over the world. The sheer number of these has provided us with a huge database. That's the information we're now sharing with you.

Ancient humans did not find food in overabundance. Lean days far outnumbered their days of plenty. In fact, they often went a day or two without any food at all. When they found sustenance, they devoured it on the spot. Rarely were all of the calories they consumed needed for immediate use. Storage capabilities were necessary to provide energy on the less bountiful days that were sure to follow. In modern times our storage facilities are kept near overflow because calories are so readily available. Every meal provides an excess that isn't needed for immediate combustion, and our bodies are designed to store it.

To have insight into hypoglycemia, first you need to understand the biochemical sequence that follows when you consume carbohydrates (sugars and starches). Blood sugar levels rise almost immediately. The more refined the carbohydrate, the faster this happens. The liver converts nearly all carbohydrates to the simple sugar glucose. Enter insulin—the only hormone that directs excess food (energy fuel) into storage and attends to the work of conservation even before a meal is completed. It's like an insurance policy that guarantees against starvation, and it's the powerful hormone that kept our ancestors alive in times of famine. It directs cells to store not only glucose, but also fat and amino acids, the building blocks of protein. Insulin sends these stores to the body's energy warehouses, primarily fat cells, but a goodly amount is also dispersed, especially, to the brain and muscles.

When all of the above are satiated, the remaining glucose is converted to fatty acid, which then gets combined with glycerol in a structure we recognize as body fat, or triglyceride. The liver packages these minuscule fat droplets for transport mainly to the storage depots in fat cells. These little packets are what coalesce into the fat accumulations we can pinch far more than we like. Fat is nothing more than surplus energy maintained in the form of triglycerides. Our mouths and insulin—the caveman's lifesaving alliance—have become, in today's world of superabundance, enemies that make us fat and ensure we stay that way.

Insulin—A hormone produced by the islets of the pancreas that is released in whatever amounts are needed to clear excess glucose from the bloodstream. It promotes the absorption of glucose into the liver and muscles, where it is stored as glycogen. It also facilitates storage of amino acids and fats, and is known, therefore, as the storage hormone. Without insulin, a person cannot gain weight.

Triglyceride—One of three "blood fats" that are known as lipids. Triglyceride is the principal constituent of body fat. It is manufactured in the liver largely from the sugar and starches that you eat.

Some individuals are unable to process carbohydrates without adverse consequences. We often use the term *hypoglycemia*, low blood sugar, to denote a whole disease. More accurately, this is a metabolic error that is really a syndrome, a cluster of symptoms that keep popping up at the same time. The condition could profit by more descriptive nomenclature, but we're accustomed to using that word and it's easily recognizable—most people have at least heard of it. Patients with this illness suffer a distressing insulin-related conflagration that's regularly ignited by eating certain carbohydrates. (See table 6.1.)

Table 6.1

Hypoglycemia Syndrome

	Male	Percentage Male	Female	Percentage Female
Number of Patients	787		7,453	
FM Only	246	31	1,877	25
FM & Craving	429	54	3,709	50
FM & Hypoglycemia	112	14	1,867	25
Number of Lean Patients	660		5,266	
FM Only	213	32	1,549	29
FM & Craving	365	55	2,411	46
FM & Hypoglycemia	82	12	1,306	25
Number of Overweight Patients	127		2,187	
FM Only	33	26	328	15
FM & Craving	64	50	1,298	59
FM & Hypoglycemia	30	24	561	26

There are two ways to cause low blood sugar. The most obvious is an excess of insulin, but it can also be induced by delayed or inadequate hormonal responses that should have applied the brakes to a rapidly falling glucose. These hormones are known as counter-regulatory, because they normally stop the overexuberant attacks of insulin. All kinds of possibilities exist, because a bit too much of this or too little of that creates a whole spectrum of stresses.

There are four important counter-regulatory hormones, but adrenaline (epinephrine) is the ultimate weapon, and the final safety net. If either insulin or adrenaline is delayed, inadequate, or excessive, another must step in to prevent hypoglycemia. They dance together, but at opposite ends of the ballroom. (See figure 6.1.) Insulin drives blood sugar down, and adrenaline pushes it up.

This is normally quite harmonious—when blood sugar drops below certain levels, hormones such as glucagon, growth hormone, and cortisol work in unison with smooth orchestration. Normally, we're not aware of the process. But in hypoglycemia, alarming drops in blood sugar alter the key, and discordant alarms are sounded. The cascade begins when sugars and heavy starches are consumed. The pancreas responds fast with inappropriate releases of insulin. This threat sets up a chemical counterpoint that, like a loud trumpet blast, wakes the dozing adrenal glands; they respond with a stupendous release of adrenaline. That's when affected individuals first realize customary fine-tuning is errant. (See figure 6.2.)

Hypoglycemia's acute symptoms, which are triggered by this release of adrenaline, are truly frightening and generally last from twenty to thirty minutes. They most often strike three to four hours after eating a meal that's heavy in carbohydrates. As we've stressed, this powerful hormone is the ultimate fail-safe weapon that copes with precipitous drops in blood sugar. When it's a bit slow in responding, it makes up for it with a supercharged attack. Unfortunately, this is a good-news/bad-news situation. It prevents fainting and may even save your life. The bad news is that it's responsible for a flock of symptoms that are quite familiar to everyone who has ever been scared, suddenly startled, or acutely

HYPOGLYCEMIA

Chronic Symptoms

- Fatigue, insomnia
- Nervousness, depression, irritability
- Dizziness, faintness
- Blurring of vision
- Ringing ears
- Gas, abdominal cramps, diarrhea
- Numbness/tingling of hands, feet, face
- Flushing/sweating
- Foot/leg cramps
- Bitemporal or frontal headaches
- Impaired memory and concentration

Acute Symptoms

- Heart pounding
- Palpitations or heart irregularities
- Panic attacks
- Nightmares and severe sleep disturbances
- Faintness or syncope
- Acute anxiety
- Hand or inner shaking/tremor
- Sweating
- Frontal headache or pressure

Figure 6.1

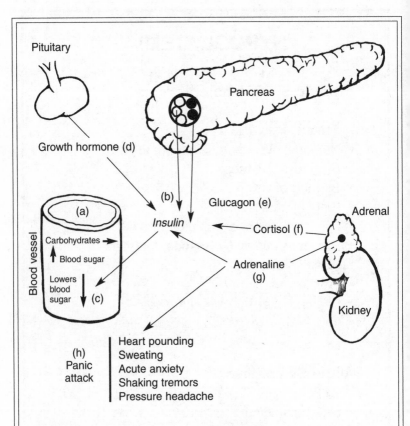

Heart pounding
Sweating
Acute anxiety
Shaking tremors
Pressure headache

(h) Panic attack

Normal	Abnormal
(a) Eating carbohydrates raises blood sugar.	Insulin lowers blood sugar too much; the brain reads "hypoglycemia" and stimulates release of:
(b) Bloodstream delivers sugar to the pancreas and releases insulin.	(d) growth hormone
	(e) glucagon
(c) Insulin enters bloodstream and lowers the blood sugar.	(f) cortisol
	(g) Adrenaline normally blocks excess drop in one or two minutes, but not fast enough in hypoglycemia.
	(h) Adrenaline penalizes the body and causes acute symptoms.

Figure 6.2

stressed. The first sensation is of heart irregularities or pounding and a feeling of severe anxiety. Shaking hand tremors, drenching sweats, faintness, and frontal pressure headaches complete the picture. Very intense reactions are labeled panic attacks. Nocturnal symptoms are often preceded by the frequent nightmares of hypoglycemia. In turn, sleep disturbances provoke daytime drowsiness and add greatly to general fatigue.

So now you can understand my level of confusion when I realized I was facing two conditions in the same patient for which nothing in my medical training had prepared me. I was forced to treat one misunderstood illness along with another that, in the eyes of my medical profession, might not even exist. This troubled me, since I didn't much enjoy veering away from the well-accepted and well-researched paths of medicine. But neither could I turn my back on suffering that I believed was real. In this situation where there was no road map to follow, I had no choice but to take, as Robert Frost named it, the road less traveled.

Adrenaline (epinephrine)—A hormone released by the adrenal glands when the body senses imminent danger. It is sometimes called the fight-or-flight hormone. It is designed to increase energy levels in emergencies. When the blood sugar falls in hypoglycemia, the body senses an emergency and releases adrenaline. This release normalizes the blood sugar within one to two minutes.

Endocrine system—This system is made up of glands that produce hormones (chemicals necessary to regulate the body's functions). They regulate or stimulate metabolism, growth, and sexual development and function, as well as maintain the body in a state of balance (known as homeostasis).

Over time, patients kept referring others. I was collecting an assortment of conditions I wasn't yet fully adept at handling. It's spine tingling in any field of work to come face-to-face with something exciting and entirely new. It was a little intimidating to find that a nameless disease was actually common, and equally astounding to realize that an existing medication could resolve the condition. I had been taught that results are what count. I remember one of my teachers during grand rounds who said emphatically: "Don't just stand there—do something!" I think this was his interpretation of the Hippocratic oath, which could be paraphrased as: "Get the patient well as best you can, but above all, do no harm." What to do seemed simple, safe, and straightforward. I would offer a diet to erase hypoglycemia, prescribe a medication to control rheumatism—or as it's now known, fibromyalgia—sit back, and enjoy my success. It was never to be: Disagreements and arguments in this field persist even though the opposing voices are getting softer.

THE DIAGNOSIS OF HYPOGLYCEMIA

In high school, my doctor ordered a glucose tolerance test. After fasting for twelve hours I had to go to his office and sit for five hours in a chair. I wasn't allowed to move around as this would cause me to release adrenaline, altering the test results. After the initial blood draw, I was given an eight-ounce bottle of glucose syrup to drink quickly without gagging. I immediately felt nauseous and dizzy, and felt a migraine coming on, but I had to remain there for the day. Blood was drawn twice every hour for a total of ten draws.

Although my results later came back as "normal," on that day I was too sick to leave the office and drive myself home. The nurse gave me a cot to lie down on, because I was too weak, sweaty, and shaky to leave! I felt like I was going to die, and in that moment,

I promised myself that I would never ever take that type of test again.

—*Chantal H., Michigan*

The five- or even six-hour glucose tolerance test has been the long-standing tool for confirming the diagnosis of hypoglycemia. Patients are given a measured amount of sugar to drink, and blood is periodically drawn to test their response to this glucose load. The party line was that if during the course of the test, a blood sugar reading fell below the magic number of 50 milligrams per deciliter (mg/dl), the diagnosis was confirmed. In my earlier days, we subjected every patient with suggestive symptoms to the rigors of this test. To our surprise, many results revealed nothing but normal levels. Despite this, they complained bitterly about a flock of hypoglycemic symptoms suffered during and after the experience.

Knowing that a spurt of adrenaline can raise blood sugar in one or two minutes, we retaliated by drawing blood more often—every half hour—hoping that added samples would catch out a low reading. This worked a little better, but was still far from satisfactory. We quickly learned that adverse symptoms were frequently not synchronous with the rigidly timed blood sampling. In other words, not everyone's blood sugar dropped at exactly the same time after drinking the sugar solution. It was obvious that technicians couldn't insert needles to draw blood fast enough to catch the rapid effects of adrenaline. No matter how hard lab personnel tried, we all too often missed the glucose nadirs. The hormone was persistently faster than we were.

Finally, because glucose testing failed to confirm our diagnosis about 50 percent of the time, we decided to try a different approach. You can never say we didn't go down trying! We had patients drink the same measured amount of glucose, but omitted blood sampling. Now subjects simply recorded their symptoms during the subsequent five hours. Most of them experienced all of the classic, acute symptoms of hypoglycemia at different times during the test. Others fell asleep, overcome by severe fatigue. Looking at countless diaries, it dawned on me that patients were simply writing down the very same symptoms they had already related in my office—symptoms that had alerted me to test in the first place. So why did we need to subject them to the ordeal and the expense? Why make them drink the horrible stuff? Why not just listen attentively to patient complaints and simply accept as diagnostic the symptoms they had so eloquently described on their initial visit?

I decided to use the test only if patients were suffering fainting spells or had an abnormally low fasting blood sugar. Either of those two factors should prompt physicians to consider the possibility of an insulin-producing pancreatic tumor. Our new system paid off. It saved patients five hours of testing, multiple needle sticks, a miserable morning, and the sick days that were sure to follow the sugar cocktail. After all, do you really need a blood sugar reading of below 50 mg/dl to tell you what you already know—eating a lot of sugar or starch makes you feel lousy?

In 1994, Drs. Genter and Ipp published some interesting findings that gave us yet another reason to abandon testing.[1] They conducted a simple and elegant experiment that explained why some patients with symptoms don't register the previously considered mandatory drop of blood sugar below 50 mg/dl. These two doctors ordered five-hour glucose tolerance tests on twenty young, healthy subjects who had no symptoms whatsoever of hypoglycemia. A catheter was placed in a vein so that blood could be sampled every ten minutes without repeated needle sticks. Samples were measured for the amounts of various counter-regulatory hormones and the timing of their release following the ingestion of the sugar load.

Surprisingly, during the test about half of the subjects developed varying degrees of the acute symptoms, such as tremors, sweating, heart pounding, anxiety, or pressure headaches. Some had only a few of these effects, but others had all of them. As expected, the battery of tests identified adrenaline release as the cause of these sensations. Very strangely, however, these responses were induced with sugar levels quite in the normal range. The lowest was at 58 mg/dl of blood, but most had levels in the 60s, 70s, and one even at 81! This flew in the face of the accepted definition of hypoglycemia: the magic number 50. This study and a later corroborating paper from France strongly suggest, at least to me, that we each have a set point for blood sugar. If it drops below our own predetermined, ever-changing level, the brain says we've got trouble, and promptly triggers hormonal and nerve impulses to prevent us from passing out.

Many physicians are unaware of these studies and order tolerance tests when a patient complains of obvious symptoms of hypoglycemia. Their normal results fool physicians into thinking patients don't have carbohydrate problems, and they tell them so. While an argument can be made that the term *hypoglycemia* should be retained for patients whose blood sugar actually drops below 50 mg/dl, we can use something else that accurately describes the group we're discussing. The simple designation *carbohydrate intolerance syndrome* wins our vote. Regardless of sugar levels or what name we use, all patients with this symptom complex respond equally well to the same dietary restrictions.

I have now been on the HG diet for over four years and it is still the most important day-to-day thing I do to keep well. Every time I fall off the diet, I suffer in various ways, including getting very anxious and emotional and having trouble thinking straight. So I get a sharp reminder every time about why I bother with the diet! It is worth tackling this issue as a blood sugar problem: It will become clear in a few days whether you are on the right track.

Take a good hard look at what you are eating and when. Do the diet as written, including watching out for the foods and ingredients on the "strictly avoid" list. Make sure you have satisfying balanced meals. Have a snack with protein and fat in between meals and make sure you never go too long without food. Make sure you carry something HG-legal with you. Wherever possible, have food cooked from scratch.

I realize this is an issue in social settings where people are sharing food, but you can make it work. People don't expect diabetics to eat any old thing and it is just as important for your health to be careful.

—*Mary, New Zealand*

Once I had a better understanding of this carbohydrate intolerance, I was much better able to discern the overlapping symptoms of fibromyalgia. (See figure 6.3.)

Unless you or your doctor can recognize the distinctive complaints that help separate the two diseases, the second diagnosis might easily be missed. The two diseases share many symptoms: fatigue, irritability, nervousness, depression, insomnia, flushing, and impaired memory and concentration. Anxieties are also common to both conditions, as are frontal or bitemporal headaches, dizziness, faintness, and weakness. Each can produce blurred vision, nasal congestion, ringing in the ears (tinnitus), numbness, and tingling of the hands, feet, or face. In addition, nausea, excessive gas, abdominal cramps, and constipation or diarrhea are frequent. Many complain of leg or foot cramps. When hypoglycemia is the cause of these chronic symptoms, they're experienced even in the presence of a normal blood sugar. That's because of the extensive endocrine and metabolic imbalances brought about by months of insulin-induced stress. There's a certain stiffness of muscles in hypoglycemia, but not the deeper pains induced by the lumps and bumps of fibromyalgia. Much confusion can be avoided by simply using our hands to map swollen areas. This type of examination makes it possible to separate the two illnesses with considerable accuracy. Lumps, bumps, and spastic tissue easily identify fibromyalgia. Fortunately, we also have the acute symptoms of carbohydrate

Relationship of Fibromyalgia and Hypoglycemia

Fibromyalgia	Overlapping Symptoms	Hypoglycemia
Skipping heartbeats (palpitations) Headaches (a) generalized 　　　　　(b) neck-occiput 　　　　　(c) one-sided Dizziness (a) imbalance 　　　　　(b) vertigo Eye irritation Salt craving Eye dryness Abnormal tastes Restless legs Constipation (IBS) Burning urination (dysuria) Bladder infections Interstitial cystitis Brittle nails Itching anywhere Rashes (a) hives 　　　　(b) eczema 　　　　(c) neurodermatitis 　　　　(d) itchy blisters 　　　　(e) acne Growing pains Vulvodynia (vaginal pain or irritation) Sensitivity to light, odor, and sound Pain (a) muscles 　　　(b) tendons 　　　(c) ligaments 　　　(d) joints	Ringing in the ears Weakness Fatigue Irritability Moodiness Nervousness Depression Insomnia Impaired memory Impaired concentration Anxiety Frontal headache Dizziness Blurred vision Numbness (face or extremities) Abdominal cramps Gas Bloating Diarrhea Sugar craving Sweating Weight gain Generalized muscle stiffness Nasal congestion Leg/foot cramps	Hunger tremors Pounding heart Panic attacks Faintness Fainting Intense hunger pangs Severe sugar cravings

Figure 6.3

intolerance to dependably point to blood sugar disturbances. These statements are important. Either disease standing alone requires its own simple approach. A two-pronged attack demands dual and simultaneous treatment.

HYPOGLYCEMIA TREATMENT: PROPER DIET

It's a good idea to stock up on food you can eat. The worst thing on any diet is when you're hungry and you go into the kitchen and you start looking and feel like there's nothing you can eat. I make a couple of big containers of sugar-free Jell-O every weekend so at least I can grab a bowl of that with whipped cream. Slices of cheese and cold cuts are good, too. On the liberal diet, nuts make a good snack, combined with string cheese or an apple. Cream cheese can be seasoned with a number of things and sliced with cucumbers. Olives and pickles sometimes hit the spot because they are flavorful. It's not a bad idea if you can get organized enough to put snack-size or small portions of things in the freezer so you can just microwave one and have something to eat in a minute or two.

—*W. M., California*

Many affected people ask if they should eat more carbohydrates, especially during bouts of hypoglycemia. The answer is an emphatic no! In fact, quite the opposite is true. Humans don't need sugars or heavy starches in their diet. The body can easily manufacture each and every type it uses in its metabolism. There exist no cases of carbohydrate deficiency for that very reason. Proteins, and to a lesser extent fats, can provide substrates that the liver can convert to glucose, albeit with a fifteen-to-twenty-minute delay. Not only that organ but also the kidneys easily convert certain amino acids into glucose.

However, we should be very clear up front: The required diet for hypoglycemia is not a zero-carbohydrate diet. Both of the diets you will read about in the remainder of this chapter restrict only certain carbohydrates, the ones that cause the blood sugar to spike and fall. Many people consume carbohydrates in the belief that they'll become super energized. It's true that healthy people compensate for rises in glucose with perfectly regulated bursts of insulin. In all honesty, however, they, too, probably admit to the late-morning, late-afternoon yawns and fatigue following carbohydrate indulgences. What rises must fall, and insulin action substantiates that axiom. Hypoglycemics have an unfortunate and exaggerated response: Their insulin surges incur overzealous carbohydrate control and induce the symptoms under discussion, but even those without hypoglycemia experience more energy without the cascade of all the hormones that results from carbohydrate loading.

Hypoglycemia can be controlled only with a perfect diet, one that eliminates all of the dangerous carbohydrates. As we previously stated, there's no need to add anything; it's what you remove that guarantees recovery. Patients must not eat table sugar, agave, corn syrup, honey, sucrose, glucose, dextrose, or maltose. Lactose (milk sugar) and the significant fructose in fruit can be consumed in rather limited amounts: Only one piece of fruit should be eaten in a four-hour period. All heavy starches must be avoided, including potatoes, rice, and pasta. Eliminate caffeine because it prolongs systemic effects of insulin. (It also paradoxically slows entry of glucose into parts of the brain.) Caffeine also helps insulin evoke or block responses to hypoglycemia, resulting in an undesirable hormonal combination that blunts release of the expected countersurge that normally brakes a rapid drop in cerebral glucose. The liver extracts quick energy from alcohol but, in just a few hours, stumbles badly from its effects and temporarily loses the ability to convert stored food residues to glucose. So sorry, but despite everything else we're stealing from your diet, no alcohol. But take heart: For most of you, these dietary restrictions aren't forever.

The elimination of sugars (simple carbohydrates) as well as heavy starches (complex carbohydrates) is mandatory because they push the body to release insulin. Avoid that response, and hypoglycemia cannot occur. It's really that simple. In time, each of the affected endocrine glands will recover. In my experience, healing begins with a display of somewhat more energy somewhere between the fourth to fifth day after starting the diet. Some patients feel more fatigue during the first few days as they change their basic energy fuels from carbohydrates to protein and fat. During this initial period, they may also experience headaches from both caffeine and carbohydrate withdrawal. The energy surge that eventually appears may be delayed for those who have been ill for a very long time. Total elimination of sugar and starch may seem like a monumental challenge, but using diligence and willpower, success is rewardingly awesome.

> When people give me a hard time about the foods I don't eat I just say, "Nothing tastes as good as healthy feels."
>
> —*Sophie, Australia*

Let's now look at the specific foods that must be completely eliminated if you are to overcome and maintain control of hypoglycemia.

Forbidden Foods List for Hypoglycemics: Foods to Strictly Avoid

Sugar in any form, including soft drinks	Black-eyed peas (cowpeas)
Caffeine from any source, including many soft drinks	Garbanzo beans (chickpeas)
	Refried beans
	Lima beans
Fruit juices and dried fruits	Lentils
	Potatoes
Baked beans	Corn
	Bananas

Barley	Dextrose, maltose, sucrose,
Rice	glucose, fructose, honey,
Pasta of any kind	corn syrup, corn sugar
Quinoa	(high-fructose corn syrup),
Burritos (flour tortillas)	molasses, cane or brown rice
Tamales	syrup (caloric sweeteners
Sweets of any kind	and starches), agave, and starch

Our diet for hypoglycemia is divided into two parts: "strict" and "liberal." They control hypoglycemia equally well. The strict diet was devised for anyone who needs to lose weight; the liberal diet was designed to maintain weight and still offset hypoglycemia. Take note: The above list, "Foods to Strictly Avoid," is applicable and, in fact, mandatory for both diets. You can't ignore that list in the beginning. Just a little cheat will certainly do you in!

DR. ST. AMAND'S STRICT DIET FOR HYPOGLYCEMIA AND WEIGHT REDUCTION

You can eat freely the foods listed below except for the few items given a quantity limit. You can eat whenever you're hungry—there is no need to starve yourself or eat on any specific schedule. If you don't see something on this list, you simply can't have it. Always check packaged and canned products by carefully studying the list of ingredients. Learn to read labels carefully every time you buy a product. Manufacturers may make changes without warning. Do your homework and don't kid yourself. The very foods that caused you to gain weight are the ones you must give up to lose it. If this appeal to your common sense doesn't succeed, go to the liberal diet. You'll remain heavy but you'll at least control hypoglycemia.

Meats

All meats are allowed, except cold cuts that contain sugar. (Check labels carefully. Low-fat or nonfat and turkey cold cuts usually have added dextrose or corn syrup. Bacon and ham are acceptable, although they do list sugar on the labels. This bit cooks off and is not a problem. Hams that are heavily coated should be washed free of sugar.)

All fowl and game, fish, and shellfish are allowed in unlimited quantities.

Dairy Products

Butter and margarine
Cottage and ricotta cheeses (½-cup limit)
Any natural cheese (cheese you slice yourself)
Cream (heavy and sour)
Eggs

Fruits

Avocado (limit ½ per day)
Cantaloupe (limit ¼ per day)
Fresh coconut
Lime or lemon juice (limit 2 teaspoons per day), for flavoring
Strawberries (limit 6–8 per day)

Vegetables

Asparagus
Bean sprouts
Broccoli
Brussels sprouts
Cabbage
Cauliflower
Celery
Chard
Chicory
Chinese cabbage (limit 1 cup per day)
Chives
Cucumber
Daikon (long, white radish)

Eggplant
Endive
Escarole
Greens (mustard, beet)
Jicama
Kale
Leeks
Lettuce
Mushrooms
Okra
Olives
Parsley
Peppers (red, green, yellow)
Pickles (dill, sour, limit 1 per day)
Pimiento
Radicchio
Radish
Rhubarb
Salad greens
Sauerkraut
Scallions (green onion)
Snow peas
Spinach
String beans (green or yellow)
Summer squash (crookneck, yellow, and green)
Tomatoes
Water chestnuts
Watercress
Zucchini

Nuts (limit 12 per day)

Almonds
Brazil nuts
Butternuts
Hazelnuts (filberts)
Hickory nuts
Macadamia nuts
Pecans
Pistachios
Sunflower seeds (small handful)
Walnuts

Desserts

Low-carbohydrate products including sugar-free chocolate with sucralose (Splenda) and sugar-free Jell-O

Custard (made with cream, egg, and artificial sweetener—no thickeners)

Cheesecake (no-crust or nut crust with cream cheese, sour cream, and artificial sweeteners)

Mousses made with whipping cream and sugar-free syrups or flavored protein powders

Beverages

Artificially sweetened drink mixes like Crystal Light, Country
　　Time, etc.
Zero-carb beverages made with stevia or any noncaloric
　　sweetener
Club soda, zero-carbohydrate flavored soda waters
Decaffeinated coffee
Mineral or bottled water
Caffeine-free diet sodas
Cocoa, sugar- and caffeine-free
After two months on a perfect diet, most hypoglycemics
　　can tolerate a bit of alcohol: bourbon, cognac, gin, rum,
　　scotch, vodka, dry wine (with noncaloric mixers is
　　okay)

Condiments and Spices

All spices including seeds (fresh or dried), all imitation flavorings,
　　and horseradish
Herbs such as garlic, rosemary, thyme, sage, etc., fresh or
　　dried
Sugar-free sauces such as hollandaise, mayonnaise, mustard,
　　ketchup, soy sauce, Worcestershire sauce
Sugar-free salad dressings
Oil and vinegar (all types)

Miscellaneous

All fats
Caviar
Tofu and soy protein products that contain no forbidden
　　sweeteners

If cholesterol is a problem, avoid cold cuts except sugar-free turkey. Trim all visible fat off meat. Remove the skin from poultry. Broil or grill foods instead of frying. Avoid full-fat cheese, heavy cream, solid margarine, hollandaise sauce, and macadamia nuts. Use egg whites or Egg Beaters instead of whole eggs. Use liquid margarine only. Nuts should be dry-roasted only. Use canola or olive oil.

DR. ST. AMAND'S LIBERAL DIET FOR HYPOGLYCEMIA AND WEIGHT MAINTENANCE

(Add these foods to the strict diet)

Fruits (limit: 1 piece of fruit every four hours; no fruit juices or dried fruit)

Apples

Apricots

Blackberries (½-cup limit)

Blueberries (½-cup limit)

Boysenberries

Casaba melon (1-wedge limit)

Grapefruit

Honeydew melon
   (1-wedge limit)

Lemons

Limes

Nectarines

Oranges

Papaya

Peaches

Pears

Plums

Raspberries

Strawberries

Tangerines

Tomato juice (unsweetened)

V8 juice

Vegetables

Artichokes

Beets

Carrots

Onions

Peas

Pumpkin

Squash, winter (such as acorn,
   butternut, fresh pumpkin,
   spaghetti, etc.)

Turnips

Nuts (no limit for those on strict list, plus add the following)

Cashews
Peanuts
Soy nuts

Dairy Products

Whole, nonfat, low-fat milk and buttermilk
Yogurt, unsweetened or made with noncaloric sweeteners
(whole milk is best)

Dessert

Sugarless diet pudding (½–cup-a-day limit)

Breads

Three slices a day of sugar-free white, whole wheat, sourdough,
or light rye. No more than two slices at one time or three
servings a day of sugar-free flat bread (no more than two
servings at a time). Low-carb tortillas—two is one serving.
Corn tortillas—two is a serving.

Other Food Items

Carob powder
Flour (gluten or soy only)
Low-carb baking mixes
Gravy made with gluten or
soy flour only
Wheat germ

Puffed rice, shredded wheat, or
other sugar-free cereals
Popped popcorn (1-cup limit)
2 tacos or 2 enchiladas
(2 corn tortillas only)

Most of the questions we are asked about the diet stem from
confusion regarding the built-in nature of various carbohydrates.

Many people have difficulty understanding why they can't eat a tiny bit of potato instead of the daily allowance of sugar-free bread permitted on the liberal diet. Most of those individuals have repeatedly tried calorie-restrictive diets. The number of calories contained in foods are simply added up, and if the total sum is kept low enough, weight loss should begin without regard for the dietary mix. So carbohydrate substitution, gram for gram, would seem logical. Wrong! That type of math won't cope with our problem, since not all carbohydrates are created equal. Since a calorie is a measure of heat, a portion of meat can be equal to a very different amount of candy. Note that a pound of feathers is larger in size than a pound of lead, but the weight's the same. A carbohydrate-restrictive diet adds up very differently: A gram of dextrose is not equal to a gram of lactose when it comes to the insulin response.

The glycemic index (GI) ranks foods on how they affect blood sugar levels in comparison with straight glucose. It's mainly used to evaluate the metabolism of carbohydrates. Protein and fat don't induce much rise in blood sugar unless eaten with carbohydrates. The GI was initially based on glucose with a number 100; the United States more commonly uses white bread as 100. (To convert to the white-bread scale, multiply by 0.7.) We'll stick with the original since white breads differ in the amount of insufflated air and the creative styles of different bakers. Tables exist to permit food comparisons by the rise in blood sugar or by the level of insulin they induce. As examples, the potato, a bunch of glucoses strung together, is assigned the GI of 98; on the other hand, fruits contain fructose, which is quickly shunted to the liver, doesn't raise the blood sugar to the same extent, and releases far less insulin; peaches have a glycemic index of 26. Perhaps you can now appreciate that, though fructose and glucose are both carbohydrates, we can't substitute their effects on GI ounce for ounce (gram for gram). In general, you'll find that foods with a high

GI are excluded from the hypoglycemia diet; lower-numbered ones can be consumed in moderation, the lowest in unlimited quantities. Please note, the glycemic index is not a perfect system. Expert studies have shown that this system is quite fallible. Individual constituents are not eaten by themselves; our foods exist in multiple combinations. A good example of this is the carrot, which we allow on our liberal diet despite its fairly high glycemic index. Its fiber content makes the difference.

When we first designed these diets, we had to rely on our patients as test subjects since the glycemic index didn't yet exist and neither did home glucose measuring devices. Any food that induced symptoms of hypoglycemia in even one patient was relegated to the forbidden list. We gradually boiled it down to the roux, the sticky residue that's the foundation for our diet listings. Sixty years later, the diets still work without much revision. In our experience, about two months of perfect dieting are needed to wipe out all the symptoms attributable to carbohydrate intolerance. Consider the dietary process as if you were building a checking account. First, you must make deposits. If you're well disciplined, you can rebuild energy reserves to the highest level allowed by your genetic makeup. Only when your account is full should you begin experimenting with other carbohydrates, and begin making withdrawals on your balance.

You may never be able to indulge in wanton spending. You should be cautious in the beginning. Uncontrolled spending, or too much cheating, produces sequential debits. You may have to push away from the banquet table now and then and take time to replenish your reserves. A negative balance will put you right back into hypoglycemia. If you permit that to happen, brace yourself for the fury of renewed adrenaline surges and panic attacks. Once you've followed the diet for a while, your body is resensitized, so when you cheat and consume too many of the wrong kind of carbohydrate, your symptoms will be magnified. If that happens, there's no choice but to go back and restart the process of restoration. It's far better to heed whatever early warning signals you're given; tighten up on your diet and avoid disaster. That's the key to damage control.

It's in your best interest to become an A student by being observant. Learn to recognize the very first symptoms that follow dietary indiscretions. Enervating fatigue often leads the way, but frontal, pressure-type headaches are almost as likely. A few setbacks from hit-and-miss dieting will develop your instinct to retreat when needed. Mental or physical stress, the premenstrual week, and injuries render you especially vulnerable. They'll sap your reserves, but if you're careful, you'll avoid fully subjugating deficits. You'll be far less fragile if you can anticipate before major symptoms resurface. In time, you'll properly ration meal contents to match energy expenditures.

Physicians or dietitians can't predict if you'll need permanent dietary restrictions. In a majority of cases, a certain amount of leeway develops, especially as fibromyalgia improves. Recall that illness causes much of your body to work day and night, expending huge quantities of energy. When the overworked, contracted tissues relax, you may be rewarded by being able to eat almost indiscriminately. Unfortunately, genetics play a part: Some patients will never be able to eat many carbohydrates. A family history of diabetes is sufficient warning that you were born with a genetically vulnerable pancreas. In that case, lifelong adherence to a low-carbohydrate diet is the safest course.

One night, I woke up in the middle of the night to my whole left arm with pins and needles. I got up to try to shake it awake and felt a flush of heat go from my head to my feet, so I went to walk down the hall to turn on the AC. Halfway down the hall I got dizzy and my vision blackened and the next thing I knew I was on the floor, with my husband over me yelling my name. After I came to, I was anxious, nauseous, cold, and had uncontrollable shivering. Eventually we went to the ER, only to be told it was syncope and I was fine. For the first time in my life, I began having panic attacks, constant anxiety, constant heartburn, and reflux. I couldn't sleep because I was terrified. It wasn't until two years later that I was told I was hypoglycemic! Suddenly it made sense and I realized all the symptoms I've had of low blood sugar all my life. I started the diet right away. The first week was rough; my body rebelled. I had major cravings, I was exhausted, my palms would get clammy, and my feet would get hot, but I pressed on. By the second week I felt less fatigue, my daily headaches had gone away, and my anxiety was nowhere to be seen! I've been on the diet six months now and it has made such a difference in how I feel! I have not had any anxiety or a single panic attack and that alone is worth continuing to eat like this for the rest of my life!

—*Erin W., California*

FIBROMYALGIA + HYPOGLYCEMIA = FIBROGLYCEMIA

Our statistics on seventy-five hundred consecutive patients with fibromyalgia are telling. Twenty-nine percent of our females and 15 percent of our males have concurrent hypoglycemia. Most of our patients began having low-blood-sugar attacks after the onset of fibromyalgia. Many other fibromyalgics feel worse depending on the amount of carbohydrate they ingest at one time. They don't get out-and-out hypoglycemic or feel severe pain, but become generally more fatigued and stiff after eating starches or sugar. They know when they've overdone it and have some degree of carbohydrate intolerance.

We wanted a single name to cover patients who have both conditions. We've chosen *fibroglycemia*. So, you might ask, why is this combination so common in our patients? Let's review a bit. We addressed our mapping system for making the diagnosis of fibromyalgia (see chapter 2). Our hands can easily identify the swollen areas of the body as contracted portions of muscles, ligaments, and tendons. Such areas are puffed up mainly because of accumulated intracellular fluid under high pressure, but they're also working tissues, as demonstrated by their spastic, constricted state. These tightened segments are steadily pulling on bones, joints, or adjacent structures twenty-four hours a day without respite. Though the effort is low-grade, these sinews eventually fatigue and begin hurting, just as would be expected from a never-ending workout. For every lump and bump we draw on our maps, there are many other affected areas too deeply hidden for us to feel. They're invisible accomplices that also contribute to the exhaustion. People who exercise stop when they get too much pain and fatigue. Fibromyalgics don't enjoy that luxury: They can never stop their muscles from working.

Remember that the currency of energy for all cells is ATP. Eighty-five to 90 percent of the food we eat is converted into this substance. Every bodily function demands huge supplies of this chemical. We can't even think without using large amounts of ATP for brain activity. Ounce for ounce, the central nervous system—especially the brain—uses more than any other tissue. Fingernail and hair growth, digestion, fat deposition, breathing, urinating, fighting infections, or healing tissue trauma all utilize ATP. The bulk of production and consumption occurs through muscle activity. As overworked tissues fatigue, they use nerves to signal the need for more fuel. The brain receives the message and immediately thinks: *I'm tired. Give me a candy bar.* When ATP production is normal, energy should be available within five minutes of eating such carbohydrates. That's no longer true in fibromyalgia. No amount of eating sweets will totally satisfy the steady or sudden demand for energy.

Most fibromyalgics fall victim to carbohydrate cravings throughout the day in an unconscious attempt to create energy. Those sugars and starches are quickly digested and converted to glucose.

Unfortunately, the carbohydrate-craving fibromyalgics quickly saturate their systems with glucose molecules, which force the pancreas to release large amounts of insulin. Such surges rapidly lower the blood sugar by driving it mainly into muscles, but also into fat cells, liver, brain, and most other hungry areas of the body. These repeated insulin surges eventually cause hypoglycemia in genetically susceptible individuals. Both the chronic and the acute symptoms of that condition are added to those of fibromyalgia. There you have it: fibroglycemia!

These are the sickest of our patients. For them, dietary modification isn't merely a good idea, it's mandatory. They face a huge metabolic chore. They must eat themselves out of hypoglycemia while simultaneously accepting the increased symptoms of fibromyalgia reversal. There can be no compromise for this group. They would continue to feel terrible on a freewheeling diet even when guaifenesin has purged much of the fibromyalgic debris from their tissues. Fibroglycemics must either choose to eat correctly or choose to remain feeling sick!

Over the years, my blood sugar has been slowly climbing as my weight rose, and now I am prediabetic. I am in a serious battle to lose weight, lower my blood sugar and my cholesterol, and not cross over the line into diabetes. I lost a lot of weight years ago on the strict HG diet, then coasted for a long time on the liberal diet, fell off the wagon a couple of times, and gained back what I'd lost, and now here I am today, trying not to become diabetic. It's not a symptom of fibromyalgia, but carb intolerance very often goes along with it, and can ultimately become diabetes. I thought it wouldn't happen to me.

Outcomes like this are what motivate us to keep harping on controlling your blood sugar and getting as much exercise as you can handle. As for me, I'm not giving up. I'm wearing a pedometer and eating from the strict HG diet. Spring is coming to

Minnesota, and cleaning up my yard and gardening will give me more opportunity for exercise.

—Anne Louise, Minnesota

Obesity sometimes offers some protection against hypoglycemia, but only in males. Once fat is overexpressed in the system, chubby cells are gradually the cause of a more serious disturbance. The larger a cell gets, the more resistant it becomes to further storage attempts by insulin. It's much more difficult to prod obese cells into opening their transport tunnels when they consider themselves already overstuffed. As a result, fewer amino acids (building blocks for protein) and fatty acids can be inserted into the usual warehouses. The pancreas, ever mindful of the waste–not–want–not principle, presumes its message is not being received. Rather than waste the digested food residues, the pancreatic islets instead increase their output of insulin. That's like hitting deafened fat and muscle cells with a hormonal two-by-four. Reawakened by this louder shouting, they dutifully respond, and storage resumes. Most structures of the body are willing to accept a bit more fatty acid, and that's what insulin orders be done. But remember that it takes higher-than-normal insulin levels to achieve that.

The battle of the bulge begins to make demands on health. Various cells including the chubby ones call upon their reserve defenses. Muscles find restrictions to satisfactory contracting when fatty acids slither into contractile elements. They fight as best they can using their biochemical weaponry.

Both muscles and fat try to repel insulin infringements on their defenses. That hormone is ever determined to find added storage facilities. Unfortunately, tissue resistance threatens to permit metabolic intolerance. Blood sugar starts to rise to slightly abnormal levels. Overweight segues into obesity; blood pressure breaches safety levels; blood triglycerides rise; so–called good lipid (HDL) gets somewhat smothered; the liver sequesters fat rather than exporting it; uric acid sneaks ever higher; the defining banner called meta-bolic syndrome is raised. Superimposed on that background, here comes the tempest and the winds of war: pre-diabetes.

As overweight becomes obesity, the bulging fat cells refuse to be fatter and fight in their refusal to follow insulin's instructions. The next step beyond simple insulin resistance (as this metabolic state is called) is type II, or adult-onset, diabetes. Cells that are unresponsive to insulin don't absorb glucose as readily as they once did. At this point, the blood sugar no longer drops abruptly; eventually it actually continues to rise. This is the way obesity sometimes corrects hypoglycemia and dupes patients into think-ing they've outgrown their sugar problem. But there's a heavy price to pay down the line. The health ravages of insulin resis-tance are many, and those of diabetes several times worse. There's a special subset of individuals who have family histories of dia-betes in parents and grandparents. They are born with insulin resistance and will invite the same fate for themselves unless they heed our warnings about carbohydrates. We won't explore those hazards any further. Nevertheless, we're adamant in warning you that neither low nor high blood sugar is healthy. And the way to avoid them both is the same: Limit your intake of sugars and starches. Many patients crave sugar due to the body's inability to make energy properly. For those of you who like statistics, here are some numbers. Not counting hypoglycemics, 43 percent of our lean and 57 percent of our obese fibromyalgic women crave carbohydrates; men don't fare much better: 44 and 48 percent, respectively. For all patients combined, including hypoglycemics, those who crave carbohydrates can be rounded out to 75 percent incidence. Just like the other patients with blood sugar fluctua-tions, they suffer all of the aches, pains, and fatigue but aren't punished by the sudden adrenaline surges of fibroglycemia. Dur-ing perverse situations, they can be pushed into that category by heavy sugar bingeing, alcohol abuse, emotional stress, infections, and even the trauma of an accident, extensive dental work, or surgery. Women are especially susceptible during the premenstrual week. It's as though they're teetering on the edge waiting for a nudge over the precipice.

Though no diet is necessary for people with fibromyalgia, those who regularly yield to their cravings could consider it. Sticking to a low-carbohydrate diet for one or two months might well provide surprises. Considerable energy and cognitive improvements are the rewards. Some encouragement is exhilarating while waiting for guaifenesin-induced improvements to begin. Even non-cravers get some of those benefits. It's great just to get rid of some of the fibrofog, getting better sleep, and avoiding the drowsiness that regularly follows carbohydrate meals. It's certainly worth a monthlong experiment. But give the diet a full month of perfect compliance to show you its benefits.

And here's why a low-carbohydrate diet can help everyone with fibromyalgia feel better even before guaifenesin has had a chance to help. A prime function of insulin is to drive glucose into cells. Especially in tissues such as fat and muscle, to accomplish this it has to tag a phosphate onto it. That's how glucose is prevented from escaping back out of the cells that it has just entered. It's a great way to lock in a substrate for quick energy needs. Insulin also signals certain kidney cells to reabsorb phosphate that was just filtered from the blood and into the urine. By sucking it back into the bloodstream, more phosphate ions are made available for glucose trapping. Muscles are especially cooperative, and some are more obedient to insulin than others. They snap to attention and soak up big phosphate loads, more than their fair share. You'll recall our theory suggests that phosphate excess is what eventually slams the brakes on energy formation. The chemistry of fibromyalgia, hypoglycemia, and the combination disease, fibroglycemia, is quite complex. But in simple terms, if you yield uncontrollably to carbohydrate cravings, your cells will get a heavy phosphate dosing—which is counterintuitive if you have fibromyalgia.

As if the picture weren't bleak enough, when insulin and glucose appear in fluids bathing the outside of cells, they insist on other visitors besides phosphates. Not too strangely, bloated fat cells, especially insulin-resistant ones, make oppressive, militant demands. Together they order cells into pulling calcium into their enclaves. Though we consider phosphate the prime villain, calcium is a steadfast accomplice. It unrelentingly goads already exhausted cells into further exertions. The low-carbohydrate diet subverts the propensity for excess calcium and phosphate to insinuate themselves into these cells. It does that by aborting excess insulin release.

As you'd surmise, fibroglycemia patients have the same salvaging dietary response as do those purely hypoglycemic. Please follow our earlier advice: Adhere to the strict diet if you're overweight and to the liberal diet if you are normal weight. If you are underweight, you will need to take special care to eat all the added foods on the liberal side. Remember, both versions of the diet prevent excessive swings in blood sugar. The added benefit of the strict one is weight reduction. It doesn't correct carbohydrate-induced hypoglycemia any better or any faster.

> I stopped all my medications cold turkey and went on the hypoglycemia diet. I started guaifenesin and went through some bad cycles. I fell off my diet and suffered for that. But slowly things have gotten much better. I'm down twenty-five pounds in weight, my mind is clearing, my muscle spasms have cleared, and I can sleep. I am not perfectly well but I can make it through the day without having to lie down for most of it. The most important thing is that I now have a life.
>
> —*Gwen, California*

When we begin treating fibroglycemia, we don't wait for the dietary benefits to kick in before starting guaifenesin. These people are very sick, so we can't think of any reason for delay. Once the hypoglycemia part of the combined disease clears (usually within two months), patients can judiciously add more carbohydrates. We discussed how to do that earlier in this chapter. Since people are genetically different, they each have to find their ultimate dietary limitations. There's a spectrum of possibilities ranging from permanent restrictions to none whatsoever.

There are no current modalities other than proper diet and guaifenesin treatment to reverse the mix of fibromyalgia and hypoglycemia. Success in chronic conditions depends greatly on the tandem efforts of individuals and their physicians, but the patient is the primary player in this recovery game. Though the demands are great, the appearance of the first good hours and days makes it all worthwhile.

We're offering you, the patient, a ladder to recovery. You'll have to climb it rung by rung or else you'll not likely even stay where you are, but continue the descent into your personal hell. Those of us who've recovered urge you to resurface and join us in living.

YOUR HOUSE GUESTS

What kind of host are you? Do you know you've had belly guests since birth? They've thrived under your sponsorship as provider of room and board. You've supplied them with luscious meals and plush living quarters. Your largesse helped them multiply to an estimated ten trillion inhabitants. Smug in their residential status, they've invited a flock of family members, visitors, and permanent subtenants.

Early invitees were gifted by your mother at your inception and others at your birth. Her placenta and your intestinal system became conduits for the new invitees. Some were transients, but many stayed on for the continuous banquet that you've catered. You've been colonized with some friendly, some subservient, some obnoxious, and some totally repulsive bacteria of all description. You almost ritualistically altered your food mixtures, people contacts, animal encounters, and living environment. Your prolific fellow passengers have readily adapted to each lifestyle change.

Insidious characters now live among them. Unfortunately, that includes innately combative playmates who initiate, abet, and perpetuate conflicts. The malicious ones are dedicated to prolonging civil warfare. They even recruit allies to terrorize the once-stable cohabitants you welcomed. They gradually expand their territories and force pacifist cohorts into sharing their sanctuary nooks. Not only do they usurp space, they likely settle into the most comfortable places. From within their ghettos they do the biblical thing: They go forth and multiply. Invasion by this immigrant colony not only dislodges, but often destroys some of your protective residents.

Internecine warfare distresses the entire system and seriously impacts health. Friendly bacteria must and do retaliate. Facing-off encampments foment clashes, recurrent skirmishes, and ultimately outright war. Repetitive onslaughts promote alternating winners and permanent enemies. Unfortunately, the good guys don't always win. Bad guys in ascendency make internal sanitation precarious at best.

Sometimes a stalemate arises on the intestinal battleground and mandates a reluctant truce. Such is made to be broken. Confronting militants are itching to break ranks and launch unpredictable battles. Such repetitive conflicts make for cumulative debris from damaged weaponry, wounded combatants, and decay from the dead. Surviving winners and losers also spread malignant toxins throughout your hosted war zone. These massive messes are strewn all over the contested field that just happens to be your gut. This is a scourge that produces gut malaise or major illnesses that spread even to remote tissues.

Breaking peace requires very little provocation, just because formidable you is on the sidelines acting the erratic prompter.

You, the unwitting accomplice, have too often subverted each armistice. Your interventions have been capricious and you've frequently switched sides. You're not aware how whimsical you've been in breaking allegiances. Your volatile habits have projected mixed signals to the battling forces to the detriment of your refugee bowel.

Once you shed family dietary disciplines of your youth, you just had to experiment on your own. Freed from constraints, you could eat whatever you designated as comfort food. Self-indulgence all too frequently broke through barriers that once dampened eating orgies. Hedonistically, you ignored red-flag warnings registering on your bathroom scale. You chose not to decipher belly-bulge signals about the major battle raging within your abdomen. You've been a chameleon-like traitor to your salubrious denizens and continued nurturing the wrong contestants.

In fairness to you, you may not realize you've been a co-aggressor. Nevertheless, you've manipulated and interfered with what was a fair fight. Some medical professionals and dietitians proffered their ill-informed advice. Weren't you counseled that fats were your undoing? They long condoned savory, starchy feeding frenzies, thereby urging some caloric moderation. For three decades, like a mantra, they coerced you into avoiding fats and perhaps excess sugary stuff. That was certainly false advertising and never a sound promotion. Your pantry and refrigerator refuges are likely stocked with evidence of your mutual ignorance.

We've outlined the low-carbohydrate diet and told you it's mandatory for correcting hypoglycemia. We also mentioned that most fibromyalgic people have felt considerably better on such dietary restrictions. The rise and fall of blood sugar created by meals and snacks were making energy demands that further taxed an existing fatigue. We also stated that the irritable bowel syndrome would dampen some 60 percent by omitting sugars and starches. In following sentences, let's detail other benefits of the diet just coming to light.

First, let's get back to the warring bacterial nations. There are many fighter ethnicities within the ranks. The muster list of enrollees carries an altogether formidable list of names. We'll ignore most of them to avoid confusion, and simply induct the leaders into your vocabulary. But keep in mind that there are lots of warriors from many clans, any of which can gain ascendency at various times. Their allegiances are insecure and alliances are transient at best. Combatants switch sides, alter the tide of battle, and lurch your gut into a revolt aimed at you.

It's enough for our purposes to write about the three "phyla." Those are like surnames. Tribal chiefs have been baptized "Bacteroidetes," "Firmicutes," and "Proteobacteriaceae." There are three others that intersperse among them but have as-yet-unknown significance in our tale. No need for you to memorize such monikers. Let's nickname the main players as "ditties," "cuties," and "aces." Ditties and cuties are the dominant types in your gut. They account for 90 percent of your resident bacteria. When aces accumulate in excess numbers, they're a warning you've reached a dysbiotic status. That means this group has grown to unsafe limits and intends to upset your innards, your so-called milieu. Sufficiently disrupted, you're sick.

When the ditties are in charge, they make pleasant, harmonious vibes and the belly is in repose. There are a few renegades among them, but they're kept in check by their elders. Many of the cuties are anything but and they should never be allowed to dominate. Aces are even more sinister: They're always at the ready to disturb the peaceful truces enacted by the other two. Among their kind are some true marauders. For our discussion it's best to think that tolerance between ditties and cuties promotes a smoothly performing gut. Cuties and aces must never get elected into leadership: It's their MO to cause insurrections, turmoil, and downright chaos.

It's amazing that these assorted breeds can actually live together harmoniously. In prime health they do just that, however, each contributing something to our health. We're gathering circumstantial evidence to condemn many in their numbers, even though some have redeeming virtues. A huge number among the trillions, good and bad guys alike, have work skills and talents we don't ignore. You probably know that vitamins are entities we cannot manufacture for ourselves. Most of them are care packets we extract from our foods. But when diet alone doesn't contribute enough, bacterial guests come to the rescue. They can and do produce most kinds of vitamins since they need them for their own livelihood. Their skills overproduce a bit, and they generously share surpluses with us as little treats.

So nobody is all bad, and even unsavory co-habitants atone for some of their nefarious ways. They break down and digest vegetable fiber into component morsels. They reassemble those and synthesize anew some leftovers into defensive weaponry. From their productive threshers they extract chaff known as butyric, propionic, and acetoacetic acids. We cherish those for various purposes. The highly nourishing "butaryl" comes off bacterial cultivators in great abundance. Lining cells of the intestine savor that by-product as a favorite food. They thrive thereby and add to our protection by shoring up their cellular walls. Normally, those become resistant enough to keep out the undesirables lurking nearby in surrounding moats. They can then safeguard the cell's innards that produce protective mucus and digestive equipment.

The cuties and aces can mass-produce toxins. Those chemicals break down the protective mucous lining inside the bowel. Most times that favorable goo is sufficiently sticky to trap both the bacteria and their noxious secretions. That's often sufficient to halt the invasion, but not when overwhelming amounts are unleashed by the assailants. Intestinal cells are on constant alert and diligently seal any lesser breaches. Yet the ruffians sometimes succeed and wedge into unprotected little crevasses they uncover. Realizing the danger, the defenders call a general muster of friendly forces. Most times only a minor scuffle ensues, the breaks are sealed, and major warfare is averted.

If burrowing succeeds in making a deeper penetration, surface structures get roughed up. Those cells are overcome and require help. They retaliate by firing chemical flares as alarm signals. Even distant, system-wide reserves recognize that SOS. They rush in to rescue resident, watchdog white blood cells and shore up their weakening defenses. Together they attract an augmented blood flow and extract required resources to hopefully dominate the fray.

Converging defenders have multiple sophisticated weapons to hurl at the attackers. Among those are little grenade-like elements, chemokines and cytokines that we visited in chapter 5. They hurl those at the evil upstarts and try to neutralize them. Brigades of larger, more dominant responders are alerted by messages from guard post observers. Those well-trained warriors carry lethal antibodies that are poisonous for the enemy. Foot soldiers from the same battalion unleash a deadly fusillade. This coordinated array of allies usually overwhelms the cutie hordes and their fellow travelers, the battle-prone aces.

Anti-rebellion efforts are constant. The defense team usually stands alone since you're not aware of the battles raging within you. It knows too well your propensity to be inimical to the wrong bacterial alliance. Your erring judgment leads you to starve would-be saviors yet feed and shelter enemy legions. You pamper them and they make you sick. They provide you with gas, bloating, abdominal pain, constipation, and diarrhea as trophies of your wanton behavior. If convicted at court-martial, you'll serve time with irritable bowel syndrome, mucous colitis, spastic colon, and leaky gut!

Once your sentence is mitigated, consider atonement. Alter your ways and give succor to your friend-defenders. Favorably adjusting your diet can foster growth of friendly battalions within just two or three days of healthy feeding. Extra millions of ditties can flourish even in so short a time. Simply choose weapon-victuals that help ditties flourish and simultaneously starve cutie regiments. For a change, let the would-be felons march on empty stomachs. That should blunt their morale before they can launch another charge.

So how do you begin a food embargo? Cuties and aces love and thrive on carbohydrates. They're adept at harvesting energy from those goodies. They even convert them into fats in case of future shortage. Their mischievous contract with fat cells invites the greasy stuff into scattered reservoirs, but especially pudgy bellies. So why not deprive them of those gluttonous morsels and serve them nothing but large portions of starvation? Our austere low-carbohydrate diet is suitably designed to stunt their growth.

On the other hand, ditties thrive on animal products: proteins and fats. They well deserve rewards for their long-standing vigilance. Invite them to a testimonial feast and promise them ample future supplies of their favored goodies. They indeed prefer meats, fish, chicken, olive oil, and any kind of fat, even saturated. To them sugars and starches are distasteful. Isn't that exactly what makes up our low-carbohydrate diet? Make friends and purge enemies: Happy food for your buddies is exactly what's stinky stuff for the others.

Your bowel tries to converse with you. Please listen despite the language barrier. Its jargon is in the "symptoms" tongue. You do have to interpret a bit. It goes silent when cutie-dittie dances go smoothly. But it's morose and strident when improperly fed. It pouts and weeps when an antibiotic kills off too many ditties. It hums along if a probiotic restores harmony. It's mellow in a cuties-controlled belly that's toxin-free. It would be thrilled if it knew how much research is being directed to understanding its microbiota. It likes to think of itself as your intestinal tract. As such it would like you to be a bit more friendly.

By now you should have a pretty clear picture why that diet is so salubrious. Let's count the many ways it loves thee. It corrects hypoglycemia; stabilizes blood sugar in diabetes; corrects most of the metabolic syndrome; defuses some fatigue of fibromyalgia; trims weight; improves about 60 percent of the irritable bowel syndrome (IBS, or "leaky gut"). Add all that to victory over Firmicutes (cuties) and Enterobacteriaceae (aces). You may not get a medal, but you'll surely be pleased with yourself. And bring along your festive gut.

Enough with the war zones. Here's a quick summary of what a new study has shown. It totally supports previous research, our multiyear stance on diet, the years-ago Atkins publication, and more. It was named the PURE study. It tabulated data from 125,287 residents from eighteen countries observed for an average of 7.4 years. Dietary surveys were broken down into categories of food intake. Plasma lipids, sugar, and, by a bit, blood pressure were lowered into more desirable or favorable values. Those eating larger amounts of carbohydrate had overall increased mortality. People ingesting larger amounts of any kind of fat, saturated, polyunsaturated, and mono-unsaturated, actually had decreased all-cause mortality. Even saturated fats led to a distinctly lower incidence of stroke. This is not the first report that fats are not villains, but this one seems large enough to placate most people.

We've harped on the beneficial aspects of low-carbohydrate diets for many years and in all editions of our books. Olive oil, nuts, and fish might contain slightly healthier ones, but all fats are friendly. This huge study definitely condemns sugar and heavy starches. The study did not drill this home, but particularly detrimental is the mixing of fats and carbohydrates. I've warned of this to anyone who would listen, including the young doctors I've been privileged to teach for more than sixty-two years. Carbs produce a killer metabolism that is early and well advertised by weight gain. As we urge in chapter 6, judiciously choose your fruit and vegetables: They're not created equal.

Thank yourself if you're already nutritiously feeding your bowel flora. You should have cleared up a lot of irritable bowel symptoms. But that still leaves the gut awash in fibrogut remnants, the diet-resistant 40 percent. Now you need to deploy your long-range missiles. You've got the properly mixed rocket fuel in the guaifenesin protocol. Handled right, it ignites the final salvo and rarely misfires. It's programmed to cleanse the fibromyalgic deposits lurking within those three-layered muscles of the intestinal tract. So in summation: Get rid of the unwanted phosphate detritus, feed the ditties, tame the cuties, then champion the cause. Be the hero to your tamed-down, docile, and ever well-behaved gut.

LIVING LOW-CARB: THE FIBROGLYCEMIA AND HYPOGLYCEMIA DIET

In the fourth and fifth months on the guaifenesin protocol I started to cycle fatigue. I found this very annoying and disruptive to my daily routine. So I decided to go on Dr. St. Amand's HG diet to see if that would help. After forty-eight hours I was amazed at the difference this change in diet had made in how I felt and realized I had been severely carbohydrate intolerant for a long time. While a minority of fibromyalgics are hypoglycemic and must eat for HG, the vast majority of us will do better eating this way, too, due to the metabolic relationship between FMS and carbohydrate intolerance. It's a very healthy choice of foods, so I encourage all who suffer from FMS to go on this diet and see if it makes a difference with certain symptoms, especially fatigue, brain fog, and IBS. For those who are hypoglycemic it's imperative to eat for HG to be well, so it's not a choice, but for the rest of us it's worth giving it a try. If you need to lose weight, do the strict, if underweight or normal weight, do the liberal diet. What we eat every day can have a profound impact on how we feel, as food can be healing medicine or poison to a person with FMS depending on that person's food choices.

—*Janet T., New Mexico*

Down to Specifics

The good news is that low-carbohydrate dieting has become very popular. Where choices were once rare, there are now hundreds of them. Products are better labeled, and restaurants from fast-food joints to the fanciest easily accommodate low-carb dieters. There are cookbooks, Facebook pages, low-carb sections in stores, websites, and bakeries that compete for your money. New medical studies are published monthly about its benefits for the current diabetes epidemic, and most doctors no longer pooh-pooh it as a fad or fringe diet. More than any other thing we've taught over the years, our use of the low-carb diet has been vindicated.

Most people begin their new diet reluctantly and timidly, quite afraid of making mistakes. That's the way it should be. Earlier in the chapter, we stressed that a certain reverence must be applied to the required restrictions. Errors are costly, and early on, gains are easily erased. Unlike the sequences necessary to determine guaifenesin dosages for fibromyalgia, the low-carbohydrate diet can be presented in black and white. Your predecessors have done all the work: *This you can have and that you can't*. Be dedicated and accurate. Don't even consider cheating or getting creative for the first two months.

For most people, breakfast is the most difficult meal. Yet there are plenty of choices. By habit, we tend to define only certain items as being "breakfast foods." But really, it's all the same to your digestive tract. Even if you don't want to consider anything out of the usual, just look around you. On both the strict and liberal diets, eggs can be prepared any style: fried, boiled, or scrambled. Omelets are a bit more work but can be made with any of the usual additions—cheese, bell peppers, sour cream, tomatoes, avocado, and sprinkled herbs. You can eat any kind of meat such as breakfast steaks or pork chops and even sugar-cured bacon, since frying burns off that bit of carbohydrate. (Watch out for sausages, though: Most mulch in some kind of sugar.) Hams frequently have honey or other sweeteners that should be washed off. You can make mini-quiches in a muffin tin and pop them out for a quick breakfast on the go.

Breakfast drinks can be made with unsweetened protein powders, egg, or soy. There are even ready-made choices, including sugar-free Breakfast Essentials. Toss in strawberries unless you want to spare your quota for later in the day if you're on the strict diet. Clever thinking creates other possibilities—say, making a smoothie using fruit, tofu, milk, and sugar-free syrups. There's nothing wrong with a scoop of cottage cheese, a serving of unsweetened yogurt, a slice of cantaloupe, and an added piece of sugar-free flatbread if you're on the liberal diet. Smoked salmon and cream cheese aren't bad choices, either. Egg custards are particularly refreshing, especially on warm, summer days. They can be made in batches using heavy cream, eggs, vanilla extract, and sugar substitutes. The liberal diet permits you to spread unsugared peanut butter on toast made with sugar-free bread. A tiny spoonful of sugar-free jelly is a nice addition. On the liberal diet, unsweetened cereal or oatmeal with sugar-free sweetener is allowed. On both diets, you can find recipes for acceptable quiches, or breakfast casseroles. Yep! We keep repeating this, and we're still not done: Your diet should be *sugar-free*.

Lunch on the strict diet could include vegetables with or without meat. Deviled eggs make wonderful snacks; they're safe if made with sugar-free mayonnaise and aren't stuffed with sweet relish. When I wanted to lose a few pounds, I used two cabbage leaves as my "bread." Large lettuce leaves can be used to form wraps, and now you can even buy them premade. A bit stickier, but slices of roast beef or cheese can substitute. Liberal dieters might well get by with sandwiches that use the thinner types of sugar-free breads, corn tortillas, sugar-free wraps, crackers, or flatbreads. Composition salads are great with added bits of beef, chicken, shell- or other fish, cheese, egg, sour cream, and avocado. Taco salads can be made with low-carb tortillas and bean-free chili on the liberal diet. There are many sugar-free salsas you can buy already prepared. Inspire yourself by creating your own versions, including variations on the traditional Cobb or Caesar salad, as long as you keep dressings sugar-free. You can always eat hamburgers and cheeseburgers with a fork after tossing out the bun or using a lettuce wrap if you are on the diet's strict side.

Just by custom, we usually conjure a different vision for the components of our evening meal—we're usually less interested in eggs and sandwiches. We also tend to prepare our food somewhat differently, using a lot more grilling, broiling, and baking. Fish is less often eaten at lunch but is something we can add to our dinner menu. Vegetables may be marinated, stir-fried, roasted, baked, or grilled along with meats or separately using the same oils and sauces. Steamed vegetables with cheese and nuts are delicious. On the strict diet, it doesn't take much imagination to use al dente cauliflower, daikon cubes, or chunks of summer squash as replacements for potatoes in certain recipes. You can purchase packaged cauliflower rice, "faux tatoes," and pizza crusts for the strict diet. Just check the ingredients as you would for any other packaged foods. You can find these now at markets from Walmart to the highest-end ones. Or you can make your own. Celery root or cauliflower can be cooked and whipped into faux mashed potatoes with butter, sour cream, and a little garlic or blue cheese. Artichoke appetizers dress well with butter or sugar-free mayonnaise, sauces, and shrimp. Slip in curry or hot paprika. Batter is easily made from eggs and crushed pork rinds or drier cheeses such as Parmesan to coat meat such as chicken on the strict diet. Nut flours make delicious piecrusts or coatings for chicken or fish on the liberal diet. Your taste buds might like the dramatic change offered by blackened meats. You could stuff large mushroom caps or green peppers with spinach, cheese, or bits of anything you dream up. Spareribs made with sugar-free barbecue sauce or meat loaves that have been stuffed with cheese or topped with sugar-free ketchup make a nice change. Stir-fry shrimp with bell peppers, mushrooms, and scallions; lace scampi with extra butter, garlic, and a few gourmet herbs to avoid menu ennui. Chopped cauliflower or shredded lettuce can serve as a replacement for rice. Many vegetables and salads are pre-packaged for easy preparation. When it comes to the salads, just make your own dressing if the packaged version comes with one that contains sugar. It's easy to make a delicious dressing from oil, lemon juice or vinegar, and Dijon mustard.

There's a world of flavors just waiting for your creativity. There are no restrictions on spices; garlic, mustard, and chili powders; sugar-free sauces; Liquid Smoke; horseradish or garlic paste; or piquant Thai dressings. These ingredients add great zest to whatever you're preparing. The liberal diet certainly provides more variety, and once your weight is normal, you'll graduate to it. Use unusual items such as spaghetti squash as a replacement for pasta on the liberal side; on the strict side, zucchini or summer squash ribbons can fake pasta dishes. There are many types of appliances to help you make those noodles in a few minutes, from simple handheld blades you twist to fully electric versions. Once made, they require only a moment in hot water to prepare. Toss with any of your favorite (sugar-free) sauces or serve it simply with butter and Parmesan cheese. You gourmet people are still permitted favorite escargot preparations and caviars.

Several desserts work in nicely on either diet. Whip up egg custards, sugar-free cheesecakes (nut flour shell) on the liberal side, and sugar-free Jell-Os. There are plenty of other delicious concoctions, even ice creams, now being made with artificial sweeteners such as sucralose (Splenda) or simply the no-sugar-added products. Mousse can be easily made with whipping cream and a flavored protein powder. Would you perhaps consider floating sugar-free ice cream or whipping cream on top of a diet root beer? One patient melted sucralose-sweetened chocolate bars in her microwave oven and poured them on her strawberries. Check carefully before you buy any sugar-free cookies or desserts. Many don't simply contain table sugar, but may be sweetened with other sugars forbidden on our diet.

Eating out is getting safer as more restaurants are responding to the growing demand for low-carbohydrate fare. Most readily substitute vegetables in place of rice or potato. Cottage cheese or sliced tomatoes provide suitable options. Fibroglycemics should bring decaffeinated coffee in packets, order a pot of hot water, and make their own brew because a stressed waiter might mix up coffeepots and serve you the real thing. The main courses are usually as safe as what you would have eaten at home. Ask the waiter if the Caesar or blue cheese dressings are sugar-free (they usually are). If not, use oil and vinegar with or without a squeeze of lemon juice or a little mustard. Occasionally, restaurants have flavored olive oil sitting on the table or will at least honor your request for some. In Mexican restaurants you can order various fajitas, ropas viejas, machaca, or even the chiles rellenos if they're only lightly floured. Italian restaurants usually offer veal or chicken piccata, bistecca, osso buco, and assorted seafoods including scampi and calamari. Satisfy your tastes but choose restaurants with cooperative chefs who'll tell you what's in their sauces.

It's not within the scope of this book to cover in depth the merits of fats versus carbohydrates as fuel sources. Many persuasive arguments are made for the fact that our modern diet is not what we were designed to eat. This may be why caffeine and carbohydrates are such potent problems when it comes to blood sugar. And we have to say, the battle is finally disengaging: Heavy carbohydrates are more often implicated as dietary villains in current medical literature, and certain fats as okay guys.

As a result of this change of attitude, it's impossible to list all the low-carb resources at your fingertips. The internet is full of recipe sites from the original Atkins.com to hundreds of newer ones. Those geared toward weight loss tend to be more suitable for the strict diet, while others are more liberal. It will be your responsibility to check the recipes against your list of ingredients you must avoid, but as with checking your products for salicylates, this becomes very easy over time. You will quickly learn to make simple substitutions to traditional recipes using noncaloric sweeteners and reducing sauces instead of adding flour. There are online stores such as Netrition that in their low-carb section have hundreds of products suitable for both strict and liberal diets, including products to thicken sauces, sugar-free sauces for flavor, condiments and dressings, and many more items.

Though the hormone cortisol can store belly (visceral) fat, only one hormone can store lipids in all fat cells, and that's insulin. It's predominantly released in response to carbohydrates, as we've already discussed; fats beg for insignificant amounts and proteins only a bit more unless they're eaten along with carbohydrates. Our strict diet permits weight reduction for three main reasons:

1. It avoids heavy insulin outputs.
2. Protein digestion and storage require more caloric expenditures than that particular food contains.
3. In the absence of surplus carbohydrates, metabolism must burn fat for energy. Fats are loosely divided into two categories: cis and trans fats. Many products now show on the label which one(s) they contain. It's easy to remember which are the good ones with the phrase "I love my SIS-ter," which reminds you that trans are the bad ones. There aren't many concerns about unsaturated fats from olive oil, vegetable oils, and liquid margarines.

Most popular weight reduction diets are simply variations on the original theme. Well-executed studies are accumulating that back the safety of low-carbohydrate diets and contradict the notion that it's the fat in the Western diet that's making you obese. Our diet is indeed healthy. Put the blame where it belongs: Look to the carbohydrates and their buddy insulin. Most are killers, and their weapon is insulin.

We are all witnesses to the explosion of obesity and adult-onset diabetes that low-fat, high-carb eating has fostered, and most sources realize that now. They are accompanied by high blood pressure, heart disease, and hardening of the arteries.

Weight reduction is easily and comfortably achieved with sufficiently low carbohydrate intake. Those who've been unsuccessfully trying to lose by shunning fats instead of carbohydrates have been seriously duped. What you've been eating is what's made you fat, hypoglycemic, or diabetic. In deference to my colleagues, I'm not your doctor and can't impose my recommendations over those of your personal physician. But if you have a weight problem, you owe it to yourself to do some research and ask hard questions. Although my patients don't always follow my advice, they'll certainly continue hearing from me on this subject.

I've been on the low-carbohydrate diet for more than fifty years. I confine myself to the strict diet during the week. It prevents late-morning and afternoon energy depletion. It also drops my weight one or two pounds below my desired level. By the weekend, I go into my liberal mode, and I confine my cheating to eating pizza, bread, or rarely rice. My eating style keeps me contented—though it might not do so for you. Each of you may eventually develop your own ritualistic system of dieting and cheating. But first, you must get out of your hypoglycemic funk. In that process, if you need to, why not take your weight down to a healthier level? After you've reached your goal, allow yourself only enough cheats to keep you on friendly terms with your bathroom scale.

Take your guai, eat right if hypoglycemia is an issue, do whatever kind of exercise you can tolerate (and keep ratcheting it up when you can), continually check your purchases for the no-nos, stay positive even when it seems impossible. Most importantly, watch the life you had before you started get better with each hour, day, month, and year.

GUAI WORKS! One of my favorite quotes from someone was about those days when everything hurts, the brain isn't working, etc. etc. "So that's where I'm healing today." Guai gave me a life back that I thought was stolen by fibromyalgia.

I now realize we all have issues we never expect. Be thankful for every minute, hour, day, month, and year ahead. You are on the right track, and coming through to the other side of the fibro experience will only make you stronger, happier, and healthier. I have been on guaifenesin and the diet for over twenty years.

—*Jeri Lynn K., California*

CHAPTER 7

THE PROTOCOL

I was diagnosed with MPS [myofascial pain syndrome] after multiple injuries working as a machinist. Although I was under the care of a doctor who was a local expert, over the next three years my condition worsened and the pain spread to all points of my body. I was diagnosed with fibromyalgia. My quality of life was horrible. A pattern emerged where I would work during the week and spend the weekend in bed recovering. During this time I frequently asked God to please cure me or take me home, as I had nothing to look forward to. I was in my forties and essentially my life was over. If not for my three wonderful children, I would have self-terminated by 1999.

I was surfing the web and ran across Dr. St. Amand's paper. After checking the toxicity of guaifenesin, which is about zero, and talking to my PCP, I quickly started out on the protocol as I had nothing to lose and everything to gain. The first few days, I felt the effects of the guai and grew hopeful. My PCP was kind enough to write prescriptions for guai until it went over the counter.

I was very sick when I started out, but day by day there were changes. At the two-year mark I knew my future was bright. During the three-to-four-year period I was about eighty percent well. Pain and muscle spasms had disappeared and strength and stamina were returning. At the

156

four-to-five-year mark I felt like I had a brand-new body, which is very nice. Today, at the age of sixty-four, I enjoy walks, riding my mountain bike, and motorcycles. I can ride the mountain bike twelve to fifteen miles when I'm in the mood. I sometimes talk to other fibromyalgics about the protocol and I tell them not to sell themselves short, to hang in there for at least a year or two before giving up on it.

—*Michael I., Illinois*

It's time to take a closer look at our protocol. We're going to lay out each step carefully. We've tried to write this chapter as clearly and concisely as we could. We'll skip over some explanations that we've already detailed in previous pages or will subsequently outline. Please digest what we say and don't allow yourself seemingly harmless deviations from what is a proven path. Some ten thousand patients have scouted the way: Take advantage of the trail they've blazed. You're about to benefit from both their successes and their mistakes. Please do it exactly our way.

FIND A DOCTOR WHO'LL MAKE THE DIAGNOSIS

Obvious as it sounds, first make sure you have fibromyalgia and only fibromyalgia. That sounds silly, but it's important to rule out more dangerous or potentially lethal conditions with overlapping symptoms. If you haven't been diagnosed, pointedly ask your doctor. Don't be shy. Explain when you make your appointments that you suspect what you have, but you'd like expert confirmation. You get the wrong vibes? Choose another doctor. Fibromyalgia is difficult enough as it is. Without an ally, it's just too stressful.

General practitioners or internists are perfectly qualified to help you precisely because they're generalists and not super-specialists. They're less likely to squeeze most of your symptoms into the smaller-size container of their limited specialty or order extensive testing. When we first wrote about it, finding a physician who believed fibromyalgia existed was a challenge that's been almost completely overcome these days. With near-constant television advertising for medications, hundreds of medical journal articles in all publications, and the fact that it is now taught in medical school and has its own ICD-10 diagnostic code, you'll find that most physicians are versed in the basics. But it doesn't hurt to ask when you make your appointment to be checked.

Face-to-face with a doctor, what should you expect? If you haven't had recent blood tests, expect that some will be ordered. This workup will survey your body for adverse conditions, since many diseases have symptoms in common. Some tests are altered by recent food or drink, so be prepared to give fasting samples. Normally included will be a blood count looking for anemia, infection, or inflammation; a chemistry panel will check organ function, lipid abnormalities, diabetes, and the chemical composition of your plasma.

It's true that 85 percent of fibromyalgics are women. Equally so, 5 to 10 percent of women develop thyroid dysfunction, mostly low (hypothyroidism). Expect the two illnesses to overlap, just by chance. It's also a fact that each condition will make the other worse. They're not otherwise linked, though they cause a mutual intensification of symptoms—as you'd surmise from the superimposition of any second disease. The ultrasensitive test TSH (thyroid-stimulating hormone) is mandatory since it's outstandingly accurate for detecting thyroid glandular dysfunction. In some areas of the country, Lyme disease is rampant. Extensive foreign travel might have exposed you to diseases such as hepatitis or parasites.

Some new patients come to us sporting the diagnosis "chronic Lyme disease." Because some symptoms don't quite fit, they wonder if they might also have something else such as "fibromyalgia." Deeper in their internet search, the possibility of chronic hypoglycemia syndrome also makes sense. Like layered house shingles, the multitude of symptoms totally overlap, and we extract one or more diagnoses from the occult mixture.

Knotted medical problems start unwinding just by listening to symptom litanies. Hypoglycemia has its own little package of complaints, as we described in chapter 6. There are key disturbances that allow us to open that particular Pandora's box. The introductory words: "When I'm hungry, delay eating too long, or overdose with carbohydrates, I get shaky, clammy, irritable, weak, confused, feel faint, and sometimes my heart starts pounding." That symptom complex is so unique to low blood sugar that the diagnosis is readily secured. There is no need to perform the very arduous, punitive, five-hour blood sugar test.

Next, we map the generally achy for whatever we can find. Our fingers "map" the person and discern the many lumps and bumps of fibromyalgia. Those are not present in hypoglycemia nor in Lyme disease. Simple? Yes, we can define and separate two of those unsavory diagnoses by listening and using our fingers for the disentanglement. That leaves us to deal with the problem of the Lyme vector.

These patients have been told they have Lyme disease based on a positive blood test. Some of them have had the confirmatory and more diagnostic Western blot test. Quite likely, they were then treated with a battery of the appropriate antibiotics. If symptoms continued despite responsible treatment, "chronic" Lyme disease was then suspected.

Many authors agree that the chronic form is greatly overdiagnosed. That likelihood has been stressed in the *New England Journal of Medicine*, which is published from an area where Lyme is endemic and widespread. An erroneous diagnosis leads to unnecessary and sometimes dangerous use of various antibiotics. Frequently an array of worthless supplements are also prescribed. Delay in sorting out the illnesses could have been avoided by just listening to the patients and then palpating their bodies. Thus, if you have been labeled with chronic Lyme disease, you have every right to question the diagnosis.

When you complain of aches and pains, your doctor will probably include an arthritis panel to help uncover the presence of lupus or rheumatoid arthritis. If you're over fifty, a woman, and have a particular distribution of pain, testing should be expanded to include the CRP (C-reactive protein) and the ESR (erythrocyte sedimentation rate). If they're markedly elevated, the diagnosis of polymyalgia rheumatica will be considered. If found, it requires immediate treatment. Polymyalgia reaches emergency status because of the threats it poses, including blindness and strokes.

At your initial appointment, give your doctor a list of all of your medications and supplements. This is no time for trying to avoid a professional opinion on the merit of such combinations. Include any over-the-counter products you take. Certain herbs and nonprescription items can seriously affect liver enzymes and kidney function. That's why your honesty coupled with appropriate blood tests could expose problems while they're still minor and correctible. In short, there's nothing ever gained by playing games with your doctor.

We remind you that there are no distinguishing tests for fibromyalgia. The tests being ordered are to reassure you and your physician that something more urgent does not exist co-expressed with fibromyalgia. When such entities are excluded, you and your doctor will feel far safer and can get on with this protocol.

The diagnosis of fibromyalgia is properly made in two parts. The doctor begins by taking a detailed medical history that includes a full systems review. Since fibromyalgia causes fatigue, pain, depression, irritable bowel syndrome, irritable bladder, numbness, leg cramps, headaches, palpitations, and a host of other diverse symptoms, your doctor will explore them, sometimes in detail. Many doctors use check sheets for baselines that itemize symptoms and, later, to track changes. Refresh your memory ahead of time so you can help establish a chronology of your complaints, including onset and progression. This sequencing will also provide you a rough guide as to when and in which order you should expect the reversal of your symptoms.

After your doctor is satisfied that your complaints and medical history suggest fibromyalgia, there will probably be an abbreviated exam. He or she may not feel comfortable "mapping" as we do, but at the very least should do a hands-on search for the so-called tender points (although with the new questionnaires to diagnose fibromyalgia, you may be examined extensively for all of them). As we explained earlier in this book, tender points have become less central to the diagnosis these days. (We think physicians should also feel places where you hurt even if they're not included in those predetermined zones.)

Finally, armed with normal blood tests, educated questioning, and tender-point or mapping results, both of you should feel secure with your diagnosis. At the same time, you should also be assured that nothing else is wrong and that organs like your liver and thyroid are functioning normally.

ADDRESS THE CARBOHYDRATE INTOLERANCE/ HYPOGLYCEMIA FACTOR

Once you've been diagnosed with fibromyalgia, you have another important thing to explore. As we explained in the previous chapter, there's no reliable blood test for hypoglycemia or carbohydrate intolerance. Your personal experience is really sufficient. You're very well aware of what happens when you eat foods high in sugar, or potatoes, rice, pasta, and other heavy carbohydrates. As much as you'd like to deny it, you've actually done the best test in existence, over and over again. Take your own symptom inventory and trust what you feel.

Remember how symptoms cluster into two fairly separate batches, the chronic and the acute? To review: The latter are the scary ones and typically strike two to four hours after eating, often during the night. They're sudden in onset and sometimes violent enough to be labeled panic attacks. Hand or inner shaking, sweating or clamminess, headache, heart flip-flopping or pounding, anxiety, irritability, weakness, dizziness, faintness, or occasional passing out are the rest of the litany. Like all the other symptoms, these may not all appear at once or as intensely in everyone. If eating makes them go away, but they recur when you're hungry, hypoglycemia is the likely culprit. Eating doesn't change the symptoms of fibromyalgia.

The chronic symptoms are more generalized. They're with you most of the time no matter what the blood or brain sugar levels. They don't materialize because of any drastic fall in circulating sugar or surges of counter-regulatory hormones. They're due to metabolic fatigue from so many fluctuations. Blood sugar headaches are frontal, suggesting sinus problems, or disposed like a contracting rubber crown, wrapped circumferentially around the head. Fatigue, irritability, nervousness, flushing, impaired memory and concentration, tight muscles, abdominal pain, bloating, excess gas, and diarrhea are part of the not-too-pretty chronic picture. This symptom complex isn't helped by eating, unlike the acute ones. Treatment requires the longer and more determined dietary effort.

If you're hypoglycemic, you have no choice but to follow our dietary advice. We discussed carbohydrate intolerance in chapter 6, but it bears repeating that if you feel worse when you eat a lot of carbs you should give the diet a try and see how it makes you feel. Reread chapter 6 and make a couple of copies of the diet. When you're first getting acquainted with its variations, keep one in your wallet or on your smartphone and another taped to your refrigerator door. It might be best to slip one into your desk at work or even your car. Before you eat anything, make sure it's on the approved list and doesn't contain any of the foods to strictly avoid. This will be much easier if you prepare your own food and don't buy packaged items. You can't afford mistakes. You should follow the diet perfectly for two months before you begin experimenting with off-list foods. When you begin to experiment, start slowly and with sensible cheats.

If you're heavy, you belong on the strict diet. Proper behavior will provide striking rewards: You reduce weight and simultaneously battle hypoglycemia. Carbohydrate craving starts to ease in about ten to twelve days, and that makes it easier to stay the course. You won't get all of the foods you previously enjoyed, but at least you can eat all you want and not go hungry. Once you've shed the weight you need to lose, you're free to add everything on the liberal diet.

Normal-weight hypoglycemics should go on the liberal diet, since it restores blood sugar control just as quickly as the strict diet. You should experience an inspiring boost in energy beginning about the fourth or fifth day, the brain fog lifts appreciably, and soon the irritable bowel eases greatly. This applies to almost all fibromyalgics even if they're not out-and-out carbohydrate-intolerant or hypoglycemic.

If you're underweight, you may have some difficulty maintaining your weight even on the liberal program. Eat more volume of the foods on that diet as best you tolerate if your scale starts dipping into lower numbers. Concentrate on fruits, nuts, dairy products, sugar-free grains, and the higher-carb vegetables listed on the liberal diet. Try sugar-free (or no-sugar-added) ice cream, and if necessary add a cup of brown rice with a meal.

I have been on the guai protocol for almost four years and have been following the HG diet. At the time I started the diet, my pain and fatigue were extreme. My level of whole body pain averaged 7 to 8 out of 10 every day, with no reprieve. I never experienced any good days or even good hours. I had never thought of myself as having typical HG symptoms, but I was hoping the diet would help my fatigue. Instead it helped my pain. I now have very little whole body pain, between 0 (most days) and 2. I am sleeping better, which I attribute to being diligent about the diet. Too much carb = restless night.

—*Carol, Canada*

You may feel more tired and irritable for the first several days after you start ditching carbohydrates and of course caffeine. It takes about one week before you glimpse a few rewards. Some of your symptoms begin to ease, and a bit of energy pops out through the snowed-under feeling. Within six to eight weeks, assuming you haven't cheated, you'll get most of the benefits the diet can provide and then you can start adding foods in moderation as we described in the HG chapter.

MAP YOUR LUMPS AND BUMPS

Mapping, as you know by now, is our term for our manual evaluation of a patient. Recall that we look for lesions: the swollen tissues of fibromyalgia (spastic muscles, tendons, ligaments, and some joints). We draw our findings on a printed caricature of the body. We depict the size, shape, and location of each and shade it according to the degree of hardness. The first one is your baseline for future maps that we'll compare for progress under treatment.

If your physician doesn't feel confident doing this, you have a few alternatives that may even be better. Ask for a referral to a physical therapist, chiropractor, or licensed massage therapist whom your doctor considers adept. Any practitioner who is familiar with what normal muscles feel like will notice the difference. Preferably, you will visit someone who is at least somewhat familiar with fibromyalgia and has good hands to feel the lumps and bumps. Show that person a copy of one of our body map illustrations, and remember that you can purchase a DVD of a mapping demonstration on our website: www.fibromyalgiatreat ment.com.

The examiner should use the pads of the fingers as though smoothing out tissue wrinkles, not digging into them, thereby creating ripples of flesh. We draw the size and location of lesions as we find them and press a bit harder or lighten up on the pen to illustrate the hardness of each lump. It's not mandatory for examiners to use our exact system. Variations can be introduced as long as the same examination is conducted on all subsequent evaluations. Would-be mapmakers should only record objective evidence to illustrate nothing but the swellings they palpate. They mustn't be swayed by subjective expressions of tenderness, since dominant pain sites change from day to day and obscure others. If your doctor has no suggestions for potential mapmakers, ask friends for someone they've used. Hospitals and orthopedists usually have a staff of physiotherapists or can refer you. Massage therapists are often excellent choices.

Go to your first appointment with a blank copy of the body map from our website, and give it to the professional who will do the examination. You can get it from this book, but it might be better to download it from the website so it's full size. This way, the experienced or novice mapper can quickly scan what you want done and make a reasonably similar search of your body.

The first map is very important and should be done before you begin guaifenesin. It's the baseline that will provide a startling reminder of where you were and will help substantiate progress when you compare subsequent maps. Copies of your first and subsequent maps can be sent to your doctor's office for professional monitoring of your progress if your physician didn't make them.

All of the professionals we mentioned are quite accomplished in palpating muscles and tendons. They know the feel of tissues and have to make only minor adjustments in their techniques to accurately sense the lumps and bumps of fibromyalgia. We happily allow anyone to copy the caricature we use for mapping purposes. Patients should be checked lying in the supine position.

Now we really need your attention. Be you patient or practitioner, here is an extremely valuable clue—probably the most significant one in this book. Read this over and over until you've mastered it. This is a fibromyalgia holiday gift for you and your mapper: a rare no-brainer in medicine. Value it! The quadriceps muscle in the front of each thigh holds signs that are easily read by discerning fingers. The left thigh is the code breaker. The outside portion is called the vastus lateralis; the front part the rectus femoris.

The outer vastus lateralis presents as a very long, tender, spastic single or two-part structure in 100 percent of adults with fibromyalgia. Its spastic portion is quite long, smooth, and only occasionally felt in separated bundles. This is generally the tenderest of the muscles of all the involved muscles in fibromyalgia. *And that easily the diagnosis is made!*

The left side of the rectus femoris (thigh front) displays six (occasionally five) discrete swollen bundles that are easily palpated when the muscle is pressed gently and stroked with the pads of the fingers in a single-direction sweep as if smoothing wrinkles out of a cloth. They feel firmer, undulated, and progressively tenderer going from the top down to just above the knee.

The right thigh is also affected but usually will show only one small patch on the outside and only one or two swollen places on the front. The hamstring muscles in the back of the right thigh are often spastic, but never on the left. The differences between the two sides are striking.

Equally fascinating is that these structures clear completely within the first month on an adequate guaifenesin dosage. It's highly encouraging for everyone involved to look at serial drawings that visually document clearing. Barring permanent tissue injury, most of those graphic lumps and bumps should become just unpleasant memories. (Figure 7.1 shows a blank map.) But as you will learn, your dosage could change.

BLANK BODY MAP

FIGURE 7.1

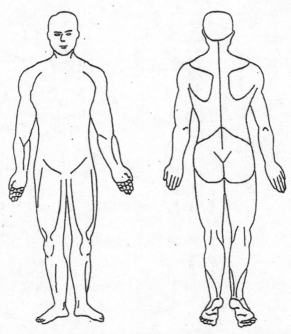

FATIGUE	HUNGER TREMORS	EYE IRRITATION	BLOATING	ITCHING
IRRITABILITY	PALPITATIONS	NASAL CONGESTION	CONSTIPATION	RASHES
NERVOUSNESS	PANIC ATTACKS	ABNORMAL TASTES	DIARRHEA	SENSITIVITIES
DEPRESSION	FRONTAL HEADACHES	a) BAD	DYSURIA	a) CHEMICAL
INSOMNIA	OCCIPITAL HEADACHES	b) METALLIC	PUNGENT URINE	b) LIGHT
IMPAIRED CONCENTRATION	GENERAL HEADACHES	RINGING EARS	BLADDER INFECTIONS	c) SOUNDS
IMPAIRED MEMORY	DIZZINESS	NUMBNESS	VULVODYNIA	d) ODOR
ANXIETY	a) VERTIGO	RESTLESS LEGS	WEIGHT CHANGES	ALLERGIES
SALT CRAVING	b) IMBALANCE	LEG CRAMPS	BRITTLE NAILS	GROWING PAINS
SUGAR CRAVING	c) FAINTNESS	NAUSEA	BRUISING	PAIN
SWEATING	BLURRED VISION	GAS	SKIN SENSATIONS	

ACTUAL PATIENT: INITIAL BODY MAPPING

FIGURE 7.1A

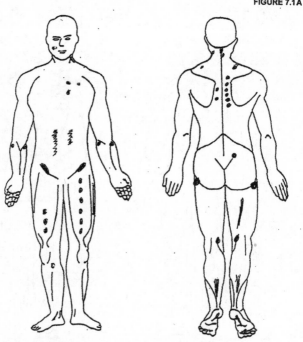

FATIGUE	HUNGER TREMORS	EYE IRRITATION	BLOATING	ITCHING
IRRITABILITY	PALPITATIONS	NASAL CONGESTION	CONSTIPATION	RASHES
NERVOUSNESS	PANIC ATTACKS	ABNORMAL TASTES	DIARRHEA	SENSITIVITIES
DEPRESSION	FRONTAL HEADACHES	a) BAD	DYSURIA	a) CHEMICAL
INSOMNIA	OCCIPITAL HEADACHES	b) METALLIC	PUNGENT URINE	b) LIGHT
IMPAIRED CONCENTRATION	GENERAL HEADACHES	RINGING EARS	BLADDER INFECTIONS	c) SOUNDS
IMPAIRED MEMORY	DIZZINESS	NUMBNESS	VULVODYNIA	d) ODOR
ANXIETY	a) VERTIGO	RESTLESS LEGS	WEIGHT CHANGES	ALLERGIES
SALT CRAVING	b) IMBALANCE	LEG CRAMPS	BRITTLE NAILS	GROWING PAINS
SUGAR CRAVING	c) FAINTNESS	NAUSEA	BRUISING	PAIN
SWEATING	BLURRED VISION	GAS	SKIN SENSATIONS	

ELIMINATE ALL SOURCES OF SALICYLATES

> Learn how to check for salicylates on your own. Stay 100 percent salicylate-free. Don't try to gamble with the protocol's rules. You will lose! "If in doubt...leave it out!" Make sure you are on your correct dose and then "ride out the storm." Follow the diet if you need it. Exercise when you can. Don't look for instant success, but instead, enjoy the small improvements that occur as time goes on. The last piece of advice I will share is for you to "live your life to the fullest now." Don't wait to get better. Life is too short. Try to find the joy in your day!
>
> —*Cheryl K., Canada*

Before you begin the protocol, you have one last but very crucial task. If you don't accomplish it successfully, you won't succeed with the protocol. It is your responsibility to do a thorough search for salicylates in your products. We provided extensive material in chapter 4 to guide you. There are no shortcuts—you must check everything! We've repeatedly seen minuscule amounts stop all progress dead in its tracks. If you're going to ignore this warning, don't waste your time reading the rest of this book.

Get a big box or bag and gather up everything you use on your body. If you have products at your work or in your car, don't forget those. Set aside undisturbed time. You may need a magnifying glass and access to the internet. Open this book to the salicylates chapter, and get busy doing your homework.

You should end up with three piles: products you can keep using, some you need to replace, and others that require deeper investigation. This latter group could have incomplete descriptions (products that list only the active ingredients) or no ingredients at all and must be researched or simply dumped. Use no product in which you can't identify every ingredient. If you want to continue with any of these, you'll have to get on the internet, go back to the store, or call the manufacturer. When you do, never rely on the person at the other end of the phone to check for you. Always get a list of ingredients. Customer service representatives are not trained in the chemistry of plants or chemical sunscreens.

Check anything you take as a medication: prescription or non-prescription, vitamins or supplements in any form. Also look at things such as nasal sprays, patches, eye drops, suppositories, and enemas. Don't forget what you're looking for: any plant name and the bioflavonoids quercetin, hesperiden, and rutin. Compounded topical hormones such as estrogen, progesterone, and DHEA are fine, but you must check the cream base, which may contain a plant oil or extract. Any product you use topically on your skin is next. This includes everything from mouthwashes, toothpastes, soaps, and shampoos, to razors, deodorants, skin care products, and all your cosmetics. Carefully check rubs or creams for relief of muscular pain that may contain menthol or methyl salicylate, camphor or plant oils. Antifungal products and any products that exfoliate should be checked as well as any products with a sunscreen (SPF), which need to be scanned for octisalate, homosalate, mexoryl, and meradimate. When you see the word *flavor* on a label, you need to make sure it doesn't contain mint or menthol—artificial or natural.

Remember: All plants make salicylate; it is part of their immune system. Come in contact only with their intact surfaces. When their saps or juices are absorbed by your skin, you will block your guaifenesin. Year after year we go on summer alert since we know a bunch of our patients will begin working in the garden. Be sure the gloves you wear are waterproof so you don't absorb salicylates through them. Your biggest task will be to keep the gloves handy where you can find them easily and not forget to put them on.

And now to address something we have recently discovered. In the third edition of this book, we mentioned that we had encountered failures using the bilayered Mucinex 600 mg guaifenesin tablet. We thought it might have something to do with the interface or the combination or not getting the full 600 mg in the long-acting formulation. But now we know differently.

I had directed three patients who drove together to their appointments to purchase their short-acting guaifenesin from a box store where it was much less expensive. This guaifenesin wasn't white like the one they had been taking from Marina del Rey Pharmacy; it was blue. When they came for their next mapping, all three had not progressed as expected. Three people all at one time? Since they had made no other changes, I quickly zeroed in on the guaifenesin itself and switched them back to their white tables. On the next trip all three had resumed their clearing.

After quite a bit of searching I found an FDA paper written in 1994 reporting that Blue Dye #1 actually entered mitochondria and reduced the production of energy. They had previously pulled a red dye off the market because of more intense energy problems but did not remove the blue one. Now we warn people to avoid ingesting medications colored with Blue Dye #1. Dyes are added to medications just to make them pretty. Rarely, they cause nausea. So we suggest you use colorless capsules or tablets whenever possible.

BEGIN TAKING GUAIFENESIN

As we stated earlier, guaifenesin is for sale over the counter. It is found on the shelf in the cough and cold aisle of pharmacies and of course online. You will want to make sure you begin with a long-acting or extended-release guaifenesin, which by definition has sustained twelve-hour action. In stores there are two strengths available, 600 and 1,200 mg. Be sure to get white tablets. Online, Fibropharmacy (Marina del Rey Pharmacy) has 300 and 600 mg specially compounded capsules and a 600 mg tablet. Most patients find it easier to start with their 300 mg capsule, which does not require you to break it and simply hope to end up with the exact dose. You can break (but don't crush) extended-release tablets.

We instruct patients to take two doses a day, roughly twelve hours apart.

Short-acting tablets or some encapsulated powders are probably effective for four or five hours, but this could vary greatly depending on the patient. They're more rapidly absorbed, stimulate the kidneys faster, and quickly fade away. We have found they're often ineffective when taken solo without added longer-acting stuff. (High-dosage patients do better by using short and long guaifenesin preparations in combination, both of which are available over the counter). Some short-acting tablets or powders come in poorly sealed capsules, and some companies sell powder for patients to stuff their own, which is problematic for several reasons. Due to the many variables, we do not endorse the use of short-acting guaifenesin as a stand-alone product. We have seen too many failures and we are determined to see you succeed and not take chances with your recovery. Since our repeated mapping documents progress, we can accurately confirm a formulation's efficacy for fibromyalgia. There are always uninformed persons who'll dash in with brash suggestions. That often includes patients who've attained alleged expertise though they've only treated one case, their own! Ignore anything contrary to these paragraphs.

FIND YOUR DOSE

> My first cycle lasted twelve days. The second one lasted eleven days. And so it went, slowly, slowly getting better. If I had to make a graph of the first several years, it wouldn't be a smooth straight line going upward. It would be more like a staircase. Every winter I felt worse, but not quite as bad as the previous winter. Every summer was a little bit better than the summer before.
>
> —*Anne Louise, Minnesota*

Please be systematic and stay at dosages for the times we specify. Stick with our outline until your basic need is confirmed.

Trust us—though it's tempting to bounce the medication up and down according to how you feel or you think you should feel, don't do it! Otherwise, you'll only succeed in confusing yourself and whoever is trying to help.

We're going to spell it out as we've learned from the past several thousand patients. In the early reversal period, mapping provides a perfect directional signal. But if you are unsure of your mapper's skills or don't have one, it is very important to keep a symptom journal or calendar to track your progress along with your own observations. You probably won't be able to confirm progress as quickly as you might with a map by an experienced mapper, but it will work just as well in the long run.

Brevity is the key to a successful symptom journal. You might keep it as simple as entries on a calendar or daily log pad—enough to jog your memory when you need to look back. It's tempting to create 1-to-10 ratings for each symptom, especially pain. That's okay in the beginning, but over time it's difficult to equate today's knee pain with the severity of last year's headache. Fatigue is still fatigue, but is it now less? Once you've experienced runs of several good weeks, a numerical rating system falls apart. How bad was bad? During treatment, worse days may become better than the good days were before you started treatment. Keep notations simple: for instance, bad, good, lousy, horrible, same, or so-so. Other possible entries might read: "headache half day," "neck very sore," "more energy a.m.," "back better," or "shoulder stopped hurting." Soon you'll decipher progress.

The brand-name guaifenesin, Mucinex, is marked extended release but we don't suggest using it, and there are two reasons for that. First is that the most convenient dose of 600 mg is a bilayered tablet, and one layer is blue. (The 1,200 mg has a green layer.) Second, the short-acting layer can cause an exacerbation of symptoms in patients that is substantially worse than the extended release. Fast-acting guaifenesin alone may initiate reversal too abruptly, especially in patients with unusual sensitivity to drugs. Such intensity is highly impacting on individuals with low pain thresholds. Since people absorb drugs at different rates, we usually begin with 300 mg tablets or capsules that work long enough for our purposes. We like to use preparations that work somewhat longer than a short-acting tablet, even though they may have a less determinate duration of action. We can thereby avoid the heavy assault of short-acting guaifenesin. With a less heavy hand, we begin at low dosages—300 mg twice a day—then increase later if we must according to our needs. Since the drug has no known toxicity, we have the luxury of moving slowly upward until we begin and sustain reversal.

Hold your beginning dosage for just one week. If you become distinctly worse, you've likely found your correct dose. Three hundred milligrams twice a day—the lowest dose we use—is sufficient for only 20 percent of patients, so don't worry if you don't notice any changes.

Please remember, nearly all of you will get recognizably worse when you take the dose that will start your reversal. If you're already tired, you may become exhausted; if you ache, you'll hurt more. Symptoms that were mild or barely noticeable may suddenly demand your attention. Briefly, symptoms reverse much faster than they set in, so you could sense some entirely new ones. You may experience what seem to be new symptoms, and the reason for that is rather simple. If these were not sufficiently bothersome, you may not have noticed them; when reversal makes them distinctly worse, you will.

If you're not worse during this first week, double your dose to 600 mg twice a day, for a daily total of 1,200 mg of longer-acting tablets or capsules. If this increased dosage proves effective, you'll notice an exacerbation of symptoms within three to ten days. Most readers will find this new amount sufficient: 80 percent of patients begin reversing at this level. You should hold here for a full month before further challenging yourself. Then, if you're unchanged, you're one of the less fortunate 20 percent

who need more guaifenesin, or you're blocking, or you're lucky
and don't hurt more while reversing. Raising your dose higher
with no increased symptoms should prompt you to reexamine all
your products and seek help from one of our online resources if
necessary to confirm that all your products are salicylate-free. A
symptom diary should tell you if are making progress. If you are a
lucky one who doesn't notice much in the way of increased complaints, raising your dose will do no harm and it will clear your
fibromyalgia faster. Since the drug has no known toxicity, we
have the luxury of moving progressively upward until we begin
to see sustained reversal.

Where do you go from there? If you're sure you're not blocking, raise the dosage to 1,800 mg per day. (That's Dr. St. Amand's
dosage: 600 mg in the morning and 1,200 at night. Claudia's is
higher.) You don't have to split the tablet or try to remember a
midday dose. You've now reached an amount that offers a 91 percent success rate. Some patients improve faster by adding short-
acting to the longer-acting medication—for instance, 200 mg,
400 mg, or 600 mg twice daily taken at the same time. If you
keep to 1,800 mg a day for another month and get neither worse
nor better days—suspect blocking. Because success rates are so
high at 1,800 mg, it's time for a thorough, repeat search. We ask
our patients to "bag their groceries" and bring us all their topicals
and supplements for staff inspection. We can offer faraway people
only the online support group to guide them through the maze.
In our office we have the luxury of individualizing dosages for
our slower responders.

If the anticipated worsening of symptoms doesn't appear and
the next map shows no change for the better, we again raise the
dosage, with two options. We could pump in an extra 600 mg to
1,800 mg of the more prolonged, gentler-acting tablets or capsules
as we offered in the previous paragraph. We could alternatively
add faster, short-acting guaifenesin. Short-acting is available in
most pharmacies as 200 or 400 mg tablets. When we attach such

to the daily dosage, we begin with 200 mg twice daily, to be taken with the longer-working product. If we still need more down the line, we can keep adding 200 mg in monthly increments up to patient tolerance or hold at any satisfactory level of map clearing.

The majority of people find their cycling dosage with relative

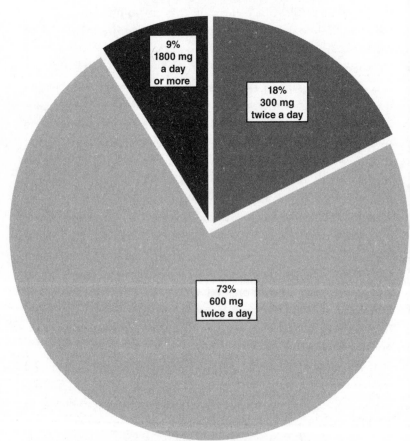

GUAIFENESIN DOSAGE TO INITIATE REVERSAL
(Extended-release formula only)

9%
1800 mg
a day
or more

18%
300 mg
twice a day

73%
600 mg
twice a day

Based on 6,000 consecutive patients

Figure 7.2

ease. They get worse and they get better. They forge ahead, whether slowly or quickly, and soon determine the direction of their recovery. By now you've guessed that it's not so simple for everyone. A small number of patients, possibly 5 percent, get barely perceptible symptomatic increase during treatment. They erroneously think they have to get hammered with pain when they reach healing levels. For those lucky people, it's not so. If mapping is not available, this group may unwittingly keep raising their dosages by unnecessary amounts in a quest for dramatic reversal symptoms. There's no real downside to this error (except expense), and those who push the dosage do get well at accelerated rates. We should also mention that a significant number of patients get better for a few days after beginning guaifenesin and start to cycle later than most. That's why we hold patients at specified dosages for a designated time. Until we find a blood test for fibromyalgia, mapping is the best method we have to determine patient status. We highly recommend that examination for anyone who can find talented hands. (See figure 7.2.)

REMAPPING WHILE ON GUAIFENESIN

Remapping is best done by the same person who did the initial exam using the same technique to ensure that an exact comparison can be made. Certain tissues clear fastest, and the lumps and bumps will disappear first in these areas. Even when considerable improvement has been achieved, remapping remains important because lesser remnants make percentage changes difficult to quantify. This especially applies to the delayed retreat of tendons and ligaments. Those structures have marginal blood supplies and only reluctantly release their accumulated debris. The trained mapper will detect subtleties that others could easily miss.

During our office revisits, we query our patients about their observations, good or bad. We remap them at every visit. We hide previous maps and refer to them only after completing the new one. This is the best and most objective procedure we can suggest to monitor activity. Lumps and bumps should get progressively smaller, softer, or more mobile. Larger lesions such as those at the hips, tops of shoulders, and shoulder blade areas may split into two or more smaller bumps. Once you're sure of dosages and reversal rates, you and your mapping professional should agree on the frequency of examinations—whatever scheduling makes you both comfortable.

Don't overlook an important fact: Until late in the reversal game, mapping adroitly detects blocking by some source of salicylate. New lesions are obvious on a deteriorating map. Blocked patients are finally alerted when they get sufficiently worse, something that mapping will sooner determine. The earlier people report setbacks, the quicker we can help recheck products or adjust dosages. We've effectively used our system for many years. Thanks to astute teacher-patients, we can identify most occult sources of salicylate. (Figure 7.3 shows maps of a patient before and after starting treatment.)

Patients usually ask how long they should continue taking guaifenesin. Once symptoms are gone, some are tempted to stop. There's a simple answer: The genetic defects that cause the illness are unchanged by medication, so stop the drug and symptoms will resume. Your symptoms won't reappear all at once or overnight, but come back they will! In time, a better medication will surely be discovered. But for now, rather dependably, the dosage that reversed you may be what you'll need into the distant future.

If you increased your medication just to speed up the reversal, lowering your intake to the originally effective dosage is proper. But if you try dropping too far, below your therapeutic level, brace yourself for the gradual return of your complaints. There's no harm experimenting if you want to, since the reversing amounts were not all that precisely measured. When you're well, you might be tempted to seek the least amount that will get you by. But remember this: If you take just one eighth of a tablet

These maps show results in a patient whose clearing dose is 600 mg of extended-release guaifenesin twice a day. The first figure shows her follow-up map after one month (note the absence of the thigh lesions). The second map shows her six-month follow-up.

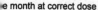
e month at correct dose

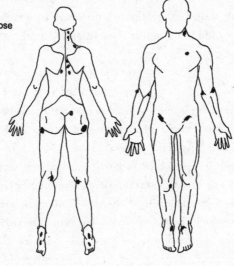

6 months

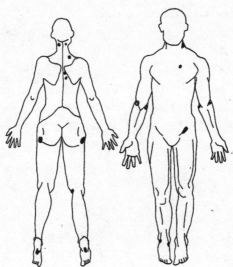

Figure 7.3

less than your fundamental requirements for the rest of your life, you'll eventually get worse. An ineffective amount is ineffective! Be scientifically inclined; remember that your body is your only laboratory, so remain alert and watch for the earliest clues that symptoms are resurfacing. There's no sense in letting the illness regain full ascendency when it is easily headed off by taking your proper dosage of guaifenesin.

> I remember when I first contemplated the protocol I panicked because there was no one qualified to map me near where I live. I couldn't see how I could possibly track my progress. However, as suggested I faithfully kept a journal. Some days I could succinctly write what kind of pain I felt, where it was, and how severe it was. However, I also had days, particularly during the first year, with some entries only containing the words "Today was horrible!" As time went on and I began to notice days when the pain was less, I began rereading my journal entries and could see that I really was making progress. It also gave me a sense of gratitude for the emerging new life I had been given.
>
> —*Laura S., Ohio*

PART II

DISTINGUISHING THE MANY FACES OF FIBROMYALGIA

Part 1 of this book provided a sweeping overview of fibromyalgia. We've given you some of the historical background and the experiences that led to our current treatment. We touched upon the medications we used in the early years, and explained how we found guaifenesin. We went through the details of the theory behind our approach, explained what we think goes wrong in fibromyalgia, and told you how you can fix it. We hope that in the process we gave you a solid explanation for your symptoms and validated the reason for all of your complaints.

Now we're going to delve into a little more detail. We want to focus on your symptoms, explore the causes, and give you some ideas about how to handle them. In the process, we will cluster them together to structure syndromes simply for convenience and easy reference. We're aware that this creates an artificial set of divisions and suggests a series of different diseases. Please don't be led astray. All you feel is related and fundamentally interconnected. We ask that you keep this in mind when reading through this part. We've also included quotes from other patients who've shared their experiences at various stages of reversal. As you'd expect, we've included mostly favorable statements, but believe us, they're the norm and not the exceptions.

I call fibromyalgia the "blind men and the elephant disease." In my case a cardiologist was unable to determine why I went through cycles of my heart skipping a beat when I was a young child. In high school, a gastroenterologist was clueless about my IBS. In college, another MD was perplexed when my big toe had serious pain. Later, a urologist was unable to find a reason for my frequent urinary tract infections. My ophthalmologist did not know why I got sudden onsets of jagged auras making it difficult to see. When I learned I had FMS and read *What Your Doctor May* Not *Tell You About Fibromyalgia*, I learned why I had all these symptoms and more. Dr. St. Amand put together all the pieces of this large, complicated puzzle and figured out how to get patients well. My hope is this new edition of the book will reach even more people suffering from the "blind men and the elephant disease," providing them with answers to get well, too.

—*Janet T., New Mexico*

CHAPTER 8

THE BRAIN SYMPTOMS

Chronic Fatigue and Fibrofog

I thought I was developing Alzheimer's at a young age due to the mental fogginess of fibro. I've never taken narcotics or any medication that affects mental function, but I once stopped at a red light as if it were a stop sign and proceeded through the intersection. People were honking, tires were squealing on the pavement, and my youngest daughter screamed at me that I was gonna get us killed. Luckily, we escaped this incident without injury or even a scratch to my SUV. She asked me why I did it and I honestly didn't have an answer. I had also experienced very short-lived disorientation. Once while driving, for a split second, I had no recollection of how I had gotten to where I was or why I was even behind the wheel driving. Once I identified familiar landmarks, I regained my memory of where I was going and why. It was such a scary experience, that I wondered if I should be driving at all.

—*Deb B., South Dakota*

The cerebral cycles of fibromyalgia entered medical literature somewhat late in the game. Descriptions of the older disease, fibrositis, made no mention of brain involvement. When this term was replaced with the name *fibromyalgia*, problems with gray matter were still overlooked in the official description of the illness. Fairly rapidly, however, academic researchers began connecting the physical pains and brain aberrations as facets of one disease. About that time, a few psychiatrists bravely took a defiant stance against their colleagues and flatly stated that the mental disturbances were not psychologically based. In 1996, when Devin Starlanyl wrote her landmark book, *Fibromyalgia and Chronic Myofascial Pain Syndrome: A Survival Manual*, she unhesitatingly described the toll the disease had taken on her energy and cognitive abilities. The term *fibrofog* was patient-invented and driven into descriptions of the disease by patient insistence.

The overall change in medical attitude was very refreshing for patients who had been repeatedly embarrassed by past it's-all-in-your-head verdicts. Yet it did nothing to help them understand the illness or to offer relief of symptoms. One author summed it up: "Fibromyalgia was often considered to be a manifestation of hysteria and was equated with psychogenic rheumatism in the 1950s and '60s. However, with recent controlled studies it became evident that patients with this syndrome had uniform, stable and reproducible symptoms and signs rather than the bizarre and changeable symptoms of hysteria."[1]

Dr. St. Amand saved my life. I was quite depressed as I previously was diagnosed with relapsing remitting multiple sclerosis three weeks before a hysterectomy (2015) that was already scheduled for endometriosis, in addition to interstitial cystitis, trigeminal neuralgia, and finally fibromyalgia. My pain level was at least an 8 on the 1–10 pain scale, 24/7. Nothing worked. No pain meds, CBD gels, physical therapy, nothing worked, much to my chagrin. I was missing four to five days of work a week due to the pain and fatigue and was using a cane. I was suicidal and tried to kill myself, but my body was so fatigued I couldn't even do that (thank God). I saw Dr. St. Amand and followed the treatments very strictly from the very first day. Only two weeks later I was off the cane, my pain level has dropped from 8 to 2 or 3, and I have loads of energy now. For the first time in years I have hope.

—*Kristen W., California*

CHRONIC FATIGUE SYNDROME—FIBROFATIGUE

When I got sick with pain all over my body I thought I had bone cancer. My aunt had died from it and I thought I'd developed it, too, even though I was almost forty years younger. I would wake multiple times during the night in excruciating pain and couldn't sit for more than an hour. Thankfully, I had a savvy internist who strongly doubted I had cancer, and after sitting in his office describing my medical issues, he told me he thought I had fibromyalgia.

I went home and started reading up on FMS, as I knew nothing about it. I amassed a collection of books that all said it was incurable, the cause was unknown. My savvy internist was very good at diagnosing FMS but was clueless about how to treat it.

After a number of serendipitous events, I met Dr. Flora Stay, the founder of the company Cleure. She gave me a copy of *What Your Doctor May* Not *Tell You About Fibromyalgia*, and halfway through the book I decided to become a patient of Dr. St. Amand and get well—what I read in that book made so much sense to me.

Each of us have different guaifenesin journeys. Some of us are much sicker than others and some of us have been very sick for a very long time. I feel very fortunate to have gotten on my guai journey much sooner than many others, and I was fortunate in that I felt better the first two months on the protocol, which made it possible to drive 850 miles by myself to our new home in New Mexico. So now I fly back to see Dr. St. Amand each year, and each year, one by one, all the oddball FMS symptoms have been going away. Some take longer than others but they all do go away.

—*Janet T., New Mexico*

Sixty years ago when I began working with the disease now named fibromyalgia, it was the fact that so many people had the same symptoms that convinced me there was a real disease waiting to be defined. Yet often enough to keep me on my toes, there was considerable individual variability. We speak in medicine of the "chief complaint," which is the single worst symptom that brings a patient to us. Many complained bitterly about the intense, widespread pain they were experiencing. Others launched into a series of descriptive words trying to make me grasp how severe was their continuous and numbing fatigue. Yet most of the time, there was that inexorable duet, both pain and exhaustion. In the end, it didn't much matter which of their complaints brought these people to my office; when I examined them, they all had the same widely scattered, easily palpable lumps and bumps in muscles, tendons, and ligaments. All I had to do was connect those physical findings together with the roster of symptoms patients provided to finally convince me this was a single, bad disease!

Table 8.1

Central Nervous System

	Male	Percentage Male	Female	Percentage Female
Number of Patients	835		4,601	
Fatigue	780	93	4,467	97
Irritability	698	84	4,049	88
Nervousness	571	68	3,509	76
Depression	633	76	3,880	84
Insomnia	665	80	4,075	88
Impaired Concentration	654	78	4,007	87
Impaired Memory	665	80	4,114	89
Anxiety	615	74	3,579	78

Medical literature is full of well-detailed studies defining both fibromyalgia and chronic fatigue syndrome. But now, most physicians believe they are the same illness. We've treated more than ten thousand patients in these categories, and we can assertively say that we've never seen a case of pure chronic fatigue syndrome. Notwithstanding the variations in history, body mapping reliably ties complaints to physical changes and amply satisfies the criteria of fibromyalgia. Fatigue is simply the dominant complaint of people with high pain thresholds. Carefully questioned, they relate the symptoms of irritable bowel, bladder or vulvar pain, and musculoskeletal complaints, however minor they may seem. The worst map we ever created was of a woman who swore she had no pain at all, only mild stiffness. Later she admitted that she'd had dental work and delivered babies without anesthesia. While most patients have a combination of hurting and fatigue, they can lie at opposite ends of the bell-shaped curve and experience very little else. Once we pulled one hundred random charts of our patients and found that fatigue beat out pain as the primary complaint by a narrow margin. More commonly we hear patients say that while they can deal with the pain most of the time, the symptoms of fatigue and fibrofog are more disturbing and disruptive to their lives.

Most patients suffer daytime drowsiness, which is accompanied by nocturnal sleeplessness and nonrestorative sleep. Even in healthy people, insomnia results in impaired mental function. Fibromyalgics may or may not get to sleep easily, but most of them wake frequently throughout the night. That's even more likely to happen during more intense pain cycles. There just aren't enough comfortable spots left on the mattress, so the brain orders an intermittent roll from side to side seeking a better position. Once woken by such exercise, how can one find a comfortable spot and get back to sleep? When these symptoms occur on sequential nights, patients are sorely tempted to increase their dosage of sleeping medications. Adding hangover effects to an already exhausted body and brain further hinders next-day mental clarity.

Sleep deprivation isn't the fundamental cause of fibromyalgia as it was once believed, but it certainly makes all other symptoms worse.

> As of yesterday, I have been following this protocol for twenty-one years. I wish that it had been around when I was younger. My children would've had the benefit of a real mother who would've had energy and no pain so we could've enjoyed activities PAIN-FREE!
>
> Before I began this protocol, my life consisted of sitting on a couch watching the world go by! I pretty much was not a participant other than saving my energy to work full-time as an RN in a stressful forty-plus-hour-a-week job. My weekends consisted of naps and just resting so I could go back to work on Monday.
>
> I'm more active today than I was before I began this endeavor! The list of things I have given up (and am glad I have done so) are: IBS, migraine headaches, insomnia, chronic pain, fatigue, mental fogginess, and I'm not nearly as clumsy as I used to be! If I didn't have arthritis in my hands and feet, I wouldn't have a pain in the world! Celecoxib manages the arthritis pain, and when needed, Thermacare wraps are also very helpful. Staying on the HG diet is also helpful, as sugar is extremely inflammatory and I can tell when I have consumed a dietary indiscretion.
>
> Hope you all have pain- and other fibrosymptom-free days in your very near future! Feeling normal is a strange thing when you are fully reversed as am I, but you'll get used to it—it's wonderful!
>
> —*Deb B., South Dakota*

The omnipresent fatigue of fibromyalgia is scary enough, but it becomes terrifying during flare-ups when concentration and memory vanish. Together they create the perfect profile of the early stages of Alzheimer's disease, and this causes many patients to panic. To say the least, it's a bit difficult to combat this trio, especially when you add to them irritability, nervousness, depression, apathy, and surges of anxiety. If you can indulge yourself with a nap, you can improve a bit, but an intended short doze might easily extend into lifelessness for several hours, which makes it even more difficult to sleep at night. Exhaustion puts you to sleep on the couch despite the blaring TV. Unfortunately, that wreaks further havoc with your internal clock. You almost hate going to bed early since you know you'll be just as tired in the morning and you'll face the pains of your nightly muscular thrashing.

The good news is that guaifenesin will reverse the fatigue and insomnia of fibromyalgia. They will yield to the same cyclic purging as the rest of your body. Eventually, fewer and fewer days of exhaustion will hound you; the positive rewards are startling. There will be energy to fit your lifestyle and enough left over for your social enjoyment. At first these will appear as isolated hours, half days, and then single days. A glimmer of hope of what lies ahead is enough to keep most people on the protocol. If you are like the rest of us, you will never forget your first energized day.

In the meantime, what can you do about the combination of fatigue and poor sleep patterns that plague fibromyalgics? So prevalent were these that, at one time, they were thought of as the malfunctions that induced the disease. There are pharmaceuticals to help you, of course, and those will be discussed later, in chapter 15. But the problem with this solution is that sleeping medications make you tired and diminish mental clarity. Should you use them every night? No, but you may have to anyhow. Are they acceptable occasionally when you absolutely need them? Yes. But that doesn't solve the every-night problem, and many people can't tolerate the side effects.

The first thing that helps sleep is exercise. Getting some during the day will ease stiffness, increase the right kind of fatigue, and even help clear your mind. Endorphin release will cause drowsy, pleasurable feelings, and exercise promotes that. So will pleasant thoughts and peaceful meditation, funny movies, or enjoyable activities. Do anything you can to relax your muscles and mind—mild stretching to beautiful music, for example, done early in the evening might help considerably.

Yoga's relaxing poses and stretches, as well as the calming breathing exercises that accompany them, may be helpful. In studies, patients with insomnia who did yoga daily for eight weeks were likely to fall asleep faster and increase the amount of time that they spent sleeping. Studies also found that a bout of moderate-intensity aerobic exercise (walking) reduced the time it took to fall asleep and increased the length of sleep on the days it was done. You don't have to spend a lot of time to reap the benefits; as little as ten minutes a day can make a difference. Early-morning and afternoon exercise may also help reset the sleep-wake cycle by raising body temperature slightly, then allowing it to drop and trigger sleepiness a few hours later. It can be especially helpful if you are able to exercise outdoors and let your body absorb natural sunlight during the daytime hours. Strenuous exercise (running or lifting weights) did not improve sleep. Don't expect immediate results, because it takes from four to twenty-four weeks of exercise for patients to fall asleep more quickly, sleep slightly longer, and experience better sleep quality than before they began exercising. As with everything, slow and steady is the key. You can find various internet resources if you search for topics like "stretches to help you sleep better." Remember that you can experiment with timing to see what works for you.

Comfortable mattresses, dark rooms, and fewer distractions are also helpful. Some people derive a great deal of help from sound machines at night. Noise can make the bedroom more peaceful.

FRUSTRATIONS OF FIBROFOG

These bad periods creep up. You think you're handling everything and then the pain starts to increase and suddenly you are in a panic...When the pain starts, I think I can still continue doing what I have been doing. What creeps up on me is the brain confusion. I get so frustrated trying to sort out the simplest things, until I give up and then I get depressed.

How do I handle it? Recognizing it for what it is comes first. Then I just have to let go of everything I don't have to do, and keep things very simple, rest a lot, baby myself. Get a massage, physical therapy, pool therapy for pain, or take whatever medications help.

It is interesting for me to watch this cycle towards depression and see how it is based on brain dysfunction and expectations. The mood swings go with the cycling, too...You can't expect too much of yourself when you don't feel well. Your brain is just trying to tell you that.

—*L. N., Massachusetts*

Physicians who treat fibromyalgia regularly hear, "I can stand pain, but I need a brain." Someone other than us aptly coined the term *fibrofog*. The term connotes a deep overcast that prevents brain-body interactions, and one in which phrases, thoughts, and words get lost. Equally disconcerting, it renders patients partially unresponsive to the rest of the world. So bad is short-term memory that it's not uncommon for patients to forget something while it's being told. Sense of place and direction are sadly disrupted. How many of us have lost the way home and suddenly found ourselves in a strange location? You forget what you're doing midtask or what you're saying midsentence. Reasoning and deduction may range from difficult to impossible; math becomes a challenge even with a calculator in hand. Patients read without seeing the words—and why bother anyhow if they can't absorb the material, follow a plot, or remember the characters? Words stumble out of the mouth in strange sequences as though letters were glued together. They're frequently misspelled or look that way even when correctly written. Patients attempt to use dictionaries for assistance, but during bad fibrofog, there's no conception of letter sequences or recall of the alphabet. Names are interchanged and children become each other; floor may become desk.

Put yourself in the shoes of family members who are forced to play hide-and-seek with various items. Where in blazes are the car keys? For that matter, where's the car? Where did you leave your purse or did you donate it to some charity? Are the groceries out there fermenting in the trunk? The corollary: Patients can't see what they're looking at directly. What's the point of looking for something when you know it won't be there? Patients forget to pay bills, honor appointments, and meet friends; some have even left their kids stranded at school waiting for the delinquent parental chauffeur. Inability to count on your own brain is demoralizing and doesn't do much for irritability, nervousness, anxiety, and sense of isolation. Go through just a few such experiences and you'll understand why we won't even bother to define *fibrofrustration*.

During brain cycles, it's common especially for female patients to experience oversensitivity to sounds, lights, odors, and other external stimuli. Women already have more highly tuned senses; now the intensity gets kicked up an octave. Ordinary TV sounds may cause severe discomfort; fluorescent lighting can be intolerable, and even expensive perfume can cause nausea. Not too surprisingly, the same factors may also induce headaches. Such symptom combinations have erroneously led some doctors to look for strange allergies or chemical sensitivities. Many patients go through extensive testing in an attempt to uncover unusual responses to the environment. Patients are quick to tell us, "It's not the chemical I touch; it's the odor that gets me." In our experience, as patients improve, these symptoms usually recede along with all of the other expressions of a totally upset metabolism.

It's up to you, the patient, to learn skills for coping with fibrofog. Understanding its nature and fundamental cause certainly helps anxiety and, in turn, fibrofrustration. With reversal, temporary cycles of cognitive impairment become more bearable. In the meantime, certain tricks soften the blow. They'll help erase the fear of forgetting important items when you well know you can't rely on your memory.

- Practice being methodical, so that it becomes second nature. Convince yourself to put things in the same place every time. For example, car keys should have their own peg by the door. If you work at always putting them there, eventually you'll do it automatically. Mailbox keys, glasses, unpaid bills, mail needing responses, shopping lists should all have special, designated places. No matter how exhausted you are, each time you have one of those things in hand, go to the predetermined site to hang or file it. If it takes just an extra minute, you can force yourself to do that no matter how exhausted or overstimulated you are.

- Post a big calendar in a prominent place—say, on your refrigerator. Write down every appointment the minute you make it. Every morning and every night, check what's written there. Do it at two specific times: just before you go to bed and when you have your breakfast. If you're afraid you'll forget something during the day, hang a note where you're sure to see it. You can also enter the information into your computer or smartphone and set it to notify you. Having it on a written calendar as well is important if you forget to charge your batteries or don't check your electronic gadgets regularly. Have your devices set to update, sync, and back up regularly without your command. Use the notification feature for important things that need to be done at a certain time.

- Make a daily or weekly list of what you have to do. Then train yourself to check it routinely several times a day. Do it on a small pad you can carry with you or on your phone. When you wake, scrutinize it carefully. Each time you complete a task, cross it off immediately—if you wait, you won't remember having done the chore. Never leave the house without checking that bunch of to-dos. Before you head out, make sure you have a list of which errands you have in mind. Don't trust yourself with the master list— you'll surely misplace it.

- If you use a landline, keep a pad and a pen near the phone and leave them there. Don't walk off with them. When you take a message, write it down right now! When the fog is exceptionally bad, cradle the phone (poor neck!) and make notes as you're talking. If things are really bad, scribble the name of the person to whom you're speaking. Keep notes concise and meaningful enough so that you'll actually grasp what you were trying to recall.

- Post notes somewhere and everywhere. Even if you carry a tablet or smartphone, it will only help you if you're looking at it. We've heard of people who hang notes reminding them to turn off lights, lock doors, water plants, remember shopping items, and even to pick up their kids at school! Make sure you carry a copy of children's schedules, including when they need to be at extracurricular activities. Buy one of those small clipboards that attach to dashboards so that you can write memos when sitting in your car (but not while driving) without having to fumble for your phone. There are many calendar programs for computers and smartphones that will drop in the appointments and obligations of all your family members. Though it may take an extra minute or two to enter them when they are being made, add this to your list of things that take under a minute to accomplish and don't postpone it.

- Make lists to take to appointments. When meeting with a teacher, boss, repairman, or client, prepare notes of pertinent topics. Prior to a doctor's appointment, itemize your questions and concerns before you leave home. We usually allocate enough time per patient, but we get frustrated when we try to walk out of the examining room and get stopped a few times with an "Oh, Doctor, I forgot..." Jot down pithy phrases to remind you of the answers you've just been given. Do the same for meetings at your children's schools or when making dates with family and friends. When discussing business matters, such as with your insurance company, get the name of the person with whom you spoke. These rituals might save you embarrassing repeat phoning and the frustration of trying to find the right person to refresh your faulty memory.

• When you're suffering from intense fibrofog, limit your driving. At the most, run one errand at a time and save the more complicated tasks for a better day. Turn off the radio while driving and concentrate on the bigger task at hand. It's not polite, but apologize in advance and ask your children or other passengers to keep as quiet as possible. If noisy children confuse or distract you, pull over and firmly review your current status. If necessary, you can use your phone or navigation program to find a park or open space where everyone can take a break. It's easy to miss a freeway exit, so use local roads for shorter excursions. Navigation programs on phones or in cars can be a lifesaver when running errands. Take that extra moment before you leave home to enter your destinations. Most will even put them into a logical order for you. And if you get lost despite using one, just find a safe place to pull over and wait until your program finds you. Be patient with yourself and don't perform complicated maneuvers like U-turns on busy streets; your program will find and redirect you. Another very important point about driving is to always have at least half a tank of gas. If you don't have that when you leave home, stop as soon as possible and fill up. This can greatly reduce your stress if you get lost or stuck in traffic. These small steps are not time wasters; they can amount to lifesavers if you adhere to them.

- At home and at work when you are in a flare, decrease sensory inputs as much as possible. Many patients find they absolutely can't function well with even minor distractions. For good, fibromyalgic reasons, they lose the ability to tune them out or relegate them to the background. Turn off music while you're working. During bad cycles, even soothing sounds can put you into overload after a while. Close the door to filter outside noise from a room where you're working: It's a small luxury to concentrate in silence. Sound-muffling earphones can help if you need to work in a crowded area, but if those are inappropriate you can purchase small wax plugs that you shape to fit in your ears. These will muffle sounds but you will still be able to hear people speak to you.

- Start working on projects early. Some take you longer than normal to perform. Don't fight it. On adverse days, your ability to absorb information has gone to La-La Land. If the task seems insurmountable at the moment, give it up and try later. Move to the next task on your list and return to the one in question when you are up to it. Sometimes you'll have no alternative but to take a break and dry that clammy little sweat that signals frustration.

MOOD SWINGS (FIBROFLUX)

There are days like today when I feel as if my ears could explode. Every single noise is so intensified. I have to walk around with either ear plugs or fingers in my ears. My husband just does not get it. It takes every bit of energy I have to go about the day without going into a nervous breakdown.

—*Tracy, Washington*

Some horrifying facets of brain cycling are the sweeping mood swings. For the most part, patients are acutely aware of them but feel powerless to exercise control. Anger, frustration, fear, depression, and self-pity can attack with great intensity then disappear in a matter of minutes. Unfortunately, their negative effects linger. How do you retract some of the horrible things you've just said? How will your spouse, friends, or family members retract what they said in response? Female patients often cry buckets with minimal upsets; both sexes can become uncontrollably angry at the slightest provocation.

Try to recognize what your seesawing moods are like during times when the teeter-totter is level. During an outburst, you may grasp how irrational you're being, but you're neither able to stop nor admit how wrong you are. On a calmer day, chat with your partner and children. Tell them you're sorry for your outbursts and beg them to ignore the past and, unfortunately, any future displays. As a modest excuse, remind them that you're sick and your brain is involved in the illness. Stress that you're firming up a plan for getting well. Not a bad idea to affirm the same message to everyone else in your life. So confess your past and pre-regret your future.

Pause when you start feeling super emotional. Try meditation plus warm showers or baths: Both can soothe your daily stresses. Imbue yourself with the old strategy of counting to ten before reacting; take a walk. Sneaking away from a problem before it fully surfaces isn't always feasible, but practice the technique and it might save you confrontations. When you know the situation is getting out of hand, say to your inner self, "I'll stop now and deal with this later." You'll calm down.

Recognize that cognitive impairment and emotional overreaction are abnormal normals of fibromyalgia. They're experienced to some degree by all who suffer its ravages. It's okay to be patient and understanding of self, but not altogether forgiving. You must acknowledge and try to be better when you apologize for your angry outbursts and overreactions to minor provocations. You know why those happen, but it's not always apparent to the person at whom you directed your dragon fire. Laugh when your fibrofog causes you to do something slapstick. Laughter is therapeutic and closes the gap between people. Try to feel your triggers and turn away from them. You can tell others that you need some time and space before you revisit the situation because you feel like you are losing control.

Six years ago I battled breast cancer, and just when I thought things would get better, fibromyalgia reared its ugly head. I had headaches all the time, and when I walked I felt like a hundred-year-old woman who could barely shuffle from one place to another. I hurt all the time and my body was weak from muscle fatigue. I got to the point that I needed help dressing myself. I spent my days on the couch just trying to find a semi-comfortable position.

I tried physical therapy, but that made things worse. I tried a chiropractor, but as soon as he put things where they should be, my tight muscles would pull them out of alignment again.

I spent a year trying to find some kind of relief. I was put on Cymbalta, Gabapentin, and Tramadol to help control the pain, and even that didn't seem enough at times. Then I was introduced to the guaifenesin protocol.

Fast-forward to today. I have been on the protocol now for three and a half years and I have my life back. I am off all the previous medicines. I'm active and in warm weather would hardly know I have fibromyalgia. I marvel when I go back and read my journal. What a difference there is! I have noticed more cycling this winter, but it's more of a fatigue with mild headache. It doesn't stop me. Just a couple of weeks ago I went cross-country skiing. I was tired afterward (I'm nearly sixty-seven), but had no ill effects from using all that energy.

I guess I'm here to say, I believe the protocol has given me a new lease on life. It is not easy to begin with, but perseverance yields great blessings. The Protocol is SO WORTH IT! If you have fears that may put you off from starting the protocol, let us help "hold your hand" through it. There really is a silver lining to those dark clouds around you.

—*Laura S., Iowa*

CHAPTER 9

MUSCULOSKELETAL SYNDROME

Pain, fatigue, brain fog, never knowing if you will feel well enough to be included in family gatherings or if you will end up on the couch or in bed because that is all you can manage, are issues all of us with FMS deal with. Then we hear about a protocol that promises to give us a new life. The hardest parts are (1) accepting that this is not a quick fix and (2) learning how to be patient with the protocol and ourselves. Just because you're not feeling lots better after three months or perhaps even after a year doesn't mean the protocol is not working. Have faith in the protocol, have faith in your ability to cope with your symptoms, have faith in what you record in your journal. Faith is moving forward with something even though you cannot see immediate results. The protocol does work for those willing to be patient and have faith.

—*Laura S., Ohio*

Muscles, tendons, and ligaments combine to keep us erect as bipeds, motor us to our destinations, and not least of all, help us raise food, prepare it, and carry it to our tables. They're also involved in the digestion and elimination of nutrients, and even play a role in reproduction. They're the largest structures of the body and outweigh the skeleton. They're constantly supporting, pulling, yanking—and in fibromyalgia they hurt! Muscles and their cohorts, tendons and ligaments, are dedicated to physical work. They never get the downtime and the relative rest enjoyed by bladders, stomachs, and fingernails. These hardest-working tissues are often first to be affected by fibromyalgia.

Table 9.1

Musculoskeletal System

	Male	Percentage Male	Female	Percentage Female
Number of Patients	835	20	4,601	80
Numbness	600	72	3,688	80
Restless Legs	516	62	3,044	66
Leg Cramps	481	58	3,253	88
Pain	827	99	4,526	98
Growing Pains	357	43	2,090	45

All muscles are not the same. They have somewhat different physiology and are affected differently by fibromyalgia. There are two fundamental types of muscle fiber (along with some subgroups that we'll ignore for the purpose of this discussion). Most animals, including humans, have red (type I) and white (type II) meat. The red strands are particularly germane to our discussion since they're the ones most involved in fibromyalgia. Fiber distribution on the left side of the body is different from the right. The same muscle on the alternate side may have more type I or type II. The differences in composition alter function, which is why aches and pains can differ so greatly from person to person.

In this discussion, we'll largely ignore white meat. Its fibers are designed for speed and short-lived action. They don't have sufficient energy for a long haul, but they're great for sprints. Fibromyalgia barely glances at them and brushes them with only a light stroke: It fixates on far better prospects. Red meat is that color because it has a much richer blood supply. It contains far more mitochondria since red needs to make energy for sustained action. As you'll recall, these little powerhouses convert food-stuff to energy, the protein ATP. Type I fibers are hardworking muscle components with many functions that ensure survival. They are literally our strongest supporters, the hold-you-up and balance muscles. Workaholics, they turn us from side to side and shuffle our arms and legs from uncomfortable to comfortable positions all night long.

Aerobic workouts, running, and distance walking actually develop red fibers. Anaerobic, resistance exercises such as weight lifting produce mainly white fibers. You can see why pain and fatigue are so prominent in fibromyalgia. It's a disease with red overtones, right smack in the heart of our most productive energy factories. Selected muscles are the first to suffer from ATP deficiencies and, for safety reasons, remain in a partially contracted state. Calcium promotes this sort of hibernation because it can't escape from the site where it was assigned to duty. It just goads muscles into continuous working. We've surely got a problem with pump failure—it's not performing its ejection function that should limit residual metabolic debris to an acceptable level. Guess the problem? Fibromyalgics just don't have enough energy (ATP) to work the pumps.

We've already given you an extensive outline depicting what percentage of the time any given muscle, left or right, was involved at the time we see an untreated patient. We extracted data from body maps of two hundred adult females. Our compilation was averaged by including recent-onset as well as advanced patients to produce a midcourse look at fibromyalgia. When we applied the same technique to the children's group, our findings on the 187 maps was truly revealing: We had a few two-year-olds, with the rest scattered up to our cutoff age, sixteen. We learned not only which muscles would be first affected at discovery, but also the pecking order of sequential involvement. That was of great help in transposing expectations for what we should always palpate in adults.

The left side of the neck, tops of shoulders, and intershoulder blade muscles are swollen in 96 percent of the kids; 84 percent on the right. Better still, the inside and outside elbows had bumps in all the children we examined, 100 percent of the time. Those are good areas to begin a search for fibromyalgic changes in the youngest patients. They're where muscles attach (called entheses), and will be present in kids without many other defective sites. The older they get, the more muscles, tendons, and ligaments will develop swollen segments.

There are lots of other places where adults display their fibro-myalgia. The most rewarding diagnostic muscle group in anyone past age fifteen or sixteen is the left thigh, the quadriceps muscle. It's involved in 100 percent of adults on both the front and the outside. The lateral part, the vastus lateralis, is distinctly tender even using only moderate digital pressure. The less sensitive front of the thigh, the rectus femoris, is also affected. It's not a long-structured smooth band like the outer thigh, but is made up of sequential, separate bundles. Since the left quadriceps is always involved, it should be considered the hallmark, present in all untreated adult patients. It's not only diagnostic of fibromyalgia, but better yet, it totally clears within a month on the correct dose of guaifenesin.

The next logical question would be if a would-be mapper could ignore checking anywhere but at the muscles we've just delineated. That is a tempting shortcut, but since under treatment the thigh clears within a month, what's left for follow-up exams? The answer is simple: More extensive mapping is required to continue to document progress. The more thorough the initial examination, the more tissue will be available for future monitoring.

Sequential mapping can then assure ongoing recovery as lumps keep vanishing in concert with patient symptoms.

We can't ignore the body's many ropy connectors. There are two main types. Tendons blend with partner muscles and hook on to bones at the other end. Ligaments, on the other hand, connect bone to bone. These widely distributed structures are deeply involved in fibromyalgia. They're responsible for causing most of the pains. We urge examiners to roll their fingers over these cord-like structures and feel for unusual hardness and, particularly, for swollen segments. Patients respond during this search by expressing considerable tenderness, so it needs to be done gently but with uniform pressure. Rolling them gently rather than poking at them will make the examination less painful.

Let's point out just a few places where those members of the musculoskeletal system are usually ignored or misdiagnosed. Pain from the deltoid tendon on the outside of the shoulder, most often the right, is sometimes attributed to the rotator cuff. Inguinal ligaments connect the front part of the hip bone to the pubic bone. They're actually formed from the abdominal muscles that curl under themselves to make the cordlike structure we can palpate. The outer portion is almost always swollen, especially in women. It produces pain at anchorage across the lowest part of the abdomen by constantly pulling and irritating where it splays like Saran Wrap across the pubic bone. If doctors fail to put their hands on that ligament and examine it for swelling, they'll erroneously suspect ovarian or bladder problems. The peroneus muscle is on the outside of the lower leg; it begins at the outer knee and goes all the way to the foot. It curls around the ankle and joins another muscle to create a tendon that hooks onto the top of the arch. The right one is much more affected by fibromyalgia than the left. They may both visibly swell just below the outer anklebone and suggest water retention. The sole of the foot is more commonly involved than not. Invariably, doctors say the pain is due to "plantar fasciitis" when it's actually due to a swollen tendon. *Itis* implies inflammation: There isn't any in fibromyalgia. Structural abnormalities and swellings described in this paragraph are easily palpated with just a bit of practice. Simple hands-on efforts can quickly expose the cause of the pain at such locations and save a lot of anguish and investigative costs.

Patients often ask us to guess how long it will take for their maps to clear. I usually reply, "I don't know," because there are often very deep deposits that will only surface late in the game. But in general we can approximate a certain order of clearing, which can help to identify where a patient is on the time line. For example, fast clearing are the lumps and bumps in the thighs. We've mentioned how we can determine the diagnosis since they're always present; and the dosage since they disappear within a month of finding the proper guaifenesin dosage. Midspeed for clearing are the areas between the shoulder blades, top of the shoulders, right side of the neck, and the left lowermost back. Last to leave are the inside and outer elbows, back of the hips, left side of neck, and groin ligaments. The first in are apparently the deepest and hardest to clear out.

FIBROMYALGIA AND OSTEOARTHRITIS

Seven years ago I barely functioned. I went to work, stopped to pick up fast food on the way home, and went to bed. I called my home my fibro-home because I let everything go. It was a disaster. I missed paying bills and could not clean up the clutter, which kept getting worse. I lost friends because I kept canceling activities. Now I feel twenty years younger than when I started this journey. Much of my medical problems were predicted by Dr. St. Amand in his book. I don't feel any fibro issues, but I do have severe arthritis. So it is better to get on this journey sooner, rather than later. I feel well enough to now begin attacking my weight—to cut the blood pressure and cholesterol issues. This will also dramatically help my arthritis.

—*Gail H., Illinois*

In our minds, fibromyalgia is only the beginning of a long, miserable progression that ultimately leads to osteoarthritis. This isn't the kind that causes crippling deformities, though it can gnarl joints a bit and cause enough damage to require knee, hip, or other joint replacement. Most people accept aches and stiffness as a normal part of growing older, so osteoarthritis is considered "wear-and-tear arthritis" and natural for the elderly. Don't you believe it!

You recall we tease a lot of history out of patients on our first meeting. We ask if their parents and grandparents had similar fibromyalgic symptoms or arthritis. We don't ask about rheumatoid arthritis (RA), which is a different disease, caused by an autoimmune reaction, or the kind of arthritis that is the result of a severe injury or accident and present only in that localized area. If we're lucky, some of those family members accompany the patient and speak for themselves. As we check off answers on our long symptom list, we often see older relatives nod as if they were being quizzed. Most of the time they eventually verbalize and suddenly explode with, "And now I've got osteoarthritis" (*osteo* is from *os*, the Latin word for "bone"). They describe X-ray findings that show spurs and degenerative bone changes that confirm their diagnosis. It's quite striking how the body manages to avoid damage to essential organs. In fibromyalgia, there's no increased cell death, muscular wasting (atrophy), or nerve damage. Kidneys perform smoothly and, with the exception of a small amount of phosphates, excrete the body's waste as they should. The liver remains completely functional and the heart pumps just fine at metronome pace. The brain thinks, remembers, and still directs traffic, although some cognitive function may be erratic in the presence of fibrofog. Cuts still heal, and the immune system remains capable of fighting disease, though perhaps a little reluctantly. Not so with the joints. The prevailing medical opinion holds that fibromyalgia is a nonarticular (nonjoint) disease, but we strongly differ. They're frequently involved early in the disease, but it takes years before damage is perceptible to a radiologist on an X-ray.

As fibromyalgia progresses, something has to give. If I were a body, here's how I'd think: *I'm getting punished with less energy and I've got to give up some less crucial functions. I sense the rising levels of phosphate. It's safer to load muscles with metabolic debris than it is to let it circulate uncontested in the bloodstream or end up in vital tissues.* It makes sense that stacking the junk into expendable structures can preserve activity in essential areas. We have ample data to underscore that protective stance by the body.

Despite how badly you feel, you've been reassured that no damage has been discovered in any organs or tissues. That's not quite true if we accept that over the years, improperly treated fibromyalgia evolves into osteoarthritis. You've probably suspected that a body so riddled with symptoms would eventually show something amiss if we knew where to look, and this is now evident.

In previous editions we stated there was no nerve damage. Wrong! Multiple scientific papers have now refuted that. Superficial, small nerve fibers are sickly. Those little filaments are analogous in appearance to the tiniest rootlets of a weed you just pulled out of your garden. However, they're not remotely close to being that big. These small fibers can only be extracted by skin biopsy and only visualized under the microscope. Reports have shown too few such fibers in thighs, calves, and lower legs in about 50 percent of fibromyalgic people. That's true for skin most remote from the trunk, but not so from samples closer to the pelvis. Using a special instrument, the confocal microscope, the cornea can be studied without biopsy. Those same dainty fibers are thinner in fibromyalgia, and there are far less of them.

Some papers have alluded to the fact that some of those hair-like nerves regenerate. I suspect that is so in fibromyalgia. Most of you have had strange rashes and sensations of hot, cold, itchy, numb, crawly, and itchy places on the skin. The disease must affect some of your small nerve fibers to produce those abnormalities. Since those symptoms eventually disappear, new nerves must grow back. We know the body is capable of healing these tiniest members of the nerve family because they routinely resuscitate after dying off from a cut or burn.

From birth, bones accept as much phosphate as their periodic growth status allows. Once they refuse more, tendons and ligaments are the next safest place to stash what the body can't use. Even with a little excess mineral, they still perform reasonably well because they're only called upon to perform short contractions. Muscles are next in the reception line and finally become receptacles in turn. These structures eventually and collectively flash messages to the brain, signaling their problem making energy. But the central nervous system can't help, and in turn it, too, capitulates: Energy, fatigue, and cognition line up. Now most patients seek professional help.

Fibromyalgia is a jerky process in affected tissues before they totally succumb. The system remains somewhat fluid, and there are better periods initially but serial failures progressively sap the tissues. Energy comes only in spurts, and in emergencies some tissues can steal it from others. At the beginning, when 25, 50, or 75 percent of the body may also be struggling, rest or minimal-load exercise improves these percentages, but it's eventually a losing proposition.

Collectively, fibromyalgic muscles and bones, the largest structures in the body, accept much more than fair shares of the circulating phosphates. Finally, generalized exhaustion forces the body to find new reservoirs for the accumulating debris. Joints are attacked and will become the ultimate repositories for calcium, phosphate, and other metabolic debris that has not been excreted by normal channels. Joints have an inexhaustible capacity and, once pressed into full service, will continue to accept deposits the rest of the fibromyalgic's life. Tartar-like crystals actually form, whereas in other tissues calcium and phosphate almost always remain in solution. Even one of these crystals contains an inordinate amount of calcium phosphate compared with the minuscule bit that disturbs metabolism in mobile cells. Fluid pulled from osteoarthritic joints consistently shows under microscopic examination every known shape of calcium phosphate crystal. Such microscopic rocks abrade and irritate cartilage, ultimately leading to bony overgrowth, spurs, erosions, and irreparable destruction. Sadly, that's permanent damage that cannot be reversed by guaifenesin. We make this a compelling argument for early diagnosis and treatment.

The body waits a very long time before resorting to this drastic solution. This scenario concludes a long-fought and gallant attempt at damage control. Because joints have such a huge capacity for accepting the offending ions, essential organs such as the heart, brain, kidneys, and liver are forever spared damage from fibromyalgia. Viewing the progression of our illness in this light, feel blessed that joints are so responsive. It's a good solution for a bad condition and allows you to stay alive, the body's first priority. Osteoarthritis may be uncomfortable and ultimately disabling, but takes years to surface. By that time, nature assumes we'll have procreated, raised our young to maturity, and are fully expendable in a biological sense.

Our protocol doesn't offer relief from osteoarthritis other than prevention before it occurs. It does clear tissues that constantly pull on or in joint surfaces. Damage begins with the first microscopic crystals that start the abrasion, but it takes time to be visible on X-rays. Patients relate joint complaints for a number of years before this validation appears. Anti-inflammatory and pain medications are the choices until sufficient damage leads to the operating table and joint replacement.

Many medications are given for muscle pain: Analgesics, muscle relaxants, nonsteroidal anti-inflammatories (NSAIDs), antidepressants, and anticonvulsants are the most offered. Heat and ice are local modalities that may help, the choice determined by which works best for the individual. Unfortunately, many muscle creams (Tiger Balm, Bengay, Icy Hot) contain salicylates, but lidocaine patches and gels do not. Topical anti-inflammatories such as Voltaren gel also do not and are easier on the stomach. The little heat pads that can be applied over painful areas won't block. Gently performed massage and other bodywork can make symptoms manageable. Acupuncture and acupressure offer relief for some. Used in tandem, various modalities blend to mutual benefit. Less reliance on medications avoids escalations in dosages and side effects.

Fibromyalgics have to be prodded into following the one piece of advice consistently given by experts: exercise. It's inexpensive, it has no enduring side effects, it never fails to show benefits, and even a little bit helps. Even the gentlest type such as stretching can temporarily soothe muscles, tendons, and ligaments. Sustained aerobics, however light, quickens the rebuilding pace for mitochondria, the ATP-making power stations we've already discussed. Increased energy production introduces stamina to push ahead even faster. For those with arthritis or severe back pain, water aerobics provide a good reintroduction to exertion. It's buoyant and combines some of the cardiovascular benefits of walking with those of resistance training initiated to overcome the water pressure. Exercise stimulates production of our natural pain-relieving compounds, endorphins, and their receptors.

We think the disease first appears because of faulty ATP production and greatly worsens by being sedentary. Inactivity causes the destruction of mitochondria. The body stops feeding what it doesn't use, and these power stations are closed down. This process can be reversed by slowly beginning any exercise program. Programs developed to begin workouts are readily available on the internet—some for sale and some free. In the beginning you can sneak them in when you're sure of your energy-limited schedule. Don't demand instant results. Over time, confidence, strength, and energy recharge their own batteries. Deconditioning is the price of inactivity, and there's no time like the present to reverse that.

There were days that at times turned into a week, when I was cycling so hard I couldn't exercise. Instead of feeling guilty, I gave myself a break. Dr. St. Amand says that after two weeks of no exercise, you pretty much lose what you've accomplished to that point. So I would discipline myself to do something as soon as I could. Many times I had to start over with very light exercise and build up to where I was before the hard cycling began. The secret is not comparing ourselves to the normal people around us that are exercising. Just do it no matter how insignificant it seems. Be patient. You will eventually see results. I have, and it's great!

—*Carol H., Texas*

CHAPTER 10

THE IRRITABLE BOWEL SYNDROME

I was never diagnosed with IBS until we arrived at the FMS [fibromyalgia syndrome] and HG [hypoglycemia] diagnosis. Everything was a mystery. I had been plagued all my life with inexplicable stomach and intestinal pains, gas, and bloating, alternating diarrhea and constipation. The most common medical advice was to "relax" and take antacids. I have been on the hypoglycemia diet, alternating between strict and liberal versions, for almost a year. It only took a month for my IBS symptoms to improve once I knew how to diet properly.

—*Gwen, California*

Some fibromyalgics are overwhelmed by their uncomfortable bowel symptoms. Their other problems seem relatively minor annoyances by comparison. This initiates a quest for answers and relief, mostly self-driven. Statistics show that the overwhelming majority of patients with gastrointestinal symptoms never see physicians for that particular issue. Those who tabulate such things write that only about 30 percent of people with IBS even seek medical help because it is embarrassing; most prefer to search the internet for ways to control their symptoms.

When a patient does visit a physician to complain of persistent aching or abdominal pain, constipation or diarrhea, gas, and/or bloating, the primary physician usually does a basic manual examination followed by some blood tests. Physicians understandably have a bit of difficulty in assessing problems deeply hidden within the abdomen unless they're given sufficient patient history and testing yields some abnormalities. For example, pain in the pit of the stomach and sour belching will result in a test for the ulcer-causing bacterium, *Helicobacter pylori*. Excess gas, nausea, diarrhea, cramps, or constipation lead to different evaluations. If these results are negative, then further testing will follow using ultrasound and X-ray. Nothing abnormal? Off goes the patient to a gastroenterologist. This specialist reviews the lab reports and other findings and confirms everything is functionally normal. Other tests might eliminate the likelihood of celiac disease. Symptoms persist, forcing the specialist to do more investigations. That segues into an endoscopy of the esophagus, stomach, and upper part of the small intestine followed by a colonoscopy to visually examine the colon. The tested subject now has a complete, certified list of normal results. It's good to have this, of course, but the lingering question, "What's really wrong?" remains unanswered. The expert's conclusion is finally, "You've got irritable bowel syndrome"—a chronic condition of the lower gastrointestinal tract. The patient will be reassured that it does not lead to more serious disease or shorten the life span; it's not inflammatory or infectious; and it does not lead to colitis or cancer.

So where does this leave you, the patient? As comforting as it is to have a name tagged onto your symptoms, and the reassurance that they aren't deadly, the next step isn't exactly clear. The usual suggested solutions are to "eat more fiber; take stool softeners; use prescription or over-the-counter medications to reduce gas, diarrhea, and cramping." This might offer some temporary relief, but it is only temporary and it's labor-intensive.

IBS is one of the overlapping FMS and HG symptoms. I don't think it pays to debate whether it's from FMS alone or HG alone. Where does that get you? And what if you're wrong? If you just do the HG diet perfectly for a couple of weeks, and it helps, that answers your question. If you do the diet perfectly and there is no difference, then it could be just FMS, or it could be a side effect of a medication you're taking.

—*Anne Louise, Minnesota*

Ultrasound—High-frequency sound waves are passed by a transducer through the area of the body to be studied, to make an image of solid organs such as the liver. These waves cannot pass through bones or make images of gas.

Endoscopy—A procedure that is done with a fiber-optic instrument, enabling direct visual examination. A long, narrow tube is inserted through the mouth, down the back of the throat into the esophagus, down into the stomach, and into the duodenum, the first part of the small intestine.

Colonoscopy—Colon probing with a similar but longer endoscope (colonoscope) inserted rectally and passed upward. The doctor then withdraws it slowly, as each part of the intestine and rectum is examined. This procedure is usually done in the doctor's office or hospital "GI lab" with the patient mildly sedated. If only the lower portion of the colon is to be examined, a shorter instrument is used for a sigmoidoscopy.

Table 10.1

Irritable Bowel Syndrome

	Male	Percentage Male	Female	Percentage Female
Number of Patients	835		4,601	
Nausea	331	40	2,723	59
Excess Gas	528	63	3,166	69
Bloating	484	58	3,391	59
Constipation	379	45	2,938	64
Diarrhea	370	44	2,521	55

Over the years, many names have been used to describe IBS, including *spastic colon*, *mucous colitis*, *nervous bowel*, *toxic gut*, *leaky bowel syndrome*, and *functional bowel disease*. We consider them all synonyms for the same condition. Most of those are inaccurate attempts at designating a cause for symptoms. For example, the term *colitis* means "inflammation of the colon." There's rarely inflammation in IBS although there is irritation. As in the rest of the body, nothing is biochemically or anatomically abnormal enough to provide diagnostic proof of disease. There's much upset, but no damage and no biochemical markers to lean back on.

As in all facets of fibromyalgia, women are affected by IBS in greater numbers than men. Expectedly, like other symptoms of the disease, intestinal complaints are usually worse premenstrually. Its clustered symptoms begin at any age, very often in children and young adults, where they may appear dramatically as the first symptoms of the disease. Adults often recall recurring bouts during early school years.

Since my teenage years I have had stomach pain and cramping...
My general practitioner would say it was "a little gastritis." He

would prescribe an antacid and send me home with a pat on the back. I suffered like this for about ten or twelve years...I went to a very eminent gastroenterologist...He pronounced "irritable bowel syndrome." When I asked him what I could do for it, he said, "Nothing. Just stay away from green vegetables."...I also experienced insomnia and some muscle pain since I was a teen. I had no idea they were all related to FMS. A few years ago, the FMS came on with a vengeance, and after seeking a diagnosis for about nine months, I finally found a doctor who told me I have FMS with gastroesophageal reflux.

—Marie, Nevada

Sixty percent of the fibromyalgics we've seen have some form of IBS. Bear in mind that the complex has many symptoms and not all patients get all of them. Some complain of intermittent difficulty in swallowing, and acid might reflux back up the esophagus from the stomach. That's so-called heartburn, the burning sensation named *gastroesophageal reflux disease*, or *GERD*. Irritation may cause esophageal spasms and produce chest pain closely mimicking angina or a heart attack. It's more common in overweight patients and often occurs at night when patients are lying prone. Waves of nausea sometimes appear out of nowhere and can last for hours or for only a few minutes, often in staccato, repetitive waves. Constipation and diarrhea can cycle on a daily basis or each can last for long periods. Nausea, gas, and bloating are disconcerting enough, but constipation and diarrhea are more alarming. Like uncontrolled traffic signals, they switch from stop to go in cycles that interfere with digestion as well as elimination. Confronted with IBS symptoms, certain doctors will order a battery of expensive blood allergy tests and find "multiple food sensitivities." These assessments may be correct, but patients often tell us they have no problem with eating foods they have been told they are sensitive to. If you inform the testing physician of this you will be instructed to do a food challenge test. Only about 2 percent of subjects who do a food challenge test in a medical setting have an actual strong allergic reaction, and 86 percent have no reaction at all. This demonstrates the large gap between skin testing and what actually bothers patients. We suggest a cheaper and far more accurate test by simply sequentially eating a tiny amount of one food at a time; in this way your own gastrointestinal tract becomes the diagnostician. If sensitivity truly exists, symptoms should get decidedly worse, and then you know to stop eating the irritating food. This is the true proof of sensitivity, because too often sensitive skin simply overreacts to an injected foreign protein.

Constipation and diarrhea can take turns in rapid shifts. It's not unusual to have one problem for months or years, and then suffer from its inverse. Those who suffer from recurrent diarrhea may undergo stool testing for candida (yeast) or parasites. Unfortunately there are over three million websites with purported tests and treatments for yeast and parasites and many alternative practitioners or friends who swear by them. Unfortunately the bulk of the sites are selling unapproved tests or dodgy treatments for things that do not exist. Stool examinations are not for novice technicians. It takes a well-practiced eye to avoid being duped into thinking food residues and mucus are cysts or parasites. Cultures are frequent sources of error since yeast is normal in stool specimens. Actual reputable scientific testing turns up ova and/or parasites in only 0 to 2 percent of those tested.

Many people cling to these "test results" and only with great difficulty can they be dissuaded from using medicinal herbs in order to try guaifenesin and have a chance for true healing.

Still others have spent months or years on antifungal (yeast) medications, such as Diflucan (fluconazole) or Mycostatin (nystatin), without experiencing much change in symptoms. There is always some danger, just as with the use of antibiotics, of what effects these drugs have on the resident gut bacteria and overall microbiome. It could greatly alter the landscape of the gut, leading to further and greater problems.

> How does it feel physically? I described it to a friend this way: "Imagine you are just recovering from a bad case of the stomach flu, where you're better but still shaky and not sure how loose your bowels still are. Now imagine you're going to try to carry on a normal life, and pretend you're fine. And imagine every day is like this." It's hard, it's uncomfortable, and the emotional component is hard, too. Cramping, urgency, a feeling of "looseness," burning pain in the lower back, nausea, acid reflux, shakiness, and weak knees. These are all symptoms I associate with IBS.
>
> —*R. A., California*

We know that fibromyalgia and undigested carbohydrates combine as preeminent forces to cause IBS. Like other cells anywhere in the body, those of the gastrointestinal tract also suffer energy deprivation. The three smooth muscle layers of the intestinal wall become dysfunctional, just as can skeletal muscle. In fact, patients with irritable bowel have been shown to have fewer muscular contractions than those without it, and these are disorganized, nonrhythmic, and appreciably more intense. This causes abdominal pain and defacatory urgency.

The small intestine has the assigned task of churning and mixing nutritive elements with digestive juices. Such activity begins the breakdown of fats, protein, and carbohydrates into absorbable components. Alternate contraction and relaxation of the intestinal wall propels raw materials to the next digestive station, where they submit to the action of various hormones and enzymes. The results are minuscule food particles that may now be assimilated and made ready for body-wide distribution. Intestinal glands share in the general problems of fibromyalgia and, along with the musculature, can't perform properly, at first in cycles and then continuously.

Food processing is mainly done in the small intestine. Bile and pancreatic enzymes massage fats into microscopic, digestible fragments. The colon (or large intestine) lies downstream, all six feet of it. Similarly affected in fibromyalgia, its glands and muscles also contribute to the irritable bowel syndrome. The main job here is to remove various salts and water from the mulch, a process that may take from many hours to a few days. It sequesters friendly bacterial residents that live in the colon, as well as not-so-friendly ones. These organisms use our food residues for their own metabolic ends and, in the process, create items for our special needs. As much as 20 percent of our ingested carbohydrates reach the large intestine undigested. There they become the main nourishment for certain bacteria that thrive when they are so abundantly nourished. These bacteria create large amounts of gas as they ferment the sugar and starch residues. This gas will cause repetitive cramping and sharp stabs anywhere in the abdomen, but mostly in the small intestine. It doesn't linger long there since it's quickly propelled forward and expelled into the much larger reception chambers of the colon. There the gas encounters forceful contractions of more powerful muscles that shove the now-hardening remnants of the digested food toward the rectum. The large bowel gets distended and bloated in places where the gas temporarily accumulates.

There are certain predictable sites where gas pools because of how our intestines are structured. First is the lower right abdomen, where air blasts out from the small intestine into the colon. Pressure builds in this area, and a bit later gas is propelled to the upper right abdomen near the edge of the liver. Remember that gas is simply air, and air rises. Cramps cut across the belly from right to left as gas is squeezed toward the highest place in the bowel, the left upper quadrant. A huge air pocket can form under the thin diaphragm muscle that pushes upward toward the heart. Sharp-stabbing or pressure pains reflected into the front of the chest can mimic a heart attack. You may ask, "Why doesn't gas move along with the forming stools?" The propulsive efforts of the intestinal muscles are a bit like grabbing a long, sausage-like balloon in the middle. The gas squeezes in both directions, but as soon as you let go, it gushes back to the center. The result is repeated pains from the same gas bubble whether it lingers some-where or rapidly shifts position. (See figures 10.1 and 10.2.)

Gas produces an amazing variety of sounds, but it's nothing more than air that's temporarily trapped. Forced to accumulate because of constipation that blocks its egress, it further dehydrates stools and makes them rock-hard. Cemented food residues even-tually plug up the rectal area like a dam. Pressure builds up behind this solid wall, and adds to the existing discomfort of bloating, nausea, and perhaps sour belching (acid reflux). Added pressure also induces painful spasms, mainly in the lower left side of the abdomen. Glands lining the colon react to surface damage by making slimy mucus just as the nasal and bronchial membranes do in response to irritation. The purpose of this mucus is to make the colon slippery so that hard stools can slither out without causing further damage to the sigmoid (the lowest segment of the colon) or rectum. At times the longer, stained mucous strings may take on the appearance of worms and lead patients to try dead-end treatments to get rid of something they never had to begin with.

The cemented head of the bowel movement is often so hard and slow to exit that it scratches the rectum, causing some bleed-ing and rectal pain. If encrusted food particles are embedded on the surface, the laceration may be deep enough to produce what we call in medical parlance a rectal fissure—a crack or tear. Higher up, small pockets (diverticula) may extrude outward from the colon. Stool contents can push into them, scratch them, and attract infection, causing diverticulitis. Rock-like stools can also push rectal veins ahead of them like an ocean wave. These get

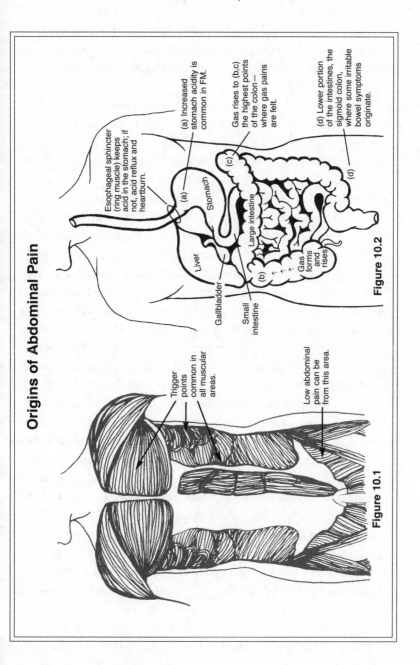

Origins of Abdominal Pain

Trigger points common in all muscular areas.

Low abdominal pain can be from this area.

Figure 10.1

Esophageal sphincter (ring muscle) keeps acid in the stomach; if not, acid reflux and heartburn.

Liver

Gallbladder

Stomach

Small intestine

Large intestine

Gas forms and rises

(a) Increased stomach acidity is common in FM.

Gas rises to (b,c) the highest points of the colon—where gas pains are felt.

(d) Lower portion of the intestines, the sigmoid colon, where some irritable bowel symptoms originate.

Figure 10.2

inflamed, sandpapered, swollen, or clotted, and become what we call hemorrhoids. Bleeding from these causes when seen on toilet paper or in the toilet bowl is often the reason doctors must order even more testing.

Patients suffering from gastrointestinal conditions are miserable, and especially when their stomachs hurt, they turn to "comfort foods," the easily digested sugars and starches. (Sixty percent of our fibromyalgics crave sweets in a vain attempt to make energy, as we've discussed.) But excessive carbohydrate consumption only makes things worse, by promoting genetic tendencies toward hypoglycemia, weight gain, and diabetes, not to mention feeding the bacteria in the digestive tract. Repetitive releases of insulin force the liver to convert carbohydrate excesses to fat. Obesity is responsible for many health problems beyond the scope of this chapter; it most certainly adds to gastrointestinal misery. Heartburn and gastroesophageal reflux occur primarily in overweight patients who carry weight around their midsection, which pushes the stomach up. "Heartburn" results when stomach acid is forced upward through the lower esophageal sphincter into the esophagus.

Pains arising from the abdominal wall cause diagnostic difficulties for doctors. A diligent physician surveys the results of testing and ascribes the discomforts of constipation and diarrhea to "IBS." The outer abdominal muscles suffer the same as other muscles throughout the body. Unrelenting spasm to the right of the pit of the stomach can instigate unnecessary testing. But the cause is quite easy to identify: Patients lie supine and simply raise their heads off the bed. The doctor should palpate both sides of the uppermost abdomen and compare the tension under the fingers. Both sides may be involved, but the right side is usually the more spastic and tender one. By this exercise the muscular cause of the pain can be easily confirmed. Patients often describe the feeling as a side-rib charley horse, a clue that it is muscular in origin.

In chapter 9, we discussed diagnostic problems caused by the inguinal ligaments. Those are the parallel double cords located on each side of the groin. They originate from the front pelvis and anchor at the pubic bone. They're actually part of the abdominal wall muscles adjacent to the lower ribs that spread downward. In the groin, they curl around each other to create rope-like structures. Those connections are what let you brace and give leverage to do a sit-up. They're almost always involved in fibromyalgia; they can be easily felt as swollen segments in the outermost parts of the ligaments. They stay tight day and night, exerting a steady pull on the attached abdominal muscles. In IBS, this can cause the feeling of rectal pressure. Sometimes irritable bowel symptoms are actually side effects of medication taken for another symptom. Narcotics such as codeine, OxyContin, and morphine and muscle relaxants like Flexeril (cyclobenzaprine) and Soma (carisoprodol) cause some degree of constipation in nearly anyone that does not resolve over time. The narcotic pain medications can also be responsible for stomach or abdominal cramps and bloating. Antianxiety drugs such as Klonopin (clonazepam) and Valium (diazepam) commonly cause constipation as well. So if you have constipation, check the side effects of your medications: Pain medications, antidepressants, antihistamines, and some blood pressure medications can be culprits. Side effects are cumulative—and added together they can grow more intense. Cholesterol drugs can cause gas, constipation, or diarrhea. Don't forget to check on your supplements: Calcium and iron are two implicated in constipation.

Antibiotics are notorious for causing diarrhea, but there are others. Protein pump inhibitors such as Prilosec (omeprazole) and Prevacid (lansoprazole) are a newer class of drugs that may add to the problem along with antacids. SSRI antidepressants such as paroxetine (Paxil), citalopram (Celexa), and escitalopram (Lexapro) are another category that list diarrhea as a common side effect. The diabetes medication metformin can cause rather severe diarrhea and gas, although generally this side effect will pass with time. Over-the-counter magnesium is sometimes touted for fibromyalgia symptoms such as tight muscles and to help with relaxation, but an excess may cause diarrhea.

Nausea is a common side effect, and many medications can be responsible. Antibiotics, anti-inflammatory drugs such as Motrin or Advil (ibuprofen), and some blood pressure medications such as the calcium-channel blockers (Procardia, Nifedical) and anti-depressants are possibilities. If the nausea is mild and occurs after taking a dose, you can try taking it with food or at least a snack.

Over-the-counter pain medications (as well as prescription ones) can be responsible for stomach pain. Some of the NSAIDs such as ibuprofen are sold in a pill that also contains another compound to protect the stomach lining. In some patients, acet-aminophen (Tylenol) is a problem. Iron supplements may cause stomach pain, and in that case a timed-release product might be more tolerable.

Constant use of laxatives is habit-forming, but even recover-ing patients are afraid to stop them and too impatient to wait for resumption of normal function. Losing what little benefit they've obtained from their drugs can't be risked; they fear their whole system will fall apart. This concern is not ill founded: They're barely coping as it is and have no emotional or physical reserves. The following story is typical.

For the last ten years or so I have been diagnosed with every-thing from colitis to food allergies to systemic candida infection because I have had so much trouble with diarrhea. Sometimes I would go for days with no bowel function and then out of the blue I'd have diarrhea...I had constant painful intestinal gas that was very embarrassing because I could not control it. I was treated for colitis and then sprue or gluten intolerance. Neither of those treatments helped. Next, an allergist diagnosed me with intes-tinal yeast infections from antibiotics. He said I had developed food allergies from the yeast and put me on an antifungal drug called nystatin. That helped a little. The next doctor... did a two-year series of European allergy shots and gave me an even stronger drug for the yeast. [He] had me injecting myself with allergy shots two to three times a week and taking doses and potions of various things by mouth four times a day. My diet was very restricted, and my weight fell from 118 to 98 pounds. The doctor had me on a high-carbohydrate diet in a failed attempt at weight gain.

In desperation and prayer I turned to the Internet and found Dr. St. Amand's information. After comparing his description of hypoglycemia and IBS to my symptoms, I hoped I had found an answer. I dropped Dr. St. Amand and Claudia an e-mail. Dr. St. Amand assured me I was on the right track. Claudia helped me get started on the diet and told me what to do in the stormy early weeks, as my body fought to adjust to the new fuel. She promised after the first six weeks things would settle down. They did. The gas and diarrhea and other symptoms are gone now as long as I stay on the diet... The good news is I can now eat anything on the HG diet and not have diarrhea or gas. I no longer look like a starved waif, having put on 14 pounds as well.

—*Gretchen, South Carolina*

Patients with irritable bowel syndrome often avoid intimate relationships, as do those with vulvodynia or bladder dysfunction. All three of these conditions isolate the individual because of the personal nature of the affected areas. Most people suffer in silence and resist explaining their illness to others because it's so vague, mysterious, and embarrassing. Studies have concluded that IBS has a serious effect on well-being; quality of life for sufferers has been found to be similar to patients who are on dialysis or suffering from heart failure. Articles love to total up the cost to the health care system but seldom dwell on what it does to lives. Support groups exist on the internet if you are so inclined.

TREATMENT FOR IBS

IBS symptoms are treated with an assortment of medications, and most patients get enough partial relief with over-the-counter products such as antacids, cathartics, and gas-reducing agents. Just as often, especially when people are treating themselves, efforts are misdirected and bypass the underlying cause. Because symptoms are confusing and changeable, suspicions arise about yeast and parasites. Prescriptions are too often added to over-the-counter stuff in a "shotgun" approach. Costs to patients mount with expensive digestive enzymes, cleansing compounds, and even colonics—things insurance does not cover. Adding this fistful of pills to those for sleep, nervousness, depression, and pain helps make their pharmacist's monthly car payments and also invites drug interaction disasters.

So how do we treat irritable bowel syndrome? These are the two simplest paragraphs we've written in this entire chapter. Begin by eliminating all sugars and complex carbohydrates. You'll find the proper diet outlined in chapter 6 and on our website. The diet is the same as for hypoglycemia except that you don't need to avoid caffeine or alcohol unless they upset your system. The diet alone will quickly eliminate 60 to 70 percent of your symptoms. Dietary restrictions will be temporary for most of you. Once you feel better, add one favorite food at a time beginning with anything but sugar, sweets, and the heavier starches, such as potato and pasta. Unsweetened grains, brown rice, and the dairy products, such as yogurt and sugar-free ice cream, are good places to start your experimentation. Be careful of products containing sugar alcohols, or the non-caloric sweeteners that end with the syllable *ol*. The most common are sorbitol, mannitol, xylitol, and erythritol. These cause diarrhea in most people, so experiment carefully to determine which (if any) you can tolerate. The newer erythritol is often the easiest on the system, with mannitol being the hardest.

It is always better to use foods with no added sugars than those sweetened with one of these.

As you diet, promptly back off if symptoms return, trusting them as reliable indicators that you've added too much, too fast, or too often. This hunt-and-peck system is the only way to learn which foods and in what quantities you can tolerate. The premenstrual week is the riskiest of the month for adverse effects. In time, you'll learn what you need to restrict, if anything, on a permanent basis. You'll dependably evolve your own personal program.

Some people are sensitive to certain carbohydrates such as fructose, fructans, lactose, and others, known as FODMAPs—fermentable oligo-, di-, and monosaccharides and polyols. FODMAPs are found in certain grains, vegetables, fruits, and dairy products. Your IBS symptoms might ease if you follow a strict low-FODMAP diet and then reintroduce foods one at a time. You can see there's quite an overlay when you compare this diet with our low-carbohydrate diet. There are many new online resources for this dietary approach.

Over-the-counter preparations work quite effectively when combined with the diet. Both charcoal and simethicone products work quite well for gas and bloating. Examples of simethicone would be Mylanta, Maalox, and Phazyme (don't use mint flavor). Calcium carbonate antacids such as Rolaids, Tums, and their many generics are good choices for an upset or acidy stomach—but use only the fruit-flavored. Prilosec is effective, but don't use those that are blue-colored. Pepcid (famotidine), Zantac (ranitidine), and other histamine-2 blockers are available in over-the-counter strengths and also counter acidity without the issue of dyes blocking energy production. Prescription strengths may be needed if the weaker ones prove inadequate. Prelief is an over-the-counter supplement that neutralizes food acids, which helps heartburn if you eat foods that trigger yours. Over-the-counter Imodium helps control cramping and diarrhea during flare-ups.

Fiber and extra fluid intake ease constipation, but you should titrate added fiber up gradually so you won't make things worse. Be sure to stick with sugar-free formulations such as those made by Metamucil, Benefiber, Fiber Choice, Konsyl, or Citrucel. Magnesium is a stand-alone supplement that should be titrated up gradually for constipation; calcium, on the other hand, might help with diarrhea.

For constipation, there are many over-the-counter choices as well. These include osmotic laxatives (such as Milk of Magnesia and nonabsorbable sugars like lactulose); polyethylene glycol (such as MiraLax); and stimulant laxatives (such as Senokot, Perdiem, Dulcolax, and Ex-Lax). Peri-Colace is both a stimulant and stool softener, a combination directed toward constipation. Magnesium is a stand-alone supplement that should be titrated up gradually for constipation. Calcium, on the other hand, may squelch diarrhea.

Titrate—To determine the proper amount of medication needed for therapeutic action by gradually and systematically raising the dosage until the desired effect has occurred.

If you're taking antibiotics, add a probiotic, which can help maintain healthy flora in the colon. It's an inexpensive insurance policy against a severe bout of diarrhea.

Rectal pressure from constipation can be relieved quite safely by inserting a glycerin suppository. Hemorrhoids may be treated with topical preparations, but beware of those containing witch hazel or other plant extracts. Over-the-counter anti-inflammatories such as naproxen or ibuprofen may help within a few days. Mineral oil is a lubricant laxative and can be taken orally or added to another drink. There are also mineral oil enemas that work similarly to the glycerin suppositories. Highly effective for constipation is good old-fashioned exercise. If you get moving, your bowels may follow suit!

There are prescription drugs on the market for IBS symptoms as well. Hopefully, you will not need to use these for long. Some patients actually get relief from diarrhea and some pain when taking tricyclic antidepressants. Unfortunately, side effects of these include dry mouth, fatigue, and weight gain. Anticholinergics (spasmotics) for cramping also have similar side effects.

> At the end of my first year, my IBS was almost gone. My energy level got better. I was able to stay out of bed when I came home from work in the evening. I was able to get a shower, dry my hair, and put on my makeup without taking several breaks. I was able to go to my grandson's football games and sit on the cold bleachers late at night. Some people never cycle severe pain but have other symptoms instead.
>
> —*Jan H., Kentucky*

Many other medications, described below, are currently used by physicians.

- Older tricyclics and anticholinergic drugs are often prescribed because they have relaxing effects on intestinal smooth muscles and ease cramping. Two commonly used for IBS symptoms are Bentyl (dicyclomine) and Levsin (hyoscyamine). Librax has similar benefits, but contains a benzodiazepine that should be used and prescribed only with caution as patients can develop a tolerance to it and may have withdrawal symptoms when it is stopped abruptly. Serotonin-reuptake inhibitors may be helpful because they keep that neurotransmitter at higher, available levels. Whereas 26 percent of patients were greatly improved by simply increasing fiber intake, 63 percent fared equally well by taking a small daily dose of the antidepressant Paxil, which has had success in the treatment of IBS. For GERD and heartburn, if over-the-counter strengths are not effective, then stronger prescription proton pump inhibitors (Protonix, Prevacid, Prilosec, Nexium) might be. For diarrhea, if the standard over-the-counter Imodium (loperamide) doesn't work, there is prescription Lomotil. These may be used whenever a problem occurs and work quickly, within an hour or so.

- Eluxadoline (Viberzi) can ease diarrhea by reducing muscle contractions and fluid secretion in the intestine, and also by increasing muscle tone in the rectum. Side effects can include nausea, abdominal pain, and mild constipation. In 2017, the FDA issued a warning that due to increased risk for serious, potentially life-threatening pancreatitis, eluxadoline should not be used in patients who do not have a gallbladder.

- Alosetron (Lotronex) is prescribed for some women who have severe diarrhea. It has actually been on and off the market in the past due to the fact that it can contribute to ischemic bowel disease. Lotronex is only prescribed under a risk management program requiring careful monitoring and education due to rare but potentially serious side effects, and only for women.

- Rifaximin (Xifaxan) is an antibiotic that was approved by the FDA for treatment of IBS with diarrhea in adults. It works by reducing or altering bacteria in the gut. It has been found to improve IBS symptoms of bloating and diarrhea after a ten-to-fourteen-day course of treatment. It is only slightly absorbed in the gut and is generally tolerated well. Not all patients respond to this approach, but we are mentioning it here because you may come across it while doing research.

- Amitiza (lubiprostone) is approved for women with severe constipation who have not responded to other treatments. It works by increasing fluid secretion in the small intestine. Side effects include nausea and abdominal pain. Before it is prescribed, patients should try stool softeners such as MiraLax or

Perdiem. Milder laxatives such as sennocides may also help. It is not FDA-approved for men.

- Linaclotide (Linzess) works by increasing the movement of contents through the GI tract and by blocking pain signals in the intestines. The medication is prescribed for adults only. In studies, patients taking linaclotide experienced improvement in multiple symptoms including pain or discomfort, bloating, and bowel function.

- Plecanatide (Trulance) was approved in 2017 by the FDA for the treatment of chronic idiopathic constipation in adults. It works by increasing intestinal transit and fluid. It was shown to be as effective as Linzess with a lower rate of diarrhea as an adverse reaction.

- There are currently new medications in development for the very large and lucrative IBS market. One that is expected to arrive soon is elobixibat, a bile acid transporter, which will be a new class of medication for IBS with constipation.

WARNING

Irritable bowel syndrome and fibromyalgia do not cause a high fever or severe pain that is persistent. If you are experiencing these symptoms, with or without nausea, diarrhea, or constipation, see a doctor to rule out more dangerous conditions such as appendicitis or diverticulitis.

As a teen I had the symptoms of what I now recognize as IBS. I never knew there was a name for the things that plagued me. Other kids dreamed of their futures and what they were going to be when they grew up. I found it hard to have those dreams. Sometimes I wondered if I was dying slowly but I never told that to anyone. All I knew was other kids my age weren't sick all the time.

—*Cris, Michigan*

As with other symptoms of fibromyalgia, stress is known to make irritable bowel worse, although of course it is not causative. The colon is actually partially controlled by the nervous system, and contains more nerve cells than the spinal cord. Any modalities that reduce stress are therefore beneficial. Yoga may help restore normal motility of the gut by calming the central nervous systems with meditation and by some targeted stretches. Certain yoga poses can help strengthen contractions or ease spasms in your intestines. Many clinics are now prescribing yoga for IBS and have posted resources on the internet.

Although among the most distressing, the symptoms of IBS will eventually cycle and go away for good with the use of guaifenesin. Dietary restrictions will have a big effect before that, so it's important to stick to the protocol.

CHAPTER 11

GENITOURINARY SYNDROMES

The bladder thing was my most serious symptom and it was guai that allowed me to get off Elmiron, a depressing (literally) medication that controlled the bladder pain. Possibly I would have committed suicide because of bladder pain because it was so bad for years. Within a couple of months on guai I was mostly free. I still have a little blood in my urine sometimes and a tendency to feel bladder irritation but nothing like the intense pain of those years.

—*Hannah, California*

The bladder, urethra, and vaginal tract share in producing some of the most overwhelmingly painful symptoms of fibromyalgia. They can induce oppressive feelings that totally overshadow brain, muscular, and intestinal complaints. This intensity leads patients to seek relief from urologists or gynecologists. Unfortunately, while most of these specialists administer local remedies, they fail to recognize the broader picture. In the end, because the underlying disease hasn't been treated, these initially helpful therapies fail. Fibromyalgia is not part of their field of expertise, and patient and physician become increasingly frustrated. Worse still, desperate patients will finally try anything with a ghost of a chance, and all too often succumb to damaging topical applications or destructive surgeries that fail to live up to promises and, worse, leave scar tissue in their wake.

Table 11.1

Genitourinary System

	Male	Percentage Male	Female	Percentage Female
Number of Patients	835		4,601	
Dysuria	214	26	1,497	32
Pungent Urine	286	34	2,089	45
Bladder Infections	91	11	2,893	63
Vulvodynia	N/A		1,755	38

THE BLADDER AND INTERSTITIAL CYSTITIS

Fifty percent of female fibromyalgics give a medical history of three or more bladder infections before we first see them. Some tell us they've had fifty or more documented attacks and other repeated episodes of painful urination when no infection could be detected. Bladder infections in males are quite uncommon and therefore require more thorough investigation.

Routine urinalysis, even in healthy individuals, often shows varieties of amorphous calcium crystals in combination with oxalate, phosphate, or carbonates. You'll recall that the entire body participates in trying to get rid of excessive phosphate. These acid particles are secreted through tears, saliva, sweat, vaginal fluids, and bowel excrements. This output is not negligible except when compared with what's excreted in the urine, which is the major dumping system.

Calcium and phosphate don't crystallize inside cells. The two substances coexist in solution. It's the same effect that's seen when you drop salt in water: It immediately enters into solution though the sodium and the chloride are still there. Sufficiently diluted, they won't form particles. Phosphate surges out of the kidneys in a dissolved state, but things change in the bladder. That reservoir holds liquid waste until sufficient volume demands voiding. While waiting in the bladder, phosphate often solidifies in combination with calcium, oxalate, or magnesium. The weight of these microscopic crystals makes them sink to the base of the bladder and at the opening of the urethra. That's similar to sand in a swimming pool that gradually migrates to the deepest area, around the drain. On urination, particles are swept out and, like liquid sandpaper, abrade the delicate lining, the mucosa. If the scraping is sufficiently injurious, the integrity of the membrane is compromised; once this is broken, bacteria is able to penetrate. The short female urethra—the tube that drains the contents of the bladder from the body—exits near the anus. Bacteria from the vagina, rectum, and skin can easily find their way up into the bladder and cause cystitis. This is the anatomical reason why women have far more problems with their urinary tracts than men. (See figure 11.1.)

Cystitis—Infection of the bladder. Symptoms include a constant urge to urinate, pain above the pubic bone, burning, searing urine, and, upon urination, producing only a small amount of urine. Antibiotics are commonly prescribed to treat the infection, as well as local analgesics that work on the urinary tract.

Under the same circumstances, intercourse is even more traumatic. Most women know about "honeymoon cystitis," which occurs during periods of heightened sexual activity. Pooled crystals damage the urethral and bladder walls from friction effects of penile strokes. The tougher vaginal lining is treated just as harshly and reacts like the bladder, as we'll discuss later when we get to that portion of the anatomy.

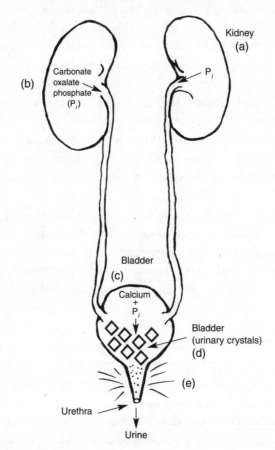

Mechanism of Bladder Infection or Irritation

(a) Kidneys retain too much but eliminate some phosphate.

(b) Kidneys release oxalates and carbonates (*anions* that, like phosphates, have two negative charges).

(c) In the bladder the anions combine mostly with calcium (*cations* that, like magnesium, have two positive charges).

(d) The combining of cations and anions forms crystals that settle to the bottom of the bladder.

(e) At the next urination the crystals scrape the bladder neck and the urethra, exposing the lining to infection.

Figure 11.1

When bladder infections are recurrent, patients are given a low-dose antibiotic for an entire year to achieve complete eradication. Infection is detected by the presence of blood or pus in the urine not visible to the naked eye. Only a microscopic examination in a laboratory can distinguish an infection from urinary tract pain. In the event of severe pain, especially pain accompanied by fever, a physician should be consulted. Without a urinalysis, even veteran patients are fooled into thinking there's infection where none exists. Antibiotics such as levofloxacin can stamp out infections in short order, making them popular choices for quick results. Because infections can travel from the bladder up into the kidneys via the ureters, it's important to treat them promptly. Prolonged use of antibiotics can cause vaginal yeast infections, or bacterial resistance. So they should be used only when testing shows the need. A urine culture done before treatment can demonstrate which antibiotic will be effective.

The symptoms of urinary tract irritation commonly occur without infection. Burning urination (dysuria) sometimes appears for only a few hours or days and resolves spontaneously. Patients may have an unbearable urge to urinate with the sensation of a full bladder, but voiding produces just a small amount of fluid. It is not uncommon during a cycle to urinate multiple times within a couple of hours.

Eventually, repeated cycles of cystitis invite more thorough investigations by urologists. When multiple urinalyses fail to expose infection, the next step is to look directly into the bladder (cystoscopy). That search almost always proves futile, so the physician resorts to a biopsy of the bladder wall. Frustration mounts if such specimens appear normal under microscopic scrutiny. Sometimes surface irritations or small clusters of certain white blood cells are found; though hardly conclusive, this at least points to a possible diagnosis.

All my life I've had recurrent vaginitis. When I had a vaginal culture, it sometimes came back no candida (I used to wonder if the lab mixed up the cultures) and yet all this irritation and discomfort continued. I used to buy Monistat cream four at a time when they were on sale. My GP even suggested I might be allergic to my own menstrual flow (if you can believe that one) and also said I might be allergic to my husband's sperm (not very helpful). Now, [after] thirteen months on guai this pain is taking a bit of a break. I actually have days when I don't have it at all.

—*Vera Lynne, Canada*

Those minimal findings or no abnormal findings earn a diagnosis of "interstitial cystitis" (IC). There is a diagnostic procedure called a potassium sensitivity test that may be done. Your doctor places (instills) two solutions—water and potassium chloride—into your bladder, one at a time. You're asked to rate on a scale of 0 to 5 the pain and urgency you feel after each solution is instilled. If you feel noticeably more pain or urgency with the potassium solution than with the water, your doctor will diagnose interstitial cystitis. People with normal bladders can't tell the difference between the two solutions.

Many doctors prefer to skip the potassium test and simply use the term based on a patient's symptoms. These include steady hurting in pelvic, pubic, or lower abdominal areas and an urgency to urinate so strong that patients might void twenty or more times a day. Urine cultures are routinely negative. Rectal pain may be intensified by hard spasms in muscles lying between the vagina and rectum, at the perineum. Decreased bladder capacity and painful intercourse are two other common complaints. A succinct description would be: It's like a ninth-month, never-terminating, pregnant-bladder condition. The diagnosis of interstitial cystitis is rarely offered to males, where the issue is often misdiagnosed as nonbacterial prostatitis, prostatodynia, or prostalgia. Only about 10 percent of those diagnosed with IC are males. Men may have the same symptoms as women, but add scrotal or penile pain. If you've been diagnosed with IC, you were 10 percent more likely to have had childhood bladder problems.

Cystoscopy—A procedure done in a doctor's office, in which the urinary tract is viewed through a cystoscope inserted through the urethra and up into the bladder. Through this fiber-optic scope, the doctor can examine the lining and structure of these organs. A patient is usually given a local anesthetic or a mild tranquilizer to help with the discomfort.

Pyridium (phenazopyridine HCL) is generic and available both in over-the-counter and prescription strengths. It numbs the bladder and relieves pain but is designed for only short-term use as it can build up in the body. Be careful when checking both over-the-counter and prescription medications for bladder pain, as many of these contain salicylate (by name). Over-the-counter Cystex and prescription medications such as Prosed and Urised will block guaifenesin.

Interstitial cystitis—A disease defined by the absence of a positive test for other bladder conditions, manifested by bladder and pelvic pain and the constant urge to urinate, which produces only a small amount of urine.

Half a teaspoon of baking soda in six ounces of water three times a day can help cut the urine's acidity. Prelief (calcium glycerophosphate) can do the same. Cranberry juice or tablets are touted as prevention from infections, but the tablets will block guaifenesin. Juice works as well as the tablets but it can raise urinary pH and create more pain. D-mannose, the active ingredient in cranberries, can be purchased as a supplement and will not.

Nonsteroidal anti-inflammatories such as Advil or Motrin (ibuprofen in over-the-counter or prescription strength) often help with the pain. As with other symptoms of fibromyalgia, the older tricyclic antidepressants such as Amitriptyline (Elavil) are prescribed for IC. This class of antidepressants acts on smooth muscle and can relax the bladder. They also cut pain perception and help with sleep. Newer antidepressants (SSRIs and SNRIs) have not demonstrated any efficacy in treating IC. Antihistamines such as loratadine (Claritin) may be taken by day. In IC, the mast cells that line the bladder are stimulated and release histamines, which cause local pain and irritation. At night, patients may prefer older antihistamines that double as sleep aids, such as Benadryl.

One oral medication, Elmiron (pentosan polysulfate), is approved for IC. It is believed to provide a protective coating inside the bladder. It has not performed well in studies but may help some patients. Other therapies include bladder instillations where various substances are inserted directly into the bladder. It is worth noting that only one, DMSO, is actually approved for this type of delivery. Other instillations include BCG, heparin, lidocaine, Elmiron, Cystistat, and sodium bicarbonate.

At this point we're sure you're not surprised to hear that there are yoga programs for IC and overactive bladder. You can find resources, videos, and books on the internet. The IC Network has resources available for both bladder and other forms of pelvic pain.

> When you're having an attack, the constant pain…the fear of sex making more pain is debilitating. It weighs down your life, your lightness, destroys spontaneity, makes you standoffish with the man you love because you just don't want to have to explain you're having problems again. That part is bad, but the symptoms that you live with night and day are even worse: never sleeping through a night, having to sleep on the outside of every bed, always worrying whether there will be a bathroom close by, stopping often on car trips, dodging into fast-food places, hoping

they won't catch you not buying anything and telling you the rest room is only for customers.

—*C. C., California*

Guaifenesin eventually clears IC complaints, but may initially worsen them like other symptoms of fibromyalgia. After the first few reversal attacks, future bouts become relatively minor and will likely disappear. Fight back early by drinking extra fluid and watching your diet and by using appropriate medications at the first hint of urinary burning. Prelief may be taken daily as a preventive measure, especially if you're traveling. Car and airplane rides are notorious triggers. It's far easier to abort an early onslaught than to subdue a well-established attack. Exercise, especially stretching, has been helpful in the long term. Take guaifenesin and begin a fitness regime sooner rather than later to help restore you to normal.

VULVAR PAIN

As a senior gynecologist with special training and expertise in vulvar disease, I have been striving to help women with the enigmatic disorder called vulvodynia, and its most common subset, vulvar vestibulitis. In recent years there has been increasing appreciation of other conditions reported as commonly associated with vulvodynia, such as irritable bowel syndrome, fibromyalgia, and interstitial cystitis. In my own practice at Scripps Clinic and Research Foundation, I've discovered that fibromyalgia is at least three times as common in vulvodynia patients as in the general population. I've also noted that vulvodynia tends not to respond to therapy until the underlying fibromyalgia is treated...Dr. St. Amand has done groundbreaking work in the evaluation and treatment of fibromyalgia as opposed to medications that only reduce or help control symptoms. His research, and that of those who follow in his footsteps, will permit fibromyalgia to become merely a painful memory for patients and their spouses. I salute his effort.

—*John Willems, MD, FRCSC, FACOG, head,*
Division of Ob-Gyn, Scripps Clinic and Research
Foundation, La Jolla, California

All too many fibromyalgic women develop extreme sensitivity and irritation of the inner vaginal lips, known as vulvitis. The problem may also involve deeper tissues of the vagina, the vestibule (vestibulitis). In the past eighteen years, we've tabulated the incidence of vulvodynia and associated symptoms. Out of 5,468 consecutive new female patients, about 40 percent had pelvic complaints.

Chronic burning and knife-like pain are common, as is low abdominal pain. Symptoms can be intermittent, localized, or diffuse. In the early stages, pain may be present only after intercourse, but later can occur without apparent provocation. Intermittent bouts are the norm initially, but in time they become chronic and symptoms become overwhelming. Vulvodynia can appear at any age, including in young girls. It's not necessarily a sign of sexual activity.

Vulvodynia or vulvar pain syndrome—Severe pain, burning, and/or itching in the vulvar area (the vulva is the area of the female's external genitalia). This area is extremely sensitive to touch, and may or may not be red and visibly irritated. Vulvar vestibulitis syndrome is less common, and applies to women who have pain only in the vestibule, a smaller area than the vulva.

Like fibromyalgia, vulvodynia is a diagnosis of exclusion. Some conditions must be ruled out, such as infection, yeast overgrowth (candidiasis), genital warts, various lichen diagnoses, sexually transmitted diseases, herpes. The appearance of the tissues is quite different from what is seen in those conditions. In regard to infection, *Candida albicans* and bacterial vaginosis (BV) are usually the first things that are considered when a patient complains of vulvar pain, but are not common causes of pain and are never causes of chronic vulvar pain. Very rarely they may cause recurrent pain that clears, at least briefly, with treatment. Yeast or candidiasis is primarily itchy, and BV produces discharge and odor. Herpes simplex virus is also a cause of recurrent but not chronic pain. Chronic lichen simplex causes itching; any pain is due to erosions from scratching. With HPV or human papillomavirus, the skin retains its normal texture although it might be slightly red, similar to a chemical burn.

Diagnosis is usually slow coming. Patients get acquainted with a few gynecologists after several pelvic exams and failed therapies, often for yeast, before the condition is suspected. Vaginal smears, cultures, or more painful testing ultimately exclude infection, nerve damage, and dermatologic abnormalities. Using a simple Q-tip can detect exquisite sensitivities in certain vaginal tissues. Physicians may also do a quite painless colposcopy to magnify and better visualize painful vulvar surfaces. The diagnosis of vulvodynia is ultimately made on the basis of pain.

Though vulvodynia can be present at any age, the diagnosis is generally made when women are in their forties. In the last edition of the book, we wrote that about two hundred thousand women had been diagnosed, but in 2018 the estimate is upward of fourteen million women, due mostly to rising awareness. That's close to our estimate that 15 percent of women in the world have fibromyalgia. From the thousands of patients we've treated, we can unhesitatingly attest that of all the symptom clusters we encounter, the vulvar pain complex produces the most consistently painful and heartbreaking impositions on a woman's life.

As we've pointed out, fibromyalgia regularly affects the inguinal ligaments that connect hip and pubic bones. They, too, cause pain in the pelvic region. We've already mentioned that spasms may occur in the perineum and add to already overwhelming symptoms. In addition, the irritable bowel syndrome with all of its lower abdominal and rectal problems is present in 60 percent of fibromyalgic women. Twenty-five percent of those with vulvodynia report recurrent bladder infections and/or IC. It's not always easy to separate bladder complaints from the vulvodynia complex given the commonality of symptoms. The same nerves affect all of those regions to spread overlapping symptoms. Because these seemingly separate conditions kept appearing in the same patients, we finally linked them into a single entity. Though we're allocating each a chapter in this section, they're all part of the one big syndrome.

Informed professionals agree that fibromyalgia and vulvodynia are often connected, but not always in the high percentages we contend. You've already read a statement from John Willems, MD, head of ob-gyn at Scripps Clinic in La Jolla, California. He continues to do pioneering work and has considerable success in easing vulvodynia, while acknowledging that those with fibromyalgia must treat that condition as well.

Oxalate—A chemical found in the human body as part of the energy production cycle. It is excreted in the urine, and is known as a topical irritant that can cause burning in the tissues. Foods of plant origin, such as fruits and vegetables, are high in oxalates.

For couples, perhaps the most horrible part of fibromyalgia is the dyspareunia or painful intercourse that is so common with the vulvar pain syndrome. Women with vulvodynia soon become conditioned to expect excruciating and long-lasting pain during and following intercourse. Soon many become afraid to initiate any contact, even cuddling, for fear that even this bit of intimacy might lead to pelvic disaster. Libido is so dulled and lubricant flow so minimal that just the thought of making love hurts. There's a high incidence of separation and divorce within this subset of fibromyalgia, often due to lack of communication that closes doors. Many women freely admit that they avoid forming new relationships knowing they must eventually perform sexually. It is important for both people in the relationship to recognize that vulvodynia doesn't affect just the vulva, but the entire perception of your sexuality. It is important that you not take too much blame on yourself and remember that your partner may be sexually frustrated, but you are both sexually frustrated and in pain. It is helpful to talk about your fears—both of you might be afraid of emotional or physical abandonment. Communication skills—being loving and clear, and creating safety and support together—can build your relationship.

A reality that's hard to face is that this condition can show the true mettle of a relationship. Not all partners will be supportive or willing to regard your problem as a problem affecting the two of you. It can be extraordinarily difficult to learn that the person you love doesn't share the degree of commitment that you do, but it's good to find this out as soon as possible, and you deserve (and can find) better.

A typical story appears below:

Prior to the guaifenesin treatments and my proper diagnosis, the most debilitating pain I would experience was the vulvar pain. The muscle pain could be significantly minimized with pain relievers but not the vulvar pain. In 1989, the vulvar pain became extreme and frequent. It was so severe at times that I would miss work. Because of this pain, I avoided intercourse with my husband and rejected the thought of having a baby.

My only relief from pain was warm baths, but I could not live in the bathtub all the time, so I sought help from my family physician. Even though [he]...was aware of my other symptoms (acne, muscle pain, insomnia), he focused on each symptom as a separate medical condition and sent me to a variety of specialists. Since he did not focus on the body as a whole and was ignorant of the existence of fibromyalgia, he did not connect my cycles of muscle pain, and fatigue... with my vulvar pain.

During the first few weeks of taking the guaifenesin I did experience vulvar pain an average of about two out of ten days, and the pain was severe. As I continued to take the guaifenesin, both the frequency and the severity of the pain decreased... Since January 1995, I have not missed work due to fibromyalgia or vulvar pain. I am not fearful of sexual intercourse, and maybe one day I will even think about having a baby.

—*Angela, California*

Given these obstacles, it's safe to say that the relationships that endure despite vulvodynia are some of the strongest we've seen. Patient and spouse must both be committed to openness and new, nonpainful ways of expressing their sexual emotions and drives. The blatant and basic assault on these women's fundamental quality of life and the toll it takes on relationships has driven many to embrace drastic "cures." Those who simply purchased miracle creams and lotions were the least harmed by these measures, because for the most part they've suffered only from a wounded purse. Others who have submitted to repeated injections of synthetic cortisone, alcohol, interferon, and local anesthetics directly into the painful areas may be left with painful scar tissue as a result. Most shocking and horrifying are the unsuccessful and sometimes mutilating surgeries women have endured. Parts of the labia or vaginal lining were excised in an attempt to eliminate pain-producing tissue. Surgery is followed by recurrences and scarring that actually intensify symptoms. In some circles, surgery remains "the thing to do," but more prudent gynecologists hesitate and cut as a last resort. This is probably the single most controversial issue on the list. The facts we all agree on: Surgery should be a last resort, not a first resort. Surgery can make you worse.

There are two types of surgery currently available: scalpel and laser. Scalpel surgery involves the "Woodruff procedure": Sensitive areas around the vestibule are cut away, and healthy skin is pulled over. Recovery can take several weeks.

More than one kind of laser is used to perform that type of surgery. The worst results are seen when doctors laser too aggressively and damage healthy tissue. Even when the operation is done carefully, recovery time is longer and more painful, and most cases of worsening after surgery result from the laser version. The currently accepted figures are that 60 percent of women will benefit from surgery and 10 percent may be made worse. This first number is lessened, however, by the chance of pain recurrence, which tends to be high. Interferon shots at the same time as the surgery seem to hurt chances of success.

As long as there is hope that another therapy can reverse symptoms and treat the root cause, it should be the preferred course. With guaifenesin, we are offering just that.

Unfortunately, vulvar pain symptoms are often subjected to treatments based on an incorrect diagnosis. It's common for women to be told (or think) they have a yeast infection that won't quite go away. It's important to remember that not everything that feels itchy is candida. If you don't see the distinctive cottage cheese discharge and your symptoms don't yield to a prescription yeast medication such as oral Diflucan or vaginally inserted boric acid capsules, further investigate the cause. As Dr. Willems says, "If the treatment doesn't work, reconsider the diagnosis." If you're prone to yeast infections, boric acid capsules can be used whenever you suspect a problem. Pharmacists will make them up for you, or you fill size 0 capsules yourself. Get them from a pharmacy or from a health food store and fill them with plain boric acid, which you can find in any pharmacy or online. You can insert them nightly for a week or so when you have an infection and once a week if you are prone to them. Some women notice a flare-up of yeast activity during the premenstrual week. If so, use boric acid prophylactically.

Dr. Willems has developed a treatment protocol that includes several therapies with refreshingly effective results. He outspokenly condemns surgery done without clear indications or done prematurely, before all else has failed. He has discovered that some compounds ease symptoms, and others even repair damage. Expert biofeedback and pelvic massage or pelvic floor therapy can make pain bearable, and he highly recommends these. His protocol uses topical estrogen Estrace cream (estradiol) to rebuild vulvar tissue.[1] It is used not to increase systemic estrogen levels, but to increase blood flow to the vulva, as well as to thicken it.

Many women experience initial irritation with Estrace, and some report itching that may actually be indicative of your skin healing—the same way that a healing scar itches. It will probably take about six weeks to notice any benefits. The Women's International Pharmacy offers estrogen preparations in more soothing bases than are normally used, and which may be considerably cheaper than your local pharmacy. If you have a local compounding pharmacy, they may be able to make an estrogen cream in a vitamin E base.

Fibromyalgic women should insist on hormones mixed with plant-free emollients to avoid undermining guaifenesin effects. There are safe commercial preparations, and compounding pharmacists can easily create them if necessary in a base of such substances as vitamin E or emu oil—both of which have also been shown to help in a stand-alone treatment.

When it comes to topical estrogen, Dr. Willems uses Estrace cream as his compound of choice. He's said that Premarin or conjugated estrogen cream can achieve the same goal, but at a significantly slower pace. We stress that vaginal estrogen creams should be used in very small, pea-size amounts so they don't significantly alter estrogen levels in the body. In this day of worry about the

Internal Female Reproductive Organs

Showing the interweave of muscles and organs responsible for pelvic pain.

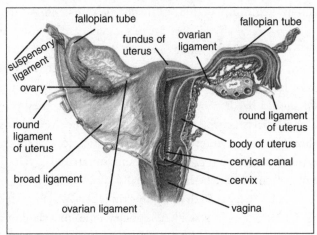

The Vulva

Showing the areas affected by vulvar pain (vulvodynia) and vulvar vestibulitis.

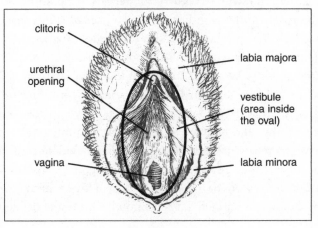

Figure 11.2

effects of hormone replacement therapies, topical compounds are not a concern when used properly. Once healing has occurred, the maintenance therapy requires lower doses still. (See figure 11.3.)

Emu oil is a natural anti–inflammatory that also has the ability to rebuild thinning, damaged tissue due to its content of fatty acids. For patients already on hormones, it can be used as an adjunct to that therapy. Lidocaine in a 2.5 percent solution can be used to deaden pain. Combinations of local anesthetics called EMLA or ELA–Max may also be okay. For some, these are irritating and should be discontinued. Unlike estrogens, they provide only symptomatic relief of symptoms and do not restore tissue. Nonhormone or nonvitamin creams (like Vaseline) can soothe by protecting the skin from physical irritants and urine.

We are often asked whether externally applied heat or ice packs are helpful. Heat packs can dry out the skin when used for extended periods. Cold packs can provide temporary relief in a flare or after intercourse, but also should be used sparingly.

Some well-meaning doctors will prescribe steroid creams, especially if you complain of itching, but these should never be used because they thin the skin. Oral steroids like prednisone may temporarily help the pain but are also powerful drugs that must be used only for short periods and as directed—usually that means tapering off them so your adrenal gland can recover.

Women who have had a history of vulvodynia at any time in their lives or have extremely fair or sensitive skin and/or skin allergies should talk to their physicians as they approach menopause. Because the body's estrogen levels plummet, this supersensitive tissue is vulnerable. Pain will not be evident until tissue damage has occurred, and then rebuilding those tissues takes time. For this reason, prophylactic therapy with a topical estrogen cream should be considered. Prevention is simple and dependably effective.

Prelief, the calcium supplement suggested earlier for interstitial cystitis, is also helpful for vaginal burning. When used for this

FIBROMYALGIA, VULVAR PAIN SYNDROME, AND BLADDER SYMPTOMS
A study of 6,928 consecutive patients

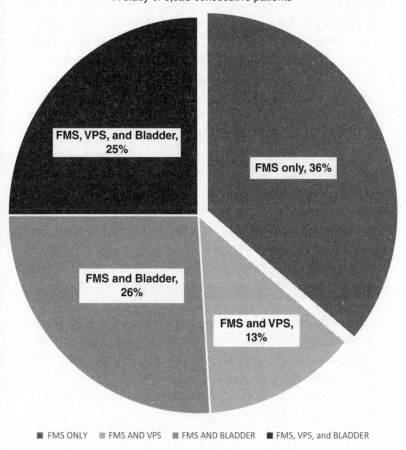

Figure 11.3

purpose, it can be taken with meals. It's available in powder form so it can be sprinkled directly onto food. It can be found in drugstores in sections displaying digestive aids such as antacids. If you can't find it locally, www.prelief.com has a list of pharmacies that carry it, and it can also be ordered online. Calcium is known to be helpful for the symptoms of vulvodynia, so this may be beneficial in other ways.

As with interstitial cystitis, mast cells are involved in the vulvar pain complex. To hinder their propensity to disgorge their irritating contents, both prescription and over-the-counter antihistamines can be used. Because it's often difficult for women with such nagging pain to sleep through the night, the over-the-counter formulas for insomnia can be used to solve two problems at once. Diphenhydramine is the active ingredient in formulas such as Simply Sleep and Sominex, as well as in generic form. It is also available in the nighttime forms of pain medication with ibuprofen. These can be taken during a flare-up or even nightly. It's safe for pregnant and nursing women, and it's not habit-forming. Effective dosages vary greatly. If morning grogginess is a problem, simply cut the amount. As with any medication, you want to use the smallest amount that works. During daytime hours, the newer nondrowsy antihistamines such as Claritin—available over the counter—are a better choice. You can add a histamine-2 blocker such as Zantac or Pepcid to see if that gives additional relief.

> I know the feeling about going for a GYN exam. They told me it hurt because I was tense. I wasn't tense until it hurt. My first exam was when I was very young, a teen. It did not hurt at all. That is how it is supposed to be. Then came the FM and so came the pain there. Every person I have had do these exams has basically blamed me. One physician's assistant used a smaller device on me, which helped a little. Ask them to use the kids' one. I think this problem should improve on guai. I do believe it is the FM. You are still young so hopefully the guai will help before marriage. Most husbands are patient with us, or ask for divorce. It is a real sad thing either way.
>
> —Karen B., Massachusetts

When simple measures don't adequately control pain, prescription medications may be used. We always view these as stopgap measures while we wait for the protocol to do its job. When it comes to prescription medications, antidepressants are often first selected as they are for other chronic pains of unknown etiology. The older tricyclics such as amitriptyline (Elavil) in dosages that vary from 10 to 50 mg daily are fairly effective because of their relaxing action on smooth muscle. Not all patients experience benefits: If so, quit and try something else. That statement applies to most other drugs, which are too often stacked up one on top of the other without thought of removing the previous, ineffective ones. The tricyclic antidepressant trazodone may help with sleep. Ativan (lorazepam) and Klonopin (clonazepam) should be used very cautiously since they are habit-forming. Neurontin (gabapentin) and Lyrica (pregabalin) are anticonvulsants that work to subdue nerve pain despite the very common side effect of weight gain. Savella and Cymbalta, members of a newer class of antidepressants, may be tried although they are much more expensive and have not been shown to be more effective than older compounds. An important note: Older drugs are safer since they've had time to show their side effect fangs; the newer the drug, the less is known about its long-term dangers. Another benefit of the older drugs, of course, is that they cost many times less.

Local anesthetics such as lidocaine ointment can provide temporary symptom relief. Your doctor might recommend applying lidocaine thirty minutes before sexual intercourse to reduce your discomfort, but it should be used very sparingly and only in the most painful spots to preserve the sensation in your better tissue. (It can cause your partner to have temporary numbness after sexual contact.) Women who have long-standing pain that doesn't respond to other treatments might benefit from local nerve block injections.

There are commonsense things you can do to ease symptoms. Avoid tight jeans, nylon underwear, and pantyhose. Seams press into the vagina and severely irritate or chafe vulnerable tissues.

Obviously, wear only clothes that are loose in the crotch, and stay away from synthetic fabrics—these are rougher and don't allow air to circulate. Use unscented white toilet paper (aloe- and dye-free) or avoid all toilet paper altogether and use distilled water spritzes (to avoid chlorine), blotting the area with a soft cloth. Urine is normally acid and therefore burns the already irritated vulva. Try pouring distilled water over the area as you urinate to wash the tissue and dilute the urine as you void. After voiding, a light coat of emu or vitamin E can protect the tissue a little.

Use dermatologically approved detergents with no dyes or fragrances, and do not use fabric softeners or dryer sheets on clothing that comes into contact with the vulva. Underwear should be double-rinsed. Do not use bubble bath or scented soaps; some experts say not to use soap at all but rather soap-free products such as Free & Clear. Simply inserting a tampon can further damage the injured tissues. Instead, use white unscented cotton menstrual pads (such as GladRags). When you're well enough to attempt intercourse, stay with water-soluble lubricants such as Astroglide that are nonirritating. Apply ice or a frozen blue gel pack (lunch box size or feminine gel packs made to fit discreetly in your underwear) wrapped in a hand towel to relieve burning after intercourse or after a long car ride. Urinate (to prevent infection) after sexual intercourse, then rinse your vulva with cool water and pat dry gently.

Do not use contraceptive creams, spermicides, douches, or freshing towelettes or sprays. Bike riding, horseback riding, and sitting for long periods without moving always make symptoms worse. If you must sit all day at work, you can use a foam rubber donut. Don't swim in highly chlorinated swimming pools, and avoid hot tubs.

Biofeedback therapy is quite often suggested and prescribed for vulvodynia. For vulvodynia, this therapy focuses on teaching you to relax your pelvic muscles. You can ask your doctor for referrals or search for a licensed, experienced practitioner. Exercise and stretching may be painful at first, but with time they'll prove beneficial. Helpful exercises and resources can be easily located on the internet. If you are practicing yoga for other conditions, there are some special positions that are known to help with vulvodynia. Videos are available, such as *Relieving Pelvic Pain* and the more specific *Yoga for Vulvodynia*.

> I have suffered from vulvar pain since 1990. I went everywhere for help. I even flew to Michigan for laser surgery from a now infamous doctor. I hooked up with The Vulvar Pain Foundation and found out about the low-oxalate diet and citrate. I began this treatment and got a little better. I added Estrace cream per Dr. Willems at Scripps Clinic in La Jolla, California...I found out about Dr. St. Amand from The VP Foundation and read up on him. I firmly believed that I did not have FMS because I didn't have the body aches and pains. But as I read through the symptoms of FMS, I was astounded. I was reading my life's history. I began the guaifenesin, and the first thing that left me was the vulvar pain. Now I do indeed have the general aches and pains (but that's due to the cycling). I also realize that I have a high pain tolerance and just tolerated the aches. I cycled fairly quickly. Dr. St. Amand recently mapped me, and I'm almost cleared out!
>
> —*Mary B., Alabama*

More than any other symptom of fibromyalgia, vulvodynia is one in which dietary triggers can be spotted. The most common triggers are cranberry juice, coffee, tea, alcohol, citrus, artificial sweeteners, hot peppers, carbonated beverages, tomatoes, and tobacco. Vitamin C is ascorbic acid and, even if buffered, can irritate the bladder, but you can get your vitamins from other sources: Half a cup of red bell peppers contains the same amount of vitamin C as an orange.

One theory—closely associated with Dr. Clive Solomons—is that plant oxalates can cause pain in women with vulvoydnia.

This theory is somewhat controversial for several reasons. Solomons was not a medical doctor, and it is not clear if oxalate content of urine is significantly different than in the general population, but quite a number of women have achieved pain reduction by following a low-oxalate diet. He also instructed women to use calcium citrate—500 mg, three times a day—to help bind the oxalates and prevent crystal formation. If you can't tolerate calcium citrate (a minority of women experience more burning with it), calcium carbonate (as is found in Tums) is the second choice. Magnesium can be added (up to 1,500 mg a day), to avoid constipation. Calcium should be taken twenty minutes before eating, and if it doesn't help could be discontinued. Women who experienced improvement on this diet reported that it began after a week or two but sometimes after six months or more.

Here are the basic things you need to know if you want to look at this diet. There is more information available on the internet, of course.

Fruits and Vegetables

Avoid many types of green leafy vegetables such as spinach, Swiss chard, leeks, okra, beet greens and beet root, collard greens, dandelion greens, and mustard greens. Among fruits, avoid elderberries, gooseberries, figs, star fruit, blackberries, raspberries, Concord grapes, and blueberries. No rhubarb, okra, or parsley. No textured vegetable protein, tofu, or soy yogurt. Stay away from citrus peels.

Nuts and Legumes

Avoid peanuts, almonds, hazelnuts, pistachios, pecans, sesame seeds, lentils, refried beans, baked beans, green beans, and kidney beans. No nut butters.

Avoid bran flakes, fiber cereals, potato chips, french fries, chocolate, and black pepper.

Beverages

For brewed beverages, the oxalate content will vary with the strength. Avoid all brewed and instant coffee, tea, and cocoa. No soy beverages. Dark, draft beer is also high in oxalate, so choose lighter bottled varieties. Drink plenty of clear fluids, especially water, to replace other beverages.

We've usually seen guaifenesin eradicate symptoms, given sufficient time. Patience and gentle management are required for healing the damaged tissue of vulvodynia. Some maintenance measures may be required for life, but none is particularly intrusive or demanding. Extremely sensitive women may wish to avoid Mucinex, the bilayered guaifenesin, because the blue dye could be a problem for them. A dye-free compounded guaifenesin is available from Marina del Rey Pharmacy (www.fibropharmacy .com), and there are white tablets available commercially.

CHAPTER 12

DERMATOLOGIC SYMPTOMS

When I first started the protocol, my face and the back of my neck and upper back broke out *realllly realllly* bad. I was so embarrassed. I wore high collars at the back and tried lots of makeup to cover up my face. But around my mouth and chin were probably 50 bumps at one time and it lasted for a good six months. It was so awful. But it takes time for those phosphates to purge out and I think that's what was going on. As a teenager (and adult), I always had problems with my oily skin. I cycled there for a couple of months, but then after those first few months, I rarely had another breakout.

—*Jan, Kentucky*

If you have fibromyalgia, you know what it's like to not feel comfortable in your own skin. When we know that fibromyalgia affects the energy production of every cell in the body, it's no wonder we notice symptoms on our largest organ, the skin, as well as on our hair and nails, things we spend a lot of time looking at. Some dermatologists estimate that about 80 percent of patients with fibromyalgia develop skin problems. Our statistics might be a little different due to what we tabulate, but it's interesting to know that specialists in that field are aware of it.

Many try to minimize the nature of the dermatologic symptoms, saying that they are not major health threats, but they can be distressing and, certainly for some people, affect quality of life.

We might laugh when we are told that we don't *look* sick, but it's also not exactly a negative thing to feel that you can still clean up well when you want to. When even that is taken from us, it is demoralizing and another loss.

SKIN

I have had this consistently since I got sick; my first symptoms being fatigue, itching rashes, and hives. I have been a notorious complainer about pins and needles, tingling, and painful burning of the skin. The itching intensified when I started the guai in November 1996. I used to use Benadryl almost every night for this. I also tried Caladryl, Benadryl cream, cortisone cream, etc. I have found several things that help: (1) dry brushing with a bath brush before a shower; (2) using a bath brush in a bath with 1 cup each of Epsom salts, sea salts, and baking soda (take a shower afterwards to wash off the salt); (3) Lac-Hydrin or Aquaphor lotion; and (4) Benadryl or prescription medications for itching or sleep at night. It has started to get better for me after a year and three months on guai.

—*Heather, Texas*

Skin is made up of layers, the dermis and the epidermis, and the subcutaneous fat directly beneath. The epidermis is constantly active and creates new cells as they push older ones up toward the surface, where they flatten to become squamous cells. Those, too, finally move farther outward to become the scaly stratum corneum that's ultimately sloughed off. The average life expectancy of a skin cell is one month. The dermis has large amounts of collagen that serves as supportive tissue. Obviously, the skin contains blood, nerve, lymph, and muscle cells along with hair follicles and sebaceous glands. As you might imagine, it takes a lot of energy to keep this huge system running properly. Fibromyalgics are energy-challenged everywhere, even in the skin.

Table 12.1

Dermatologic System

	Male	Percentage Male	Female	Percentage Female
Number of Patients	835		4,601	
Skin Hypersensitivity	283	34	2,937	33
Itching	547	66	3,234	70
Rashes	367	44	2,657	58
Brittle Nails	251	30	3,270	71
Easy Bruising	173	21	3,453	75
Excessive Sweating	471	56	2,078	65

All types of rashes appear on the skin of fibromyalgics, such as eczema, nonpustular acne, seborrhea, hives, rosacea, large red patches, tiny red bumps, scaly-dry areas, and small blisters. Skin can also simply itch, or feel sore, or have a crawling sensation without any visible changes. Numbness, tingling, and hypersensitivity to touch are common and come and go with no rhyme or reason. Diagnoses such as dermatitis and psoriasis are tossed around, but most are mysterious, unnamed eruptions that don't quite fit into existing nomenclature. Nails crack, chip, or peel and are often ridged. Cuticles shred, get thickened, and tear. Hair is usually of poor quality: dry, short-lived, and frequently breaking and falling out prematurely. Excessive sweating is also common (hyperhidrosis)—according to a Mayo Clinic study, it occurred in 32 percent of their fibromyalgic patients. In 1998, a scientific paper first reported mast cell involvement in fibromyalgia. These are highly specialized white blood cells that produce more than thirty identified chemicals and proteins. Subjects (in this case all female) underwent skin biopsies that showed mast cells disgorging their contents into the epidermis, the deepest layer of skin. Their stockpile includes histamine, a strong perpetrator of allergic reactions, including itching and hives. These cells are also involved in the immune response. People with hay fever can attest to histamine's handiwork: swelling of affected areas; itchy eyes and nose; excessive tearing; sneezing; congested sinuses; wheezy lungs; and a runny nose.

Other studies have also found higher-than-normal blood and tissue levels of histamine in fibromyalgic individuals. There it attacks the lining of bronchial tubes, lungs (asthma), bladder wall (interstitial cystitis), and vaginal tissues (vulvodynia). Mast cells are also implicated in facial flushing, cramps, and diarrhea. They gradually attract another type of white blood cell, the eosinophil, which intensifies these body-wide disruptions.

A protein, immunoglobulin G, can suddenly protrude through the wall of a stimulated mast cell. It then will stick on a receptor in the epidermis, where it is a known stimulator of autoimmune reactions. Mast cells are also activated by a brain factor called CRF (corticotropin-releasing factor) secreted into the bloodstream under stress conditions. Starting to make sense? The body triggers its cells, including the brain, to respond to anything irritating, injurious, or deemed foreign in its tissues.

Now there are many published articles detailing the variety and extent of skin symptoms in fibromyalgia. All kinds of other weird effects appear. We expect patients to report tingling sensations in their fingers, toes, or scattered areas such as the face and lips. Crawling feelings anywhere on the skin feel like errant hairs or insects that are never there. Burning can be felt anywhere on the surface of the body, commonly on the back of the neck, arms, or thighs—or sometimes the opposite, a cold swatch of skin.

Fibromyalgics routinely cut irritating tags off their clothes before putting them on for the first time. Fiery hot, itchy soles and palms can be relentless. So intense is this burning sensation that I would pull my feet out from under the covers even on a winter night. Symptoms in my hands were best relieved by holding bagged ice wrapped in a washcloth. I'm certainly not the only one who has made such improvisations.

> I have struggled with sensitive skin since childhood. I could never wear certain fabrics. They would make me itch and break out in rashes. I learned to wear only 100 percent cotton fabrics and my underwear and socks inside out, so the seams would not irritate my skin. My undergarments were always washed separately and set on extra rinse. The blankets on my bed were 100 percent cotton and very light. I kept them untucked as it was cooler that way and I never liked the weight of them on my skin. It would annoy me and make me feel very hot and itchy. Jewelry and watches were also a problem. My chest and neck area would turn bright red from my necklaces no matter what the metal. If I wore a watch, my wrist would often feel tingly and numb and then a dull, heavy ache would set in.
>
> —*Chantal H., Michigan*

Nearly all fibromyalgics experience itching. It's generally worse and spreads at night because of the warmth generated under blankets. Humid weather is also a trigger. I soon learned not to scratch. Even gentle rubbing seemed to set in motion a seven-year itch that didn't stop even when my skin was bloody from scratching. When itching began in the evening, I knew I was in for a particularly sleepless night.

Generalized hives (urticaria) are among the worst rashes. A woman flight attendant was the first to show us how intensely those could affect a person. For many years, she suffered bouts of a strange type of giant hives that oddly involved only her face and neck. Each patch was accompanied by an underlying redness and an unusual amount of swelling. She described herself as looking "like a gargoyle." We finally saw her during one of those cycles, and I reluctantly complimented her on the accuracy of her description. On hive days, she had to call in sick to cancel flights. She'd undergone exhaustive testing for allergies and autoimmune diseases. At that time, it hadn't occurred to us that this had any connection to her fibromyalgia. Under treatment, the mystery unraveled. She was not the first to realize that hives always appeared during her pain cycles, but she was the first I'd seen with such dramatic symptoms. In between attacks, her skin was clear. Cortisone or topical steroid creams are often suggested for hives, but generally are not very effective. The reason is that hives are caused by dilation of the capillaries, which allows fluid to leak into the surrounding tissue. Angioedema is the result of a similar but deeper process in which fluid seeps ever deeper, permeating the dermis, epidermis, and subcutaneous tissues. Since creams can't penetrate very deeply, they only improve the appearance of surface layers. Yet neither cortisone creams nor topical antihistamines (for example, Benadryl cream) are blockers as long as no plant derivatives have been added, and they can provide modest but welcome relief.

Hives can be acute (episodic) or chronic as mentioned above. Chronic hives are those that have appeared at least twice a week for longer than six weeks, although that number is somewhat arbitrary. In 75 percent of patients, hives last longer than one year; 50 percent, longer than five years. In 70 percent of those cases no cause is ever identified. Allergy skin testing isn't much help because people with hives react to most substances applied to their skin.

Chronic hives are less responsive to treatment and much harder to relieve. Once released, histamine effects are not easily blocked even by antihistamine taken on a regular basis. Antianxiety drugs have been used with some success in select patients, but they cause fatigue and are not used long term. Histamine-2 blockers such as Pepcid and Zantac, or Nexium and Prilosec, work by a different mechanism and may undependably benefit hives, but can be added to antihistamines such as Benadryl or Claritin because they work in different ways. One of the tricyclic drugs, doxepin, powerfully blocks histamine release, so it is often used for patients with allergic skin eruptions. Topical doxepin is marketed as Zonalon, and will not interfere with guaifenesin.

Brief courses of oral steroids may be given for particularly severe outbursts of hives, especially when itching is unbearable. Steroids are counterproductive in long-term usage because of risky side effects such as osteoporosis, immune system depression, cataracts, ulcers, diabetes, and high blood pressure. They can also disrupt sleep and so should be taken early in the day. Ephedrine is a powerful histamine blocker, but raises blood pressure and speeds up the heart. Beta-blockers help a bit (propanolol, atenolol, metoprolol, and more), but they slow the heart rate, drop blood pressure, and may cause fatigue.

Oatmeal is made from one of the plant parts that doesn't contain salicylates and is the mainstay of topical treatments for itching. Colloidal oatmeal can be pricey but is simply finely ground oatmeal suspended in water or another liquid. You can make your own to add to your bath by putting whole rolled oats into your blender and mixing them to a fine powder. You can also use this oats-and-liquid mixture as a face mask if that skin is irritated. If you prefer to purchase it, there are many products, such as Aveeno Baby Eczema Therapy Soothing Bath Treatment.

About 16 percent of patients with chronic hives can identify a physical stimulus for the rash. Exercise is one such trigger for histamine release, as is anything that induces sweating. A few people are sensitive to cold, sun, heat, and/or prolonged skin dampness.

I just got over the itching. It lasted for three weeks. All the Benadryl and prescriptions for itching didn't help it much at all. What helped me was just plain Tylenol or Advil. Heat seemed to make it worse but ice did help. I was also given a prescription for a lotion to use that would keep the skin from looking too bad from all of the scratching. It was Aquaphor ointment. After my itching was finally over, I did go into a pain cycle and am now coming out of it. In fact, today I feel pretty good. Yay Guai!

—*Katy, Alabama*

Don't forget to check your medications: Many have itching as a side effect. If you are taking one or more of these, you might want to discontinue them or swap them out for something else to see if you notice any improvement. Let's look at some of the commonly used medications for fibromyalgia (but remember to check those you take for other conditions as well) that could be adding to or causing the problem.

Acetaminophen has a rare side effect of skin rash, hives, or itching, but with ibuprofen, one of the more common side effects is itching skin. This is true of other nonsteroidal anti-inflammatories such as naproxen as well. Tramadol and other opioid pain medications list itching skin as a common side effect—this is thought to be a direct effect of them binding with their receptors. Duloxetine and milnacipran—two of the FDA-approved medications for fibromyalgia—list burning, crawling, itching, numbness, prickling, and "pins and needles," as possible side effects, but with pregabalin itching is only a rare side effect.

Most of our fibromyalgia patients have visited dermatologists and learned that their scattered dry and scaly patches are eczema or neurodermatitis. The worst case we've ever seen was in a young attorney. His entire body was affected, but most distressing were his cracked, bleeding, and scabby hands. He was so embarrassed that he stopped offering clients a handshake. His appearance so overwhelmed him that he virtually ignored his muscular aches, fatigue, and minor cognitive difficulties. Upon mapping, we found the telltale lumps and bumps of fibromyalgia. While we could at least reassure him about muscle recovery with treatment, we couldn't promise resolution of his skin issues. On guaifenesin, his rash became worse during each of the early reversing cycles. We took that as a good sign. Patchy improvement soon appeared and eventually cleared, never to return.

In my own case, patches of seborrheic dermatitis tormented me. Despite the superficial scaling, some tiny, broken skin areas constantly burned and felt raw. They were concentrated in my scalp and eyebrows, the sides of my nose, and the adjacent cheeks. I would also get intensely itchy, tiny blisters on my fingers. I deliberately burst them since I much preferred the burning of the denuded base I'd left behind. Patients have described similar eruptions on other body surfaces.

Psoriatic lesions often worsen during attacks of fibromyalgia. The issue is characterized by small areas of red–pink, flaky, itchy, and scaly patches. These occur primarily on the scalp, backs of elbows, knees, and lower spine. They're ugly to look at, but at least aren't contagious. As with many other rashes, stress, alcohol, and climate changes make symptoms worse. However, short sun exposures help. The vitamin D derivative Dovonex, as well as coal tar preparations in cleansers, shampoos, and baths, are safe to use with guaifenesin.

One night I was speaking to members of a support group and found it hard to avoid staring at one woman's face. She had been diagnosed with rosacea, which produces a distinctly red color, but hers was a deep magenta. It's another skin problem related to eosinophils, mast cells, and histamines. Eyelids and skin around the cheeks may be worst hit. Red bumps and pimples emerge, and thread–like blood vessels become visible through the skin over time. During treatment, this woman soon observed that her most intense displays cycled in step with her fibromyalgia. She's now symptom–free, and the rosacea has cleared. Dermatologists sometimes prescribe metronidazole cream for rosacea; this does not block guaifenesin.

A less dramatic, restricted, or generalized flushing of the face
or upper torso may appear only during adverse cycles. This condition is called dermatographia and is caused by a linear swelling of
capillaries that force edema into the skin. People with this problem can use a fingernail or blunt instrument to write on their skin
and leave an inscription that remains legible for several minutes.

Approximately eighteen to twenty-four months before I was
diagnosed with FMS, I was diagnosed with rosacea. I was devastated. Now looking back on it, I see that a lot of things were
going wrong back then, but it was the symptoms on my face that
got me to the doctors originally. I took tetracycline daily for three
years. I hated it, but if I stopped, I broke out so bad, and my skin
would peel away, and I was red!!! Within a few weeks of starting the guai, I gave up the tetracycline as an experiment. I have
not used it since. The symptoms have been manageable, although
stress will trigger the rosacea again. Right now I am in a bit of a
flare over a new job, but not enough to send me back to the tetracycline. My eyelashes grew back, and fell out, and grew back. I
am very confident that the longer I am on the guai, the [more the]
scare of rosacea will be behind me.

—*Dawn, California*

Many fibromyalgia patients suddenly experience outbreaks of
acne. It's not uncommon to hear, "I must be in my second childhood," or "I never even had pimples in high school." Acne, white-
heads, and blackheads may be caused by blocked pores induced
by hormonal surges of testosterone. Acne recurrences are frequent
in fibromyalgia, but not pustules or blackheads. If these are sufficiently bothersome, they may be effectively treated using a
mild antibacterial cleanser. During troublesome outbreaks, spot
treatment with benzoyl peroxide or triclosan might work. Acne
products should be carefully screened for salicylic acid, which is
regularly used in soaps, washes, cleansers, toners, scrubs, and so on.

Common sense should be exercised by those with irritated, fibromyalgic skin. Itchy eyes, facial flushing, or flushing of the upper torso and rosacea are quick reminders that mast cells are active. Avoiding triggers is an obvious suggestion. Here are just a few of the most common ones: sun exposure, excessive heat, irritant botanicals, citrus extracts, alcohol, hot drinks or foods, spices, dyes, strong fragrances, and hot baths. Treat dry, flaky skin with regular use of an alpha hydroxy acid cream or lotion. My coauthor, Claudia Marek, advocates AmLactin or Lac-Hydrin. They contain lactic acid, the skin's natural alpha hydroxy. Pamper such skin with gentle moisturizers with a few simple ingredients. Use soap washes and avoid hot water; use warm instead. Some waxy compounds seal in moisture. Prescription retinoids are also okay with guaifenesin: Both Retin-A and Renova soothe acne breakouts if your skin can tolerate them, as will alpha hydroxy products, triclosan, and benzoyl peroxide compounds if not.

FINGERNAILS

> Nearly everyone in my support group can identify with having bad fingernails that break. Lots of us have dry fingertips that are always cracking. My nails finally got so weak that I could not even wear acrylic nails because my nails would bend and break underneath them. It took several years on guai, but now my nails are much stronger. I know they will never be glamorous, but at least they are normal and look presentable.
>
> —*Janeen, Idaho*

During a new patient visit, we have a checklist of sequential questions and check off answers. That's how we get the statistics we quote in this book. That's how we can state with considerable accuracy that "among the last six thousand patients, 75 percent will have…" such-and-such a symptom. One slot on the list asks about the status of their fingernails. Thinning, chipping, and breaking nails are extremely common in fibromyalgia. Sometimes defective nails don't break but instead peel off like sheets of mica. Early in the FM game, nails do fairly well, but they eventually lay down alternating good and bad layers, and suddenly four or five of them break all at once. In long-standing fibromyalgia, they're forever broken or don't even grow. You'll understand this phenomenon by comparing nails to concentric rings in trees. During untreated fibromyalgic cycles, there's an abnormal concentration of debris in the bloodstream. These minute excesses visit all parts of the body, as you've seen in earlier chapters. Tiny clusters of calcium phosphate hunker down in the nail root as fragile and unstructured sediments. Outward growth over the next eight to ten months brings the brittle horizontal ring to the nail tip. There all it takes is minuscule pressure to chip it off from the adjacent, healthier layer like so much dried mortar. Under treatment, nails stay solid for ever-longer periods of time until they become as strong as your individual genetic makeup allows.

Hangnails are common because the softened fingernail easily tears at its edges. I also remember dry, thick, cracked skin around my nails and knuckles before I treated myself. It was hard to explain since the problem lingered throughout the seasons regardless of weather. Cuticles may get dry, irritated, or shred, and the whole area may crack and bleed. Rubbing vitamin E, lanolin, or emu oil into the affected sites is helpful. Immersing fingers into warm paraffin helps, too.

Some fibromyalgics have problems with nail fungus. It's not really related to fibromyalgia, except that the immune system might not be quite up to par. Drugstores sell topical compounds that should be checked for salicylates; the prescription drug Penlac is compatible with guaifenesin. Oral antifungal medications need to be taken for months since nails are so slow to grow out. It may be unwise for patients already on multiple oral medications to add another; it's safer to stick with topical products.

While waiting for the lengthy correction, soothe the areas by gently massaging nails, cuticles, and adjacent skin with the oily substances we mentioned above. Disguising the glaring defects with artificial nails is tempting, but lack of aeration further weakens the underlying bed. Best to let nails regain their normal strength and flexibility. It takes twelve to eighteen months for toenails to grow from the root to the free edge, and eight to ten months for fingernails. Certain paint-on nail strengtheners add synthetic fibers to hold the defective nail together. Use them as first-line treatments to protect vertical fractures from extending down into the nail bed. When you're applying expensive treatments to dead tissue, remember that the visible part of nails lacks nutritive blood supplies. Ignore extravagant claims and just accept that you're coating for cosmetic effects.

HAIR

> You will notice [after beginning guaifenesin] your hair is getting back to normal, actually better. Mine used to be dry, but got to where I could go a few days before I had to wash it (when I was sick, I didn't wash it for three days and it wasn't greasy). My hair is very healthy now. Just give it some time. I am taking 3,600 mg of guaifenesin a day, and have been totally pain free for about three months.
>
> —*Mary B., Florida*

Fibromyalgic hair is often limp, poor-textured, and slow growing; it splits easily at the ends. Defective energy production extends to hair follicles. Test results are usually normal and scalp pathology is rarely found, so we've given up referring to dermatologists unless someone needs a reassuring consultation. Hair normally falls out in cycles, but now a whole bunch may come out at one time. Maybe you understand that when you're sick, but it may also get worse in the fourth or fifth month on guaifenesin. Fibromyalgia reversal goes faster than did the slower accumulation of the compounds that cause it. Convalescence is also accelerated, but defective hairs come out faster than normal ones take their place. It's a good general rule for the entire body: Primarily, sick tissues participate in the cleansing process. Hairdressers are our allies. They're used to instructing clients about periodic hair loss. They easily spot healthy new growth to reassure patients and inspire them not to panic.

Many compounds are advertised to help hair growth, but when dealing with hair loss caused by fibromyalgia, patience is the best medicine. Gentle shampoos, conditioners, and a good stylist are the best weapons, along with time. Minoxidil (Rogaine) is the only product approved for female hair loss. It needs to be applied daily, which is a burdensome chore for someone too tired to make such efforts. New growth is abruptly lost if applications are stopped. Women with hair loss should avoid contraceptives or hormone replacements that contain testosterone or DHEA—both have masculinizing effects on the body.

Two thirds of women and most men lose hair with aging. Don't expect guaifenesin to produce the full head of lustrous hair you never had. Though quality may improve, there's a limit imposed by your age and genetic makeup. When you're reading promotional advertising, remember that, as with nails, only the roots of your hair are alive. What you apply to the hair you can touch and see can only improve surface appearances and how it feels to the touch. Lots of products accomplish exactly that, and they don't have to be pricey.

Other symptoms that fall into the category of dermatological symptoms of fibromyalgia are easy bruising, mottled skin, and painful skin (allodynia). Allodynia is simply a hypersensitivity to stimuli. The pain can be provoked by a light touch to the skin, pressure from clothing, showering, or combing or brushing your hair. Even a light breeze blowing across your skin can be painful. Tactile allodynia is caused by something touching your skin, mechanical allodynia is caused by movement such as wind blowing or clothes rubbing on your skin, and thermal allodynia is caused by heat or cold temperatures. There are no specific treatments for these, although cool compresses or ice packs (wrapped in several layers of towel) could help. Remember to stay away from very cold and very hot things applied to the skin, as they will only exacerbate the problems. Skin stinging when exposed to the sun is an example of this. In severe instances, topical lidocaine or lidocaine patches may be applied. Loose-fitting and lightweight clothes made from natural fibers (layered if necessary) are best during a flare.

With the exception of chronic hives or psoriasis, most dermatological problems are not serious. They can be managed with gentleness, routines such as using lukewarm water instead of hot, and dabbing in place of scrubbing. A few gentle, unscented products are enough. Over time, guaifenesin may render all this attention unnecessary.

I have been losing a lot of hair. The part that I minded most is all of the little hairs that are coming in. I walked in the snow the other day, and when I got home, there was all of this fuzzy dandelion fuzz sticking out—my hair is very curly-frizzy. Then I went to the hairdresser and she was pleased that I had so much healthy new hair coming in. I didn't know that it was new hair growth and that I am on my way to healthier stuff.

—*Jan, Kentucky*

CHAPTER 13

HEAD, EYE, EAR, NOSE, AND THROAT SYNDROME

Years ago in medicine, there was a specialty in head, eye, ear, nose, and throat (HEENT). Then eyes became too complicated to remain part of the grouping, and it's now a stand-alone discipline. Perhaps as a reflection of my years in medicine, this chapter will deal with the all-inclusive cluster of symptoms, all of HEENT. Most fibromyalgics find at least a few problems in their heads—but not the psychological kind, just the outer structures!

> I could always tell when my younger son, Sean, was in a cycle, although he did not complain much of pain. When I would wake him up for school in the morning, his eyes would be almost glued shut with gooky stuff. I would have to put a wet washcloth over his eyes and let it sit for a while to soak this off. The clumps in his eyelashes were stiff and incredibly hard to get out. Those were the days when he would wake up irritable and tired, and have the most trouble in school.
>
> —*C. C., California*

Fibromyalgics have problems with the inner skin, the mucosa, the name given to all moist membranes of the body. These areas are subject to the irritating effects of fibromyalgia. One reason is that the watery secretions that keep them wet become acidic and create surface burning. Eyes react with excessive tearing that dries during the night. As water evaporates, it leaves behind mucus and calcium phosphate crystals. By morning, only a sticky, sometimes gritty "sand" lies in the corners of the eyelids. It's a mistake trying to rub it away since lids get scratched and then remain irritated for a few days. It's better to rinse and gently dissolve them using a wet washcloth.

Table 13.1

Head, Eye, Ear, Nose, Throat

	Male	Percentage Male	Female	Percentage Female
Number of Patients	835		4,601	
Headaches		84		94
Frontal Headaches	465	56	3,098	67
Occipital Headaches	407	49	2,978	65
Generalized Headaches	312	37	2,078	45
Dizziness	613	73	3,881	84
Vertigo	154	18	1,781	39
Imbalance	654	78	3,633	79
Faintness	149	18	1,413	31
Blurred Vision	390	47	2,938	64
Eye Irritation	497	60	3,290	72
Nasal Congestion	580	69	3,116	68

Table 13.1 (Cont.)

Head, Eye, Ear, Nose, Throat

	Male	Percentage Male	Female	Percentage Female
Abnormal Tastes	409	49	2,848	62
Bad Taste	315	38	2,381	52
Metallic Taste	252	30	2,158	47
Ringing Ears	483	58	2,853	62
Unusual Sensitivities	234	28	2,067	45
Light	225	27	1,621	35
Odors	137	16	1,781	39
Sounds	144	17	1,384	30

It's tough not to keep fingering itchy lids. Imperceptible, soapy residuals are forced into already damaged tissue. That further removes protective mucus, and if the eyeball shares the irritation, vision blurs. Even dim light from TV screens makes patients wince, and brighter sources are downright painful. Contact lenses are extremely irritating at these times, get cloudy, and need constant cleaning. Light sensitivity occurs, and patients instinctively shove sunglasses into place, anticipating the sunlight. Ophthalmic-safe creams help the lids, and artificial tears provide a protective corneal cover. Hold something cool over the eyes; use chilled cloths or well-wrapped ice inserted into plastic bags to keep water from further irritating the lids. Tissue around the eye is thin and very sensitive and may get "burned" by anything excessively cold (or hot). Patients may also be sensitive to the bright light from televisions and computer screens, for which a blue filter can be installed for comfort. Screen light can also be dimmed. For reading, the non–backit Kindles are easier and less stressful. If oncoming headlights are painful when you drive at night, you can buy special glasses at most pharmacies that are tinted yellow.

Blurred vision can have other causes as well. There are four eye muscles attached to each eyeball. They're hooked into the orbits and coordinate eye movements. Any or all of the eight can be affected by fibromyalgia. In my early years with the disease, I could feel swelling, spasm, and tenderness in any one of them at different times. Blurred vision results when these fibromyalgic muscles tire from trying to synchronize focus.

The lens of the eye is a living gel-like structure. It participates in fluid shifts and admits nutritive substances through its membranes. Blood constituents move in and out under tight control. Just as glucose can enter to excess, so can calcium phosphate. Any ion intrusion has to be accompanied by water to guarantee safe dilutions. Extra water loads thicken the lens and alter the focal point to induce temporary nearsightedness. When it's eventually sucked out, the lens flattens to a more farsighted state. This ever-changing lens thickness causes blurring, and fibromyalgics periodically fight to maintain focus. Remember, reversing cycles reproduce symptoms, so blurring will occur whether the disease is getting better or worse.

At other times, both eyes get dry and red, or what we call injected. Tears don't stream out adequately; even the mucous channels get dammed up. When inner eyelids desiccate, patients blink excessively. It doesn't help much since few coating lubricants are there to meet the challenge. Eyelid muscles blink and twitch with rapid winking, suggesting a nervous tic. The only way to stop this is by holding light finger pressure on the lid. Since dryness may provoke this scenario, wet with artificial tears. There are many over-the-counter brands and prescription formulations, such as Bion

Tears, GenTeal, Lacri-Lube, and so on. An eye specialist who treats patients with fibromyalgia reported that tear production may be decreased by 90 percent, and this may even be worsened by many medications.

Many drugs used for fibromyalgia and other conditions list dry eyes as a side effect. Antidepressants (tricyclics and SSRIs) can cause problems, and so can antihistamines. Birth control pills and other hormones, especially estrogen, can affect how much water goes into your eyes, as can beta-blocker blood pressure medications. Other blood pressure medications may contain a diuretic such as HCTZ, which can add to the problem for more obvious reasons. It's rare but possible that anti-inflammatories can make dry eyes worse.

> I am forty-seven and have had dry eyes for what seems forever. I recently had to go to the doctor it got so bad. My left eye first turned so red I thought I had an infection. Then because the antibiotic dried it even more than normal, I scratched my eye with my own eyelid. That was corrected, but the dryness continued. My doctor gave me a prescription for an eye drop. This I use in the a.m. and p.m. In between for lubrication I use Bausch & Lomb artificial tears. My eyes still get "glued" in the a.m., but not as bad. So it has gotten somewhat better, just not cured. I do believe it is the fibro. I always had dry eyes, just not as bad. They will probably start to get better at times and worse at times.
>
> —*Christine, California*

Resting your eyes in a cool dark room can help when they itch and you have problems focusing. Many patients report that eyeshades (the kind you wear to travel) are helpful. Relaxation is the key to help with the muscle spasms, so a warm compress is a simple thing you can add.

EARS

. I, too, have noise sensitivity that comes and goes. Some days I
cannot tolerate the sound of the TV or radio. I cannot tolerate
noisy neighbors who play the radio with the bass blaring into my
home. It drives me crazy and I have been known to tell some
of them off for it. Sometimes I cannot tolerate the noise in restaurants of people talking, kitchen clattery, etc. Other days noise
does not bother me. I can say now that after these years on guai,
it is getting better. But I was raised on a farm, where there was no
noise, and to this day, I miss it.

—*Char, California*

Women have more acute senses than men, and they're kicked up
an octave or more during bad flares of fibromyalgia. Regardless of
sex, heightened sensitivities to light, sounds, and odors are common in fibromyalgia. Any of the three can trigger headaches and,
oddly enough, nausea. For some reason, television noise is sometimes unbearable, especially when shows have built-in laugh or
augmented soundtracks and loud music. Anyone with a fibromyalgic spouse is familiar with the anguished shout from the next
room: "Turn the TV down!"

Ringing in the ears can start suddenly out of nowhere. It's
almost always brief, but occasionally it persists for hours. If that
sound is steady and unchanging, it's usually not due to fibromyalgia. Less frequently there's a buzzing or the sensation of flapping
insect wings deep in the auditory canal.

Hearing is at times dulled, and momentary deafness may follow though it's usually on one side at a time. Many years ago,
I lost my hearing in one ear for two days. I was in my thirties,
and the sudden onset was frightening. A colleague looked into
the canal and found nothing. My premature deafness cleared as
quickly as it appeared and never returned—well, except from
a different cause in my eighties. Externally, the ears may turn a

glowing red like a Christmas tree ornament that's been plugged into a light socket. They feel burned and, at times, sensitive to the touch—forget about trying to wear earrings. The canals may itch and invite a Q-tip misadventure that temporarily satisfies, but usually resurrects the same discomfort within a few hours. If flakiness and dry skin are visible, you can apply a gentle oil with care so that you don't push dead skin deep into the canal. Emu oil, because of its anti-inflammatory properties, is a good choice.

Generally, the symptoms arising from the ears need little intervention because they come and go so rapidly. Tinnitus spells become most unwelcome intrusions that make it tough to get to sleep. At quiet times, noises in your ears are unnerving, especially if they're unrelenting. There are counterbalancing, noise-producing gadgets that mitigate the steady drone; quiet music may also render offensive sounds less audible.

> Someone recommended the book to me *Too Loud, Too Bright, Too Fast, Too Tight: What to Do if You Are Sensory Defensive in an Over-stimulating World*, by Sharon Heller, Ph.D. Whether my sensory defectiveness came along with the FMS, I am not sure, but this book sure helped me understand these things better. It also helped explain things to my nine-year-old son.
>
> —*Kathy, Florida*

The sensation of ear fullness and earaches are other common symptoms that may be experienced. Generally these two symptoms do not occur bilaterally at the same time. One ear may hurt or the other; rarely do they both cycle at the same time. If you are suspicious that an earache has an infectious cause—perhaps it occurred after a respiratory infection—you can have your doctor or nurse practitioner look inside. Remember that ear infections are uncommon in adults even if you've been exposed to children who have one.

NOSE

> My sinuses have cleared up considerably—I used to have a tissue
> in my hand twenty-four hours a day. Now I'm not even taking
> Allegra except during ragweed season. I used to get colds or sinus
> infections three to four times a year. I haven't been sick since I
> started guai.
>
> —*Karen, Texas*

Nasal membranes, like the body's other membranes, are not immune
to fibromyalgia. Histamine release can cause sudden bursts of liquid
mucus either externally from the nose or as postnasal drip. Waking hours may be spent sniffing, blowing noses, or clearing throats.
Mucus drainage is usually clear; the appearance of yellow or green
phlegm can indicate a superimposed infection that requires treatment. Because of the excess mucus, affected individuals mistakenly
blame their sinuses for the frontal headaches of fibromyalgia. Antihistamines may dry some of the offending discharge; during the day,
be sure to use nondrowsy varieties. We've mentioned before that the
bodily secretions of fibromyalgia are acidic. Delicate nasal membranes
are easily burned by surges of watery mucus. Inopportune bursts of
sneezing are triggered by such irritation and represent nature's effort
to blast out some particulate offender. Itching of the nasal tip emerges
out of nowhere; even with rigorous rubbing, relief is scant.

Facial rosacea also attacks the nose, causing it to light up and
swell a bit. It's slightly suggestive of Rudolph's dilemma and
requires a lot of powdering to dim the glow. Patchy areas of pimples and irritation can occur anywhere on the body but are most
annoying on the face. The dry mucosa of the nose may crack and
easily bleed. Mineral oil, vitamin E, or plain Vaseline can soothe,
coat, and protect the area. If you have sensitive skin, you may prefer a soft cloth handkerchief to nasal tissue, which can be irritating. There are some softer varieties on the market, but make sure

they don't have added lotion (which can be more irritating) or aloe (which will block your guaifenesin).

For affected patients, odors can be amazingly oppressive. Sensitive patients become ill from exposure to scented lotions, colognes, and perfumes. They don't fare much better with natural odors, from flowers with strong scents to fish to the smell of cooking oils. Headaches may spring up after a brief exposure, sometimes accompanied by nausea. It often takes some effort to find personal and household cleaning products that don't irritate or set off symptoms. It's difficult to totally avoid exposure given the prevalence of fragrances and heavy perfumes in public places, although this is much less frequent than it used to be. Some patients have to submit requests for participants at planned events to abstain from using scented products. Some patients are actually disabled because of their sensitivity. Today there are many fragrance-free and even no-masking-fragrance products available. Here's something important to know about the labeling of topical products: Products labeled fragrance-free or unscented often simply contain no perfume, whether synthetic or naturally derived. But such products might still have a scent—the ingredients' intrinsic scent. It is also true that in some cases where a product is virtually scent-free, "masking" fragrance may have been used in the product to cover up the naturally occurring smell of any of the ingredients. ("Parfum" or "fragrance" would be on the ingredients list.) Customers simply come to know that these products are not perfumy. This is common in soaps, where the raw materials have an unpleasant odor. There are product lines that label products "Fragrance-free. No masking fragrances." One of these is the line Vanicream; another is Free & Clear. A small line called Magick Botanicals also contains neither; likewise products from Cleure (www.cleure.com). All Cleure products are also salicylate-free. It's best of course if you are very sensitive to smell to stay with tried-and-true products.

THROAT

I've...found that sinus problems and IBS can both cause bad breath. For at least ten years, I've finished brushing my teeth by brushing my tongue and brush way to the back (I have no gag reflex). My daughter commented how I don't have bad breath anymore as I used to have from time to time. I don't have the chronic sinus drainage that I used to have before guai, nor the allergies and such, either. IBS is fading, too. Guai is changing my life one step at a time...or is that one pill a day?

—*Sandy, California*

The entire surface of the mouth and throat is lined with sensitive membranes. Salivary glands secrete digestively helpful but also unwanted compounds, which include phosphate (phosphoric acid). Such acidic secretions can scald like an excessively hot cup of coffee, leaving a burned sensation. We can blame similar secretions for the sour or metallic tastes that can linger for long periods of time. Saliva leaks out during sleep and causes rashes around the corners of the mouth (more often visible in small children and fair-skinned people). More distant membranes aren't impervious to the acid wash, which can cause a sore throat or dry, hacking cough. Menthol-free cough drops, such as Halls Fruit Breezers, xylitol "mints," and old-fashioned Luden's are some products that won't block guaifenesin. Avoid mint, mentholated, and medical-strength herbal lozenges.

Let's not forget dental calculus. We discussed the nature of tartar crystals very early in this book. You may remember that they're largely made up of calcium phosphate, components pouring out from saliva. These small crystals wedge between the teeth and invade surrounding tissues to cause gingivitis. Salivary glands may swell slightly, ache, and become tender when irritated by their own acid contents. It's not uncommon for gums to bleed when brushed, especially in the early stages of reversal as tartar softens.

The tongue sports the largest number of oral taste buds. Like any other muscle, it may become tender or feel as though it's been cut. Sometimes only the borders are affected, as if they'd been abraded by an emery board, and can be unduly sensitive when rubbed against the teeth. Foods may seem altered, tasteless, or distressingly foul. During fibromyalgic flare-ups, mouth sores can occur; sometimes this is a herpes (cold sore) resurgence, but often they're of unknown, not viral origin (aphthous stomatitis). Smaller sores can be chemically cauterized using an old-fashioned styptic pencil. Various compounds will shorten a true herpetic cold sore onslaught, including Abreva, the oral medications acyclovir and famciclovir, and zinc lip balms.

As a dentist who treats patients with fibromyalgia, I often get complaints of constant battles with bad breath. There are many reasons why this occurs, including medication, oral hygiene habits, the foods you're eating, the dental products you use, and old, defective fillings, crowns (caps) or dentures. Many medications have a side effect which leaves the mouth dry. This is a major contributor to bad breath. In general, bad breath is caused by sulfur gases that are given off by bacteria. If you clean your mouth thoroughly—flossing, brushing the gums and cleaning the tongue—bad breath will be history.

—*Flora Stay, DDS*

A common complaint in fibromyalgia is dry mouth, with or without dry eyes. It's sometimes part of the illness, but just as often it's a side effect of medication. Antidepressants, sleeping pills, antihistamines, hormones, blood pressure medications (especially beta-blockers), diuretics, nasal decongestants, anti-inflammatories, and muscle relaxants are among the most common. Consult a physician before altering the dosage of a causative medication. Treatments include toothpastes designed for dry mouth such as Cleure unflavored (www.cleure.com) and their nonmint xylitol breath fresheners, which increase salivary flow. Sugar-free lemon drops or other tart candies can be helpful, too. Strong flavors such as cinnamon may further irritate the oral tissue. *The Fibromyalgia Dental Handbook* by Flora Stay, DDS, addresses fibromyalgia's effects on the mouth.

Sensitive teeth haunt many patients, especially after they've had chemical bleaching. Topical fluoride gels may be painted on surfaces as a restorative treatment. Again, get a nonmint brand such as those marketed by Cleure or Colgate (PreviDent).

People who have fibromyalgia hurt all over. The pain often extends into their teeth and jaws, leading patients to believe they may need a filling or root canal. This is often caused by pressure on a nerve; a dental problem can be easily ruled out by an exam if the pain persists. The sore throat of fibromyalgia is usually unlike that of an impending infection. It's more superficial and not helped by swallowing, clearing, or coughing. Patients may raise only the usual clear mucus. Spastic outside, mid-neck muscles may impinge on nerves and cause an intense sore throat indistinguishable from a strep infection. The absence of swollen glands upon examination can distinguish between the two. Swallowing is sometimes downright painful, as though a foreign body or tablet were locked in some deep recess. This sensation can last for weeks, but causes no tissue injury.

My ENT says my larynx is swollen, but other than that couldn't find anything wrong. I've been really hoarse all this time and the left side of my throat is also swollen. (He saw that it was swollen also when he did the scope on my throat.) He is sending me to a voice specialist in Salt Lake. I've had throat problems a lot in my past. I'm fifty-six years old. My tongue has had sores on the left side and on the front that come and go. I have been diagnosed with fibromyalgia and my regular doctor says this is all part of it, maybe from a swollen tendon in my neck.

—*Elaine, Utah*

When dealing with these symptoms, recall how they came and went while you were developing the illness. On guaifenesin, they'll also resurge when you're clearing. Since they keep popping up, how will you tell whether you're improving or further regressing? Don't focus on just one problem, but survey all of the components of fibromyalgia at one time. If you can't get a decent mapping, the only method you have to evaluate any systemic benefits of treatment to date is by keeping a simple symptom diary. For example, progressively more good days and less intense down ones is a reliable indication that the treatment is working.

MISCELLANEOUS SYMPTOMS

> Profuse sweating—I'm thirty-five now, [and] this started when I was around twenty-three. I thought it was peri-perimenopause. It wasn't. I always felt like I was burning up inside from the inside out. I would be dripping with sweat. It was very embarrassing.
>
> —*Chantal, Michigan*

Every time we write a paper or book, we have leftovers, symptoms that don't fit into any category. They reflect the overall metabolic problems facing the body. Let's take a moment to look at them here.

Weight Gain

Most fibromyalgia patients gain some weight, and about 35 percent put on twenty or more pounds. We mentioned the loss of mitochondria that occurs in sedentary people. Muscle biopsies have shown up to 80 percent fewer mitochondria when compared with well-toned athletes. Lacking a full complement, we're left with fewer food-burning stations to eat up calories. Insulin to the misdirected rescue: If you don't burn it, store it. And fat cells are very accommodating. (See table 13.2.)

Table 13.2

Miscellaneous Symptoms

	Male	Percentage Male	Female	Percentage Female
Number of Patients	385		4,601	
Weight Gain	212	25	1,701	37
Allergies	196	23	1,328	29
Palpitations	370	44	2,757	60

Just about the only success we've had with weight loss in fibromyalgia is by using the strict low-carbohydrate diet that we detailed in chapter 6. Low-calorie diets may further slow metabolism, especially over time. By contrast, carbohydrate restriction doesn't have the same effect because of fat and protein substitutions. Wouldn't weight loss improve your self-image and mobility? Once you get moving, you'll re-create mitochondria and, thereby, replenish your stamina and energy storage capacity.

In the last year, my symptoms became so severe that I took matters into my own hands. I read every book I could find on the subject. When I finished *What Your Doctor May* Not *Tell You About Fibromyalgia*, I knew I found the answers I was looking for. I started the protocol in mid-August and immediately felt that my body was changing in response.

I still struggle with doctors who think I'm trying the latest fad and family who think I'm so desperate for a cure that I'm just imagining improvements. The latest neurologist I've seen thinks that fibromyalgia stems from depression. I told her I've never been depressed. I wish I would have known this when my father was still alive, because he had the same symptoms.

—*Ruta S., California*

Temperature Regulation Problems

Patients complain of low-grade fevers, and in rare cases the thermometer may register over one hundred degrees. The majority of fibromyalgics sweat excessively at any time. Even minor fevers break at night, interrupt sleep, and drench bedclothes. Hot flashes are common in both sexes—I joke that I went through menopause at age thirty-two. The body's thermostat malfunctions in various ways, and you may feel comfortable only in a very narrow temperature range. You may rapidly switch from too hot to too cold. Layer clothes that easily go on or off for fast coping; keep a jacket or shawl handy.

Water Retention

We've previously discussed water retention, so we won't review the physiology here. The body holds on to what only seems like excess water. It has to retain two or three pounds during attacks to facilitate the ionic shifts of calcium, sodium, phosphate, chloride, potassium, and magnesium as well as larger-size compounds. Water accumulation will go into either direction: depositing or reversing attacks. It's the same chemistry going forward or backward. During cycles, fibromyalgics are accustomed to swollen eyelids and hands upon waking; rings temporarily don't fit. During the daytime, gravity rules, and fluid dutifully slips out of the arms and torso to the legs. By late afternoon, shoes may not fit well. Without obvious swelling, skin is stretched from within. Internal edema tugs on millions of tiny nerve endings and indeed makes legs restless. Add foot and leg cramps for a miserable night. Vitamin E (800 mg) or magnesium at bedtime undependably ameliorates symptoms. The FDA no longer allows physicians to prescribe quinine tablets for cramping, but you may certainly drink a few ounces of sugar-free quinine water at dinner. A quarter cup of pickle juice has been shown in studies to stop foot and leg cramps. Medications should be reserved as second-line therapy because of their side effects. The first-line medications for restless legs are Requip (ropinirole), rotigotine (Neupro), and Mirapex (pramipexole). All were developed to treat Parkinson's disease. Nausea, light-headedness, and fatigue are the main side effects. These are not recommended at all for patients who have severe symptoms less than three nights a week. They do not treat or cure restless leg syndrome; they simply help control symptoms.

Dopaminergic agents are the second class of drugs approved for restless legs. As with the first category of dopamine agonists, these have rather severe side effects and are not generally prescribed in the absence of severe symptoms. These drugs, including Sinemet—a combination of levodopa and carbidopa—increase the level of dopamine in the brain and may improve restless leg sensations. However, they may actually cause a worsening of symptoms after daily use. Side effects include nausea, vomiting, hallucinations, and involuntary movements (dyskinesias).

As with other symptoms of fibromyalgia, benzodiazepines such as diazepam (Valium) may be prescribed to help with sleep. They aren't known to do much more than that. Opiates were once used when other drugs didn't work, but these days that is extremely rare because of addiction issues. An old blood pressure drug, clonidine (Catapres), may work in the brain stem to turn down the involuntary movement of the muscles. It can cause problems with your heart rate, cause weight gain and shortness of breath, dizziness and drowsiness.

As with other symptoms of fibromyalgia, it won't hurt to check the side effects of your medications. In this case, allergy and cold medications, antidepressants, and antipsychotic or anti-nausea drugs are the most common ones that make restless legs worse.

Cold compresses on the legs before bed can help, especially if you experience tingling.

Exercise and stretching can help, too. Flexing ankles to stretch your calf muscles before bedtime is a common, simple thing to do.

You'll find a lot of information and videos on the internet if you search for "yoga and restless legs." As with other uses for yoga, the stretching and the meditation and breathing are all equally beneficial and are a formidable team.

Each reader could probably add to this symptom list. Remember the sudden leg kick or arm jerk just as you're falling asleep; intermittent nightmares; boil-like tenderness of your scalp; sudden toothaches though nothing's wrong; sharp stabs that run through your ears; unexplained shivers or total-body chilling; vibrations that come out of nowhere; electric currents that zigzag down your extremities? They're all real and not figments of your imagination. Always remember that our theory supports the notion that many cells in the body are struggling to fend off the sieges of fibromyalgia.

CHAPTER 14

PEDIATRIC FIBROMYALGIA

When I was growing up, my nickname was "Slow as molasses in January." As I grew older, the sense that I was not like other children deepened; I could not stand still and hold my arms out to have my clothes fitted; I needed more sleep but could not seem to get it; I had little energy and took refuge reading, lying down on a window seat instead of playing outside. Burying myself in books, I felt the pain and difference of my childhood less acutely, but the guilt was always there; I felt that I was failing everyone around me by not being like them, by not being able to do what they did so effortlessly. My parents, after taking me to the doctor for thyroid tests, concluded that my tiredness was a character trait and not an illness, and I grew up believing them, never having heard anyone say otherwise.

—*Cynthia C., Michigan*

FACING THE PROBLEM: DID I GIVE MY CHILD FIBROMYALGIA?

As we learn more about fibromyalgia and reflect how it's affected our lives, we become aware of similar symptoms in those around

290

us. Some will confide that they have the illness by name; others we can diagnose if we just listen to their complaints. And since fibromyalgia runs in families, it's inevitable that it lurks close to home. This is exactly the reason why we have treated so many families over the years, dating from back before fibromyalgia had a name.

During the process of guaifenesin reversal, it's inevitable that we stare face-to-face at the child we once were—a child with abdominal pain and side stitches; or unexplained headaches; perhaps baffling irritable bowel syndrome; or growing pains in the lower legs and knees so we woke crying at night; wrenching charley horses the day following gym class; hours and days with fatigue and that drifting brain that just wouldn't concentrate in school. Sometimes this reminiscing is actually healing, because we can forgive our own shortcomings and understand that we suffered from a very real illness that was not understood at the time.

During this process, we may sadly realize that one or more of our children are facing the same struggles. Nearly every day, a parent asks, "My daughter has bladder infections and growing pains—is it possible she has fibromyalgia?" "My son used to love sports, but now he won't even dress for PE. Something's always bothering him—could he have fibromyalgia?" The list grows and we're asked about lethargy, headaches, former A students who suddenly don't achieve—all in the same anxious tones. Parental suspicions usually translate into accurate diagnoses.

If you or anyone in your family has fibromyalgia and you're suspicious, look as objectively as possible at your child. No doctor on earth will ever know that little person as well as you. What should you look for? We've mentioned that kids don't very often fake pain; if they do, it's usually to get out of doing something obvious. They're not seasoned actors, so the put-on is fairly transparent. Not well coached in the role they're playing, they can be easily distracted. Part of your challenge is that they may be fairly inarticulate and nondescriptive. They won't say much more than "it hurts" or "I've got a headache." Younger children, or anyone who's had the disease a long time, can't recall being without this or that symptom. As we said before, they don't identify themselves as unusual or abnormal. Always tired? Just constitutionally weaker than their peers. Having no wellness point of reference, they don't know what's unusual about growing pains and daily headaches.

Focus on your observations. Are your children exhausted some mornings even though they've had a substantial amount of sleep? Have you seen them leave off playing with friends or siblings and lie down for a spontaneous rest or nap? Have you witnessed intermittent difficulties with memory or concentration? You might notice that they easily complete tasks one day but badly fumble on the next try. Do they have abdominal pain, constipation, and diarrhea? Does your daughter have bladder infections, painful urination, or vaginal irritation? Do they complain of leg and knee pains by day and seemingly more vicious ones by night?

> It was not his aches and pains that made me realize my son had fibromyalgia. It was the simple observation that some days he could do his homework with little effort and a few days later he could not write a sentence without many errors. On those days he was easily frustrated. Tired, [he] could not see or comprehend the errors he was making or fix them. There was a desperate tone to his voice when I tried to elicit answers from him. This touched a chord in me and brought memories of my own childhood flooding back. I recalled days of not being able to spell words I knew very well. I remembered being told to look them up in the dictionary but I could not because I did not have the vaguest idea what letters I was looking for.
>
> —*Claudia Marek, Cedarpines Park, California*

We've had the opportunity to diagnose and treat hundreds of children under the age of ten. In almost all of these cases a parent with the disease, not a physician, first suspected the illness and brought the child to us for confirmation. Children with fibro-myalgia may begin adverse cycling from an early age, a few even before preschool years, but remember that initially those cycles can be far apart, making a pattern difficult to spot. The youngest kids can't articulate where they hurt, but cyclic whining, crying, sleep disturbances, and irritability speak for them. Slightly older children can at least alert their parents about pains in their knees and adjacent structures. These are often dismissed as "growing pains," especially if grandparents are consulted. Since they're often the earliest recognizable symptoms of fibromyalgia, we record them to pinpoint the onset of the disease. In children with higher pain thresholds, fatigue, irritable bowel, or bladder symptoms may be the first clues. Some little girls may begin with bladder infections, vulvar irritation, itching, or pain. One of the key ways that the symptoms of fibromyalgia are obvious in the early period is the way they appear one day and are mysteriously gone the next.

Fibromyalgia is probably easiest to spot in children aged seven to ten years because of the demands of school and extracurricular activities. Pains come and go without rhyme or reason and are recurrent for a few days at first, then months, and finally even for years. About 40 percent of the fibromyalgic adults we question recall having pains in their legs when they were young. Remember, there are no such things as growing pains! The term is actually a misnomer because the hurting begins well before the enormous growth spurt of puberty. Growth is not painful. A baby triples his or her size in the first year of life and doesn't seem to experience any discomfort in the process. Older children with fibromyalgia slowly realize they're not like other kids, but why? "Why" is recurrent: Why was schoolwork easy yesterday; why am I still tired after sleeping twelve hours; why do I have so little stamina when my friends can go and go like the Energizer Bunny?

Lacking comprehension, youngsters soon become adept at making seemingly valid excuses. By the time they're teenagers, many have really good reasons why they hurt or why they no longer want to participate in activities they once enjoyed. But look closely: Those excuses don't really hold up.

> It was with great relief that I discovered my daughter had fibromyalgia...because all the doctors were telling me there was nothing wrong with her and asking "What's going on at school?" as if her pain was some psychological problem. I am even more outraged now than I was when it happened. It can't be said often enough, get your child checked out and treated when they are young, before they are old enough to say "Oh Mom, I don't have FM and I am not listening."
>
> —Lisa W., California

Physicians depend on parents for crucial information and observations. Even then, they may not recognize the early intrusions of pediatric fibromyalgia, much less grasp that there's effective treatment. Parents are on the firing line. They must trust some instincts and long-term observations. Since we can't just sit back and watch our children suffer, discovery and the solution are up to us.

PEDIATRIC FIBROMYALGIA

The diagnosis of fibromyalgia in children started to appear in medical literature in the 1980s, when it was dubbed "juvenile primary fibromyalgia." In 2001, the American College of Rheumatology announced the diagnostic criteria. These were similar to the ones we know in adults, but children needed to have otherwise unexplained pain in only three quadrants of their bodies for greater than three months. Instead of the famous eleven out of eighteen tender points required for adult patients, children only had to have five. They also needed to have several from an additional checklist of symptoms: fatigue, anxiety, poor sleep, or IBS.

This ACR statement confirms what we found: Children do not usually have the full spectrum of symptoms. Understanding the nuances of pediatric fibromyalgia requires us to think somewhat abstractly. The illness must be viewed as a spectrum, with the least affected or youngest child offering the fewest clues.

Officially, symptoms go something like this: 96 percent of the children experience sleep disturbances (versus 75 percent of adult patients). Children have more headaches than adults (71 versus 53 percent), and a greater prevalence of depression (43 versus 32 percent). Measures of pain and fatigue are relatively equal between the juvenile patients and in the literature for adults. Anxiety and IBS are the next most common symptoms.

A significant fact is that boys and girls are equally affected before puberty. When we wrote the first edition of this book, we were just beginning to assemble statistics on our pediatric cases. Of course, since that date, many more families have come in to be examined. While working on our book *What Your Doctor May Not Tell You About Pediatric Fibromyalgia*, a chance observation by my coauthor that we were seeing as many boys as girls struck me as odd. But when we pulled the records from our charts, we documented that she was correct and the sexes were evenly represented.

Most adult patients are female, but that's not so before puberty. So what changes at that time to skew the incidence to 85 percent women in adults? What could possibly happen through the accelerated growth of postpuberty? We finally realized that adolescent muscles and bones soak up great quantities of phosphate. Though both sexes get more massive at that time, boys get much bigger and will have to sustain that size for most of their lives. They may be taking in more phosphate than they could normally excrete, but suddenly their bodies can use every bit of it.

Though the symptoms recede around puberty, the disease will regenerate later in life, sooner in women, maybe in the teenage years or later. Many factors determine how soon symptoms resume, from heredity to physical or mental stressors. Symptoms don't come back suddenly. At first, there's only a bit of nagging during the premenstrual week: Cramps, PMS, and headaches, often of migraine intensity, uptick and strike more regularly. Soon enough, it becomes impossible to keep step with peers in gym activities or on playing fields. Formerly promising athletes tire far too soon and lag behind. The thought of expending energy terrorizes these children, who know that muscular pains will surely follow within twenty-four hours. In the beginning they barely comply with compulsory physical education requirements, but that's as far as it goes.

Pain waxes; stamina ebbs. Brain haze sneaks in, and textbooks might as well be written in hieroglyphics. Without reason or warning, they're upset with dizziness and exhaustion. What good are fourteen hours of sleep? Backpacks weigh a ton. Eyes go in and out of focus; that glassy look is interpreted by teachers as deliberate inattention. We used to call them lazy teenagers, but now too commonly a parent and physician make the diagnosis of attention deficit disorder (ADD). What a rotten conclusion!

We don't have to belabor the fact that school absenteeism destroys a child's academic edge. The new information age grants little mercy in today's fierce competition for college. Slowly, the fibromyalgic youngster loses his or her perpetual catch-up race. Though determined parents may manage to wrench homeschooling tutors out of their budget-conscious school districts, it doesn't compensate for the well-rounding effects of extracurricular activities. Only social interactions with peers can provide certain skills during teenage years. The self-esteem and confidence we desire for our children is hard to come by when successes are isolated and they've been taught to believe they're too ill to compete.

It's imperative for physicians and parents to make an early diagnosis of fibromyalgia and attack the cause, not cover up the symptoms. It will take persistence to accomplish this, but the stakes are high. Our children don't really have many formative years, and it's never too early to show them how to accomplish things by determination and hard work. In general, children haven't lived long enough to see impact on many tissues, so there's less disease to reverse. Recovery is much faster than in adults.

I do not remember a time when I did not have headaches. Since my mother had always suffered from migraines, my headaches seemed to be part of my destiny. The pain in my head was, at least, taken to be real by my family. Not so by the outside world, in which, during my adolescence, I would often hear: Just relax, lie down in a dark room for a few minutes, and take an aspirin. Fasting glucose tests, an electroencephalogram, an electrocardiogram, and other tests at the university clinic showed nothing. I had migraines, and not much could be done beyond living with them. Expensive shiatsu and acupuncture gave me sporadic relief but no more than that. I lived my life around my pain, as frustrated as my doctors. I hid my pain as best I could, but I could not hide it from those closest to me. By the time my daughter was three, every week I was taking a bottle of naproxen sodium and Tylenol, and as much sumatriptan as I could get my doctors and medical plan to provide, and yet I was still helplessly spending my afternoons on the couch. I had severe headaches every day, and most of them were migraines. I felt isolated by my pain, unable to even begin to communicate to anyone what my life was like, and increasingly devastated and guilty from the effect my pain was having on my family.

—*Cynthia C., Michigan*

THE FIBROMYALGIC CHILD

Let's take a quick look at the most common symptoms in children and how they present.

Central Nervous System

Children may become oppressively cranky for no reason. We hear the words *finicky*, *fussy*, *irritable*, and *emotional*. Placating a child is difficult, but this child will also have periods of calm and go weeks or even months without symptoms in the beginning. Inappropriate sleep patterns are very common. Sometimes a youngster will wake crying and resist all consoling efforts. An older child may display fatigue by the unusual behavior of suddenly taking a nap without any urging, quite voluntarily. It is not normal for a child to break away from an activity he or she usually enjoys. An older child may be too tired to study or engage in pleasurable activities. A student who was academically proficient gradually begins to suffer from cyclic learning problems.

Musculoskeletal

Aches and pains, common complaints in adults, can escape attention in younger children for lack of verbal skills. Young children may cry and say things like "my head hurts" but not be able to explain what kind of pain or where it is located. You may hear things like "my legs hurt." Older children may only reluctantly admit to problems; many are in denial because they want to be like everyone else. They prefer melding into their peer group. As with adults, pain in any muscle, tendon, or ligament can be caused by fibromyalgia.

Irritable Bowel

She holds her bottom and says it hurts and is frequently constipated. If it hurts to have a bowel movement she will hold it in. She'll just scream because she has to poop and she is scared. Last time we went to her pediatrician she asked if there [was] any sexual abuse. That is not the case at all! We are just a good wholesome, religious, loving family with a health problem in an embarrassing spot.

—*Sandi, California*

There are few descriptive words for intestinal and excretory functions, and they are seldom among the first ones taught. So a young child's immature verbal skills may hamper his or her expression of symptoms. Many people ask if colic is a part of fibromyalgia, but we just don't know the answer. Abdominal pain, gas, burping, and diarrhea can be symptoms of fibromyalgia. So can constipation.

Genitourinary

I have never been without vulvar pain. I remember my mother putting cold cloths on my genital area and scolding me for whatever it was I was doing to irritate myself.

—*Jayne B., Clarendon, Pennsylvania*

Among the most frequent symptoms of pediatric fibromyalgia are those related to the urinary tract, especially the bladder. Infections often strike those areas even in very young children. The urine may have an intermittently pungent and rather unpleasant odor in both boys and girls. It may be very concentrated and may have a deep color.

When a child complains of any pain or burning on urination, pediatricians will suspect a bladder infection. Girls are often accused of wiping in the incorrect back-to-front direction.

Vaginal problems are less frequent in young girls than in grown women, but can certainly occur. Such symptoms cause little girls to tug at their underwear, trying to pull clothing away from where it rubs or digs into areas.

Dermatologic

We have already listed many rashes in the adult chapter. Mothers often describe one or more of these eruptions in their children. Fair-skinned children are more susceptible than darker individuals. Hives are very common; dry scaly rashes near the nose, eyebrows, and scalp may be observed. Dry, lightly scaled isolated patches may appear anywhere. These do not usually itch, but when they clear they may leave a residual slightly discolored area. The outside of the upper arms or lower legs may suggest eczema.

Miscellaneous

The dry, burning, itching eyes or eyelids of adults are not as apparent in children, but sometimes there will be redness of the whites of the eyes, and children may repeatedly rub them. Tear glands can extrude a gritty caked material from the inside corner of one or both eyes, especially at night. Irritation of the nasal membranes is frequent. The nose may run with clear mucus, and there may be chronic sinus congestion. Mucus may also back up in the inner ear, and a slight hearing impairment may ensue. Although fever always raises the suspicion of infection, adults and children often run low-grade temperatures during adverse cycles. In children, this can mean readings slightly above one hundred degrees. Because the child also becomes irritable, cries frequently, and cannot be pacified during such cycles, infection is logically suspected. Yet when fibromyalgia is the culprit, symptoms never localize to any particular system, and the fever mysteriously clears.

A good rule to remember: A young person has not had enough time to develop several diseases. In all likelihood, multiple symptoms and physical abnormalities will stem from only one condition. Alert parents and physicians should be aware of this. Fibromyalgia is not a disease of black and white. There are many color zones in between, and children change as they grow and mature. We have not given you an easy one-two-three bingo check sheet that will make the diagnosis simple. There is no such sheet. But you know what it feels like to have fibromyalgia.

TREATING CHILDREN

She was not like my other two children, who ran and played all day long. She would always sit on the sidelines watching or "holding" other people's things for them. She started to complain of constant neck and shoulder pain. We tried everything but nothing consistently worked. We watched a very profound change in her from when she was eleven through thirteen. She became very foggy in her mind and could not remember the math she had done the day before. She also got discouraged, and every day became a "burden" to her that she felt was becoming too great to bear. We started her on guaifenesin and soon she was sleeping and kept telling me how different she felt. She was able to do her schoolwork and remember what she had learned.

—*Wendy M., California*

Someone once sent us a paper written in 1928 by a family doctor. He described children with growing pains, "great mental and body fatigue," "cold extremities," and "feeble digestion." He listed so many other symptoms that the diagnosis of fibromyalgia is obvious in retrospect. He successfully treated his small patients using a tree bark extract called guaiacum. For some reason, not many pediatricians paid much attention. Sixty years ago, one ingredient was purified to guaiacolate and included in some cough preparations. Five years later, it was synthesized as guaifenesin for another brand. Thirty-five years ago, several companies pressed the compound into tablet form and marketed it in long-acting formulations.

There's no need to go into great detail about the treatment of children, since it's not much different from that of adults. As we've stated, guaifenesin is an over-the-counter medication and is available in various strengths. Tablets may be broken to create smaller doses; there are capsules that might be easier to swallow. Crushing is not advisable—without a capsule, guaifenesin lands directly in the stomach in sudden release, and nausea may follow. There are liquid guaifenesins available (make sure the one you purchase is only guaifenesin—100 mg per teaspoon) as well as pediatric sprinkles (100 mg per packet).

All guaifenesin is bitter, so it takes a bit of ingenuity to hide the taste. Liquids can be disguised in juice. Capsules may be opened and the contents hidden in applesauce or pudding. You may have to delay treatment until children can swallow tablets or mask the distasteful liquid preparations. It's very difficult to force a choking child to keep trying, especially if larger quantities are necessary. We start children at 300 mg every twelve hours and gradually raise their dosage until subsequent mapping shows reversal. With liquid or sprinkles, these should be taken every four hours—but make the total milligrams to start 300 mg twice a day.

As with adults, we remap children after a month of taking guaifenesin. If that technique is not locally available, parents have to wing it and make conclusions based on complaints and behavior. Simple notations about fatigue and pain levels on a desk calendar are really sufficient to monitor progress in most cases.

TIPS FOR MAPPING CHILDREN

Mapping is not simple when dealing with squirming children. Little children hardly submit to any examination, and the tickle factor inserts itself as a strong impediment. We use the same mapping technique, because it helps us make and confirm the diagnosis accurately. Mapping is even more important in children because of their lack of verbal skills. Squirming is not a problem because we are not trying to locate tenderness: We can examine by merely feeling gently. A soft stroking examination will suffice when one's fingers are sufficiently trained. We sometimes resort to an old pediatric trick in tickle-sensitive areas. We ask the children to play doctor and help us conduct the examination. They press firmly atop our own examining fingers as we move them. Tickling vanishes and the child seems to relish participating in the procedure.

Children display far fewer lumps and bumps. However, the left side of the neck (sternomastoid muscle), top of the shoulder (trapezius), and areas inside the shoulder blade are affected in 96 percent of kids with fibromyalgia. About 84 percent have the same lumps on the right side as well. A lump on the left side of the thigh (front and outside) is present in 100 percent of adults, but it's only present in about 75 percent of kids. When it is present, as with adults, it will clear within a month of the child taking the correct dosage of guaifenesin.

Unless the situation is desperate, it's sometimes wiser to initiate treatment at the beginning of summer vacation or the long winter break. This allows more time for rest and avoids simultaneously struggling with reversal cycles, school, and homework. Within a few weeks, most children demonstrate noticeable improvement before classes resume. Parents should not hesitate to begin guaifenesin for a student who, because of impaired memory and concentration, is getting failing grades. Initially, it may be helpful to cancel music or dance lessons for a month or two, depending on the severity of the illness and individual stamina. It's also counterproductive to remove just-for-fun activities so that a child feels left out and weird. If a temporary break is necessary, assure your child that he or she is getting well and will soon resume normal routines. It's also wise to consider resuming activities one by one without waiting for a complete response. Most children can cope just fine even when they've only partially purged. Getting back with friends prompts confidence, takes the focus off the illness, and convinces them that they're not really different from their peers.

It's true, you really do get worse before you get better, but you're going to get worse eventually anyway, so why not try the protocol and get your life back? Last summer my husband, our two young boys, and I started the protocol. It was so rough that it was almost comical, and at times we had to laugh or we were just going to end up crying. All four of us were exhausted, irritable, brain fogged, and in pain, but we set aside the summer to get through the hard beginning months, trusting it would eventually get better. The improvements were slow at first and each one of us responded differently, but as time went on we really began to notice the changes taking place. Slowly we were sleeping better, cognitive and pain symptoms eased, and we had increased energy! This summer, a year later, we have been tackling our ambitious "summer fun" list, checking activities off one by one, making up for last year's lost summer. We have been constantly stopping and taking stock of just how well we are doing, amazed at how far we have come. We are not 100 percent yet but we are so much better than we have been in years! Time on the protocol goes by slowly, yet fast at the same time. Take it one day at a time, do it as written, and you'll see that it works! You have nothing to lose and everything to gain.

—*Erin Woods, California*

HELPING YOUR CHILD DURING REVERSAL

It's tough to watch an ailing child, especially if you're the one who transmitted the defective gene(s). The first few reversal cycles are disturbing, but you should use all of your parental skills to make them tolerable. Preschoolers can rest and take warm baths; most can swallow liquid Tylenol (acetaminophen), Advil (ibuprofen), or the like for pain relief. Insomnia and frequent waking can be countered with diphenhydramine (as in Benadryl, Simply Sleep, or Sominex), which is available in various pediatric strengths.

The many over-the-counter medications for symptoms such as diarrhea, gas, and painful urination need only be checked for salicylates. In general, children's compounds don't contain aspirin because of the danger of Reye's syndrome. (Pepto-Bismol is a rare exception, but is clearly marked.)

We cannot speak out adamantly enough against using strong medications in childhood and adolescence. We have seen too many children who have ended up as quasi-invalids not because of fibromyalgia but from the horrors of habituating drugs. Parents sometimes vicariously suffer their child's pain and become over-protective. They will occasionally even demand of their physicians that narcotics be given for pain and sedatives for sleep. As their children build up drug tolerance, parents become desperate and embark upon the search for stronger drugs. The demand leads to heavy-duty drugs in addictive combinations in an attempt to totally relieve all symptoms.

The side effects of sleeping pills and narcotics take a huge toll on children's lives. Their acuity is dulled, and they may have daytime fatigue (in excess of what fibromyalgia causes) and miss even more days of school. As such times accumulate, children fall farther behind, become isolated, and eventually can no longer catch up.

Because children use fewer products than adults, older ones might actually enjoy helping you find salicylate-free items as you simultaneously teach them. Tom's of Maine makes nonmint children's toothpastes, as does a company called Hello. Kids may also enjoy the citrus flavor produced by Cleure (www.cleure .com). Oral-B's children's line, Zooth, does not contain mint, and Colgate Watermelon is also okay. Janelle Holden, DDS, created a children's line called Tanner's Tasty Paste (www.tannerstastypaste .com), which, like Cleure, contains no mint and no sodium lauryl sulfate.

Children should be encouraged to interact with friends and

stay as active as their illness allows. No matter how often you have to repeat, it's encouraging to hear that nothing's so seriously wrong that time won't fix it. Parents walk a bit of a tightrope at this point. They must display compassion while remaining resolute that some symptoms will be revisited and must be endured. They might need the wisdom of Solomon and the patience of Job to steadfastly hold a sick child to certain standards of achievement and behavior. But in truth, applying common sense and an attentive ear to the child's needs serves as an admirable substitute. Older children quickly learn how to pace themselves, working hard during better periods and resting when they feel worse. Smaller children can't be expected to understand—but then their lives are also less stressful and missed opportunities have fewer negative consequences.

As the parent of a child who may need a little extra help, it's up to you to make his or her needs known clearly and succinctly. Of course, you will also have to work within the limitations imposed by the situation. With perseverance and more than a little prodding, you can set up your child to succeed in his or her world. A tough start doesn't spell disaster, not if you remain firm in the expectation that your child will do his or her best. You will get cooperation if you persist because there are caring teachers and physicians.

One of the first moves with children is to set up a conference with each teacher. Delay is dangerous, because it will eventually become unavoidable, and at that point it may be too late to change opinions. Too many absences and poor grades and too much inattentive behavior may have already convinced some teachers that your child is an underachiever. The simple tactic of using an early approach and explanation will make a big difference. Have an outline and make a list of what needs to be said, but keep it brief. Do not overwhelm teachers with a ream of paper and medical records.

Explain that your child has fibromyalgia; if that draws a blank look, you can try chronic fatigue. A short letter from your physician might be put in your child's file. Explain that symptoms will come and go and most of the time there may be no need for special attention, but at times your child will need help. The best thing for everyone involved is to understand that you have high expectations for your child. Be realistic and don't expect all your goals to be met at this first meeting. You are simply trying to establish communication.

Most children test the system once they're feeling well. At some time or another, expect them to stop their medication. Each of our children has done exactly that; even Malcolm, the original guinea kid, has done it more than once despite his pride at being the first person treated with guaifenesin for fibromyalgia. We have to expect that, as they grow older, they feel that great surge of invincibility required to propel them into lives of their own. Rest assured, they'll grope their way back to the medicine shelf and that bottle of guaifenesin when they feel bad enough. Luckily, since they're young and haven't fallen far behind, they respond as before and quickly make up lost ground.

In summary, guaifenesin is safe at any age. The return road from fibromyalgia enjoys a higher speed limit. The journey is even shorter if begun early. For the sake of our children we, their parents, must trust ourselves to diagnose the illness perhaps sooner than physicians can. We're fortunate to have a reliable medication that so swiftly restores our youngsters to normal. Looking at our affected family, those of us with fibromyalgia will inevitably reflect on our own past. We'll always wonder how different our lives might have been had we been provided an early diagnosis and effective treatment. For most of us, life would certainly have included considerably less suffering and fewer broken relationships. Instinctively, as parents, we can surely appreciate that our sad experiences gave us insight to help our children, and were thus not entirely wasted.

Both of our boys, ages seven and ten, have fibromyalgia. Within the first three months on the protocol we noticed improvement in both of them. One of the biggest things we noticed is how their bodies responded in their tae kwon do class. They would both tire easy and get frustrated and our oldest especially hated the stretching portion because it hurt him so bad to stretch. After just three months on guaifenesin our oldest became so much more limber, stretching without complaint. They both had more energy and could handle the demands of the class without becoming frustrated. They still have bad days as they are cycling, but we have seen such an improvement!

—*Erin W., California*

PART III

STRATEGIES FOR THE ROAD BACK

CHAPTER 15

MEDICAL BAND-AIDS

Currently Promoted Treatments for Fibromyalgia—
What You Don't Know Can Hurt You

Ms. W. presents today in follow-up for depression. States she is significantly better. Feels like a different person and thinks she may have fibromyalgia and has been taking guaifenesin twice a day from a book she red [sic] and states that she is doing much better also. Patient is eager to discuss this novel or book by someone in California about the treatments of fibromyalgia, which she states "has saved her life." A/P 1) Depression: Patient is significantly better and I am happy for her.

2) Myalgias: Also better. Encouraged the patient to continue to take the guaifenesin if it is effective for her.

> *—Actual medical records of patient,*
> *Durham Medical Center*

There is no mystery to the standard approach to treating fibromyalgia. And the saddest part of that statement is that of all the chapters in this book, this one has changed the least in the years since our last edition. The party line is echoed throughout medical literature over and over, and little or no dissent is heard. Therapeutic options arise in scholarly journals such as the *Journal of Rheumatology* and work their way down into publications for general practitioners, chiropractors, nurses, and physical therapists. All footnote the same studies, and the same advice is given, tailored slightly for each target audience.

THE ACCEPTED TREATMENT

> It may well be better not to treat patients with our well-known but hardly effective armamentarium of drugs...Treatments with antidepressants, tricyclics, formal exercise programs—particularly because they do not seem to work—prolong medicalization and dependency, the opposite of what we should wish to accomplish.
>
> —*Frederick Wolfe, MD,* Journal of Rheumatology[1]

So what's the accepted treatment for fibromyalgia? We already know that at best it's only partially effective, because disability claims, alternative treatments, and self-help groups abound. To make matters worse, the deplorable choices patients are being offered by many doctors are not great improvements over simply suffering in silence.

The current party line for treating fibromyalgia is to:

- Assure patients that fibromyalgia is not going to kill or maim them.
- Advocate exercise for resurrecting energy.
- Endeavor to restore normal sleep patterns.
- Suggest physical therapy.
- Suggest relaxation modalities.
- Relieve as much pain as possible using medications the physician feels comfortable prescribing. (This varies greatly from doctor to doctor.)

- Prescribe as many other medications as the physician feels comfortable for relieving fatigue and other symptoms such as constipation (from pain medications), anxiety, and depression.
- When those fail to restore health, help patients file for disability.

On the surface, we can't imagine anyone quarreling with these noble goals. They sound simple enough, and if achievable, they'd be a solution. Or would they? Although exercise, meditation, and better sleep will help patients for a time, none of them will actually keep patients from getting worse. And it is highly unlikely that sick people can push through the pain of even a minor workout on a consistent basis. Using prescription drugs is not the answer. Over time, dosages will increase, as will the list of meds, and side effects will add more complaints to an already long list.

On top of that, the very last item—"Help a patient to file for disability"—will mire patient and doctor in a legal battle. It will require many forms to document just how ill he or she has become, and both will need to testify that there is no possibility of improvement. Generally legal help will be required by a lawyer who specializes in such cases and charges accordingly.

AN OVERVIEW OF MEDICATIONS COMMONLY USED FOR FIBROMYALGIA

The doctor who diagnosed my FMS asked if I was depressed. I was not happy about being in constant pain that seriously disrupted my life, so I said yes. He said that pain and depression are like the chicken and the egg—which came first? He explained it was a cycle, one feeding off the other. He prescribed amitriptyline because it has been known to ease pain. Simply put, I felt drugged: sluggish, detached, hollow, empty, and very unlike myself. I felt no benefit for my pain. I couldn't wait to get off it but I followed directions and tapered off. My senses gradually reawakened and I felt present in the current moment again, better able to appreciate the colors and simple sensations like the wind on my skin and the warmth of sunshine.

—*Jody D., North Carolina*

Since the mid-1980s, antidepressants have been used for fibromyalgia. The earliest of these that are still in use are amitriptyline, doxepin, nortriptyline, and trazodone. It's not really known why they help, but it's primarily through increasing the deep phase of sleep. Side effects include weight gain, dry mouth, constipation, and fatigue. Studies suggest tricyclics gave relief in only 30 to 40 percent of patients; clearly, not much better than the 30 percent accepted as placebo response.

Newer, specific serotonin-reuptake and norepinephrine-reuptake inhibitors are prescribed as though they were no more dangerous than after-dinner mints. Because antidepressants don't seem to be as dangerous as narcotics, physicians continue prescribing them despite the unpromising statistics; making combinations of the various types of antidepressants is increasingly popular. Side effects for these newer classes vary greatly, but most common are drowsiness, nausea, headache, and dry mouth. For fibromyalgics, particularly disturbing can be hair loss, significant weight gain, and lowered libido in both males and females. Papers continually surface questioning whether these drugs have any advantage over placebo. At least clinically, a significant numbers of patients have been helped. In those for whom these drugs are effective, sleep patterns are somewhat restored, depression eased, and pain perception may be diminished up to 50 percent. (However, some people get adversely wired up and suffer serious disruption of stage 4 sleep.)

Although tricyclic medications, notably low doses of amitriptyline and cyclobenzaprine, have been beneficial in controlled therapeutic trials in fibromyalgia, overall effectiveness in patients has not been impressive. Patient self-rating of medicinal therapy has been no better than such nonmedicinal treatments as physical and chiropractic therapy. Only 30 to 40 percent of our patients described medications as very effective. In the only long-term longitudinal study reported in FMS, we surveyed 39 patients for three consecutive years. Although 83 percent of them continued to take some medications, usually multiple, during the three years, only 20 percent felt well.

—*Don L. Goldenberg, MD,* Journal of Rheumatology[2]

The above paragraph is discouraging—and it gets worse! Antidepressants have no lasting benefits for fibromyalgia, even though pain and depression may be temporarily masked. Their effectiveness lessens after about nine weeks, and unfortunately, the disease marches on. Nothing has been done to alleviate the cause, and symptoms simply burst through the drug suppression at some point. Dosages should not be titrated upward. Studies show that if low potencies don't work, then higher amounts won't prove much more effective.

The new "selective" SNRIs (serotonin-and-norepinephrine-reuptake inhibitors) are now the first-line drugs for fibromyalgia pain. Studies have shown these to be ever so slightly more effective for depression than the older SSRIs, but the two classes haven't been studied head-to-head for fibromyalgia. Since these are the newest class on the market, there are fewer of them available. Both types have about the same side effects because of their similar action. These include insomnia, anxiety, sweating (especially at night), muscle pain or cramps, weight gain, fatigue, drowsiness, headache, raised blood pressure, nausea, and problems with judgment, thinking, or coordination. Another common side effect is sexual dysfunction. This might be slightly less common with newer drugs, but it remains a major reason for discontinuation.

Some male patients have reported swollen testicles when taking milnacipran.

Cymbalta (duloxetine) and Savella (milnacipran) are the only antidepressants approved by the FDA specifically for fibromyalgia. Other drugs in this class include Effexor (venlafaxine), which is an older drug and available as a generic. This brings us to the so-called discontinuation syndrome (or withdrawal), which occurs when one of these drugs is discontinued abruptly. Effexor is considered the most difficult one in this class to stop because of its relatively short half-life. But all these drugs should be stopped only under the supervision of a physician.

According to the FDA, all antidepressants have a very serious increased risk of suicidal thinking and behavior, especially in young adults. All antidepressants now carry a black box warning on their packaging. This is the strongest tool the FDA has to issue consumer safety warnings. They are almost always issued for an entire class of drugs because side effects broadly apply to all those related compounds. Unfortunately, black boxes are becoming so common that patients don't always understand their gravity. Investigators recently looked at the twenty different drug classes that made up two thirds of the two hundred top-selling drugs in America. Half of them carried these serious warnings, but the packaging wasn't always clear.

> I have tried Savella. The side effects are pretty horrible. Although it did help my pain, it was just not worth it. The nausea, sweating, hot flashes (to the point of feeling like I was cooking in my oven), fevers, and dehydration were not worth it to me. I was on it for about twenty days until I couldn't take it anymore. Everyone I know has had the same nasty side effects. I have yet to meet someone who has had good luck with this medication. Your doctor might prescribe either Lyrica or Cymbalta or maybe both. I will forewarn you that Cymbalta will give you horrible headaches for

about a week. Most doctors don't offer Lyrica because with most patients it causes serious weight gain or bloating.

—*Melissa, South Dakota*

Muscle relaxants, sedatives, and antianxiety drugs are all commonly prescribed for some of the many symptoms of fibromyalgia. Patients tolerate them only in limited quantities because of the hangover fatigue they generally induce. That and mental fogginess are two reasons patients give for discontinuing them. Confirming their value by double-blind studies is difficult, because sedative effects are too obvious compared with placebo. They don't interfere with our protocol and are helpful for those who handle them well.

Antiseizure drugs have worked their way into the fibromyalgia arsenal. Beginning with Neurontin (gabapentin), a drug designed for epileptic seizures that do not respond to other medications, these began to be used off-label for nerve pain. Lyrica (pregabalin)—a more recent tweak of the molecule—was the first medication indicated for fibromyalgia.

Topiramate (Topamax) is a medication that was originally designed for epilepsy and is now approved for the treatment of migraine headaches in adults and teenagers. It is often used off-label for nerve pain and fibromyalgia. Doses are titrated up, especially when used for controlling migraines, but the side effects of fatigue and dizziness, burning and tingling often preclude patients reaching an effective dose. A recent study linked topiramate to a fourteen-fold increase in birth defects.

MEDICATIONS APPROVED FOR FIBROMYALGIA

The first step in the currently accepted treatment ladder is to prescribe at least one of the three drugs currently FDA-approved to treat fibromyalgia. If a patient is already taking one of them, another will be piled on based on some evidence that at least for a time this will work better than either one alone.

Pregabalin (Lyrica) is not an antidepressant. It was originally approved to treat patients with seizures, and subsequently nerve pain such as from shingles, diabetes, and spinal cord injuries. Researchers aren't exactly sure how Lyrica works to help fibromyalgia symptoms, but it most likely helps decrease the number of nerve signals, which calms down overly sensitive nerve cells.

When used for fibromyalgia, Lyrica is a capsule that is taken twice a day. There's a large range in doses, from 150 to 450 mg a day. Once you start it, you can't just stop. It can start to help with pain in as early as a week but it generally takes longer and doses are usually titrated up. It actually has a modest success rate. In studies only 40 percent of patients saw a 30 percent pain reduction, compared with 29.1 percent taking placebo.

The most common side effects are mild to moderate dizziness, sleepiness, blurred vision, dry mouth, swelling of hands and feet, and commonly weight gain. There's even a term for that—*Lyrica belly*. Lyrica can also have an effect on concentration. It should not be used with many classes of medications, including some blood pressure drugs, diabetes drugs, narcotic pain relievers, sleeping pills, and alcohol. It is not known if the drug is safe for pregnant women. Lyrica carries a special warning for men, who should not take this medication. Animal studies showed lowered fertility in males, and it could cause sperm abnormalities. Birth defects were reported in some of their offspring. It is unknown if pregabalin would do the same in humans, but until further studies, it would seem prudent for men to avoid it.

The second medication that was approved for fibromyalgia was the antidepressant Cymbalta (duloxetine) in June 2008. It was originally used for major depressive disorders, anxiety disorders, and diabetic neuropathy. It belongs to a class of medications called serotonin-and-norepinephrine-reuptake inhibitors (SNRIs). It's not known how exactly it helps with fibromyalgia, but it may also decrease the number of nerve signals on the pain pathways by increasing the level of two naturally occurring substances called serotonin and norepinephrine. These affect mood and suppress feelings of pain. SNRIs block serotonin and norepinephrine from reentering cells, and therefore increase the levels of these substances in the blood.

Cymbalta is taken once a day. The basic dose of 30 mg is often doubled after the first period of treatment. In studies, duloxetine caused a 30 percent reduction of pain in 47 percent of patients (compared with 34 percent of patients in placebo). Dropout rates due to side effects in these studies was a hair under that of pregabalin.

The most common side effects are nausea, stomach pain, loss of appetite, light-headedness, agitation, hallucinations, diarrhea or constipation, and loss of muscle coordination. Suicidal thoughts and abnormal bleeding have also occurred. Drinking with duloxetine is forbidden and may cause liver damage. It has a number of drug interactions including the triptan migraine medications, tramadol, and some of the other antidepressants. It cannot be stopped abruptly; withdrawal studies led to the FDA requiring its strictest warning label.

Milnacipran (Savella) is also an SNRI antidepressant medication that was approved early in 2009 for fibromyalgia. It was originally on the market for depression and psychiatric disorders. It's believed to work by increasing the level of neurotransmitters, the same mechanism as duloxetine.

Savella is a tablet that's taken twice a day and increased over time from the starting dose of 12.5 mg up to 200 mg. Benefits in studies are rather modest: 36.4 percent of patients reported at least a 30 percent pain reduction compared with 28.1 percent on placebo. Common side effects are headache, dizziness, fatigue, swelling of the hands and feet, dry mouth, constipation, hot flashes, palpitations, increased heart rate, insomnia, and weight gain.

Savella has a large number of drug interactions, including anti-inflammatories, other antidepressants, Topamax, tramadol, benzodiazepines, and muscle relaxants. Alcohol is contraindicated, and Savella cannot be stopped without slowly weaning down the dose.

Withdrawal from discontinuing antidepressants is a hot-button topic. What is clear is that it is harder for most people to discontinue them than was initially described by their manufacturers. Information is largely anecdotal at this point, and symptoms are hard to study because many of them mimic the symptoms of depression. Those who have taken the drugs longer than six weeks will likely have some withdrawal symptoms when they are discontinued. Some will require professional help to wean off properly. Symptoms can range from mild nausea, light-headedness, vivid dreams, and headache to panic attacks, hallucinations, tremors, and electric shock sensations in the brain.

Doctors will often add an antidepressant to pregabalin to increase its effectiveness for fibromyalgia. The combining of several classes of these drugs represents a new focus for clinicians, but we urge patients to think long and hard before submitting to adding more and more things to a list with modest benefits and more side effects.

PAIN

By the time patients visit doctors, they have more pain than they can manage by themselves. The brain gives pain priority over other sensations because it is such an important warning signal. Yet as we've seen, there is no damage in fibromyalgia and the pain is chronic, or something that goes on day after day. The result is a brain that has exhausted its resources. Evidence is ample that the body responds in a different way to pain that is consistently present.

There are no medications in the *Physicians' Desk Reference* designated for long-term relief of chronic pain, defined as lasting longer than six months. That's because these medications aren't safe or devoid of serious side effects. In general, chronic pain is more difficult to treat than the acute kind. In normal responses to trauma, the brain masterminds the release of endorphins and other specific hormones to deal with hurting. Nature's idea is to blunt pain enough for the injured body to get to safety. Also, pain is a necessary warning signal that persuades the injured to rest and heal by respecting necessary limitations. The brain isn't programmed for dealing with prolonged hurting because it expects its pain to be a self-limiting messenger.

Even before their initial consultation, patients have tried over-the-counter analgesics such as aspirin, acetaminophen (Tylenol), and nonsteroidal anti-inflammatory drugs such as ibuprofen (Motrin, Advil). A physician may have already prescribed mild muscle relaxants or those that treat nerve pain like pregabalin (Lyrica). Many are already taking an antidepressant from one class or another.

The relief most patients feel with these medications quickly wears off. Before tossing up his or her hands, the doctor may have raised the doses a bit—accepting the collective medical wisdom that, in this case, a little more can be better. But still the patient is in pain and complaining. The primary care doctor has no choice but to refer the patient to a specialist.

At some point the specialist will have to confront the patient's pain with something stronger. It's time to get serious and turn to bigger guns—narcotics. They're all close cousins with different names, some natural and some synthetic, and are marketed alone or in combination with acetaminophen, ibuprofen, or, rarely, aspirin. Readers may already be closely acquainted with some of them: Vicodin, Lorcet, Lortab, hydrocodone, OxyContin, Percocet, Norco, and fentanyl, for example. At first, the pain is certainly dulled, and patients learn to deal with side effects: a little fatigue, nausea, dizziness, and constipation. With the exception of constipation, these lessen over time as the body becomes accustomed to the compound. Hormones related to the hypothalamus (such as estrogen) are reduced, which may be one of the reasons for fatigue and weight gain. A growing number of new studies are showing a link between opiate derivatives and the growth of cancer cells.

The first problem with narcotics is that the body gradually builds a tolerance to them. There's only a certain amount of time nature allows for the efficacy of any particular pain reliever. So they aren't really designed for long-term use. But faced with unyielding pain, physician and patient succumb.

And here comes the catch. When searching for relief from pain, danger lurks at every step, and patients are given contradictory information. They take what are marketed as "safer" pain pills, achieve temporary relief, develop tolerance, and move on looking for more powerful help. Unless fibromyalgia is treated at its root cause, the hourglass runs down.

After just a few weeks of using narcotics regularly, many patients aren't able to muster the willpower to stop them. The narcotic now occupies receptors in the emotional part of the brain, where it produces pleasurable feelings. The body doesn't have to work to produce its own feel-good chemicals, endorphins, anymore. A pill is doing it the easy way. When the plug is pulled, the brain becomes petulant: *You ration me and I'll give you pain like you've never felt before!* Withdrawal means greater fatigue, insomnia, cognitive wipeout, severe anxiety, and more. That's true drug dependence, a physical reaction beyond the control of the conscious mind. When it's time for another dose of narcotic endorphins, the brain reproduces every mental and physical symptom the individual has ever experienced. Fibromyalgics can't discern the difference, since their brains have been expressing identical complaints for years. Even when the patient's fibromyalgia has improved, she feels all the same symptoms. It's nevertheless brainspeak and duplicity. No longer are muscles, sinews, gut, and bladder sending distress signals; the brain now initiates them. Even after guaifenesin has sufficiently reversed the illness, the brain keeps trying to get the narcotic endorphins. Once the narcotic is discontinued, it takes months for the body to begin producing its own natural endorphins again, which makes this period very difficult. This is the reason that patients are put on even more potent and long-acting narcotics such as OxyContin or morphine. The rationale is simply that since these compounds don't wear off as quickly as, say, Vicodin, the patients are spared the discomfort of rebound pain every four to six hours.

Escalating drug use ends up badly, especially these days when opiate abuse is so prevalent and terrifying and on everyone's mind. Doctors are watched and forced to justify prescriptions to insurance companies and medical boards. Patients face intense scrutiny on all sides that even attacks those who only use modest amounts of narcotics and never increase their dose. It is hard to say where this crisis will end and how it will play out for hapless chronic pain patients left without relief.

On this emotionally charged topic, it's hard to get both sides to listen to scientific fact and reason. Narcotic side effects are certainly easier to tolerate than never-ending pain. Dependency is not the same as addiction, which by definition means that drug use is causing a problem in certain social ways. Dependency simply means that the body has come to depend on an outside chemical to fulfill a normal function. The body converts narcotic pain medications to morphine, which occupies pain receptors in the brain, ones that were designed for natural endorphins. When this happens on a daily basis, the brain is duped and cuts production levels drastically, and—especially in fibromyalgics—this can be down to next to nothing. There's no problem as long as the body continues to get the artificial supply, but when a dose is skipped or delayed, there is no longer any natural chemical to replace it. Since endorphin receptors are largely in the emotional part of the brain, depression and apathy also occur.

Long-term release of endorphins promotes desensitization to their effects. As we've seen before in other systems of the body, unrelenting messages are eventually ignored, construed as crying wolf. In this case, they wear down endorphin-producing cells, which finally refuse to respond. The brain gradually produces less, and unneeded receptors recede into the depth of cells, where many are destroyed. Steady narcotic use meets that same kind of ultimate stonewalling: Brain cells tire, reject the opiate signals, and keep right on hurting. Mounting complaints make doctors think patients must be overly sensitive to pain and obviously need heavier dosages. Counterintuitively, narcotics may actually increase pain. They can essentially reset a patient's pain threshold.

Tramadol (Ultram, Ultram ER) is a narcotic-like pain medication that has been studied and shown to be of some benefit in fibromyalgia. It is also manufactured with acetaminophen under the name Ultracet. It binds weakly to opiate receptors and is related to antidepressants. The most common side effects are drowsiness, slow heartbeat, weakness, and light-headedness. Convulsions have occurred at higher doses or in patients who have combined the drug with other medications that raise serotonin levels. Originally touted as not being habit-forming, it is now conceded that it can be, and therefore it should not be stopped abruptly.

Research has shown that low doses of an old generic drug, naltrexone, might help with fibromyalgia pain. At high dosages, it's used to treat opiate and alcohol addiction. It simply blocks opioid receptors and voids their narcotic effects. As a result, opiates and alcohol should not be taken while on naltrexone, or nausea, vomiting, cold sweats, chills, and numbness in the limbs may occur. Naltrexone may also interfere with or counteract over-the-counter NSAIDs.

Use of naltrexone initially increases pain. Side effects include vivid, bizarre dreams, fatigue, spasm, and pain; these usually recede after a few weeks. It is unlikely that large studies will be mounted to test this generic drug since little financial gain would accrue to any drug manufacturer.

Complete relief from fibromyalgia pain is not always possible. If your pain is moderate but you're living a normal life, going back to work, we've made progress.

—*Doris Cope, director of pain management at the Pittsburgh School of Medicine*

So what do you do if you don't take narcotics? Cumulative studies have clearly demonstrated that acetaminophen (Tylenol) can lead to kidney or liver damage if taken in high doses or even if regularly used over several years. That same study found no such problems with some nonsteroidal anti-inflammatory drugs (NSAIDs) such as ibuprofen or naproxen. However, this entire group may induce bleeding ulcers, liver damage, and symptoms that mimic fibromyalgia or even disrupt deep-sleep patterns. The newer anti-inflammatories (COX-1 inhibitors) that are kinder on the stomach appear to be harder on the heart. Celecoxib (Celebrex) alone of the COX-1 inhibitors remains on the market but with a warning label suggesting that it, too, may have cardiac risks.

Recent references suggest that all NSAIDs, along with acetaminophen, can interfere with energy production in mitochondria. If taken before exercise, they can actually interfere with some of its strengthening benefits. However, when compared with prescription compounds, over-the-counter medications certainly have less potential for side effects. The most important thing to remember is that the warnings for excess intake should be heeded.

The official position of the American Medical Association is to use the lowest possible dose necessary of a medication for as short a duration as possible.

Last night before going to bed I took some sleeping pills (trazodone) and an anti-inflammatory (Voltaren). By the side of the bed I put some Bonine because I was feeling a little dizzy, Ambien because I come wide awake every night between 2:30 and 5:30, and if it's earlier rather than later, I knock myself out so I can get a little rest, Tylenol because my spine aches terribly after lying in bed, Pamprin because menstrual cramps can be awful in the middle of the night, and a heating pad (because a few nights before I woke up with a severe calf cramp that crippled me for three days afterward). I ask you, is that normal? I've always hated taking pain pills; even after I ruptured a disc, I refused to take painkillers and sleeping pills. I got through it with difficulty but I survived. Now I am so worn down that I'll take anything if it will help me get some sleep. Every morning I wake up expecting to be normal again. It's a bad dream.

—*Susannah, Maryland*

ENERGY

An alarming trend has begun largely in response to the fatigue, mental slowness, and lethargy caused by narcotic pain medications, especially the more potent ones. It's becoming all too common to see patients of all ages on potent combinations of painkillers offset by a stimulant.

Prescription stimulants include medications such as methylphenidate (Ritalin, Concerta) and amphetamines (Dexedrine, Adderall). These medications are in the same class of drugs as cocaine and methamphetamine ("meth"), and normally increase alertness, energy, and attention. Most commonly used are the newer class called by the cheerful name *wakefulness promoting agents*. These are modafinil (Provigil, Alertec, Modavigil), armodafinil (Nuvigil), and adrafinil (Olmifon). Common side effects are dizziness, suppressed appetite, insomnia, agitation, and diarrhea. They can obviously increase heart rate, raise blood pressure and body temperature, and cause muscle shakes or tremors.

Even stronger stimulants, amphetamines such as methylphenidate (Ritalin, Concerta, and Metadate), amphetamine salts (Adderall), and dextroamphetamine (Dexedrine), are still used in many patients with severe fatigue of other medications. In fibromyalgia, where energy formation is faulty, these drugs are particularly problematic, especially when used for long periods. Although they'll work initially, the cells eventually become exhausted and fail to respond to even higher doses of stimulants, rather like beating a dead horse. The body's energy stores are dragged farther back into deficit spending, and it takes time to recover when the drugs are finally stopped because of lack of efficacy. Side effects of stimulants are pretty obvious: jitteriness, anxiety, and insomnia. They may also raise heart rate and blood pressure. Patients with fibromyalgia, because of the nature of the disease itself, may be more susceptible to rebound fatigue, depression, and anxiety.

Other, less potent compounds that are sometimes used to promote daytime alertness are the antidepressants fluoxetine (Prozac) and buproprion (Wellbutrin).

SLEEP

Difficulty falling asleep and staying asleep long enough to reach the stage 4 phase of restorative sleep is the first major hurdle that we face in dealing with the other symptoms of FMS. I absolutely cannot nap no matter how hard I try, and going to sleep at night requires a ritual of sleep aids, a calming atmosphere, total darkness in the room, numerous pillows piled around my body, a lightweight cover. I would like to trade a day with a normal person who goes out like a light, sleeps deeply, and wakes refreshed. Oh, I wish…

—*Elizabeth R., Georgia*

The desire for restful sleep eventually leads exhausted fibromyalgics to demand sleeping pills. By that time, an expensive mattress, contoured pillows, blackout curtains, and white-noise machines haven't made much difference. Pre-bedtime rituals that initially helped—warm baths, dimmed lights, soothing music, or meditation—no longer work. The combination of deadening fatigue by day and sleeplessness by night is a common one, and there are no easy solutions for this.

My own experience was that nighttime inactivity further stiffened my already contracted muscles, tendons, and ligaments. Every time I'd lie in one position for a few minutes, my pain mounted progressively. At first it was subliminal—just enough to make me restless. As the night progressed, I hurt enough to wake from whatever stage of sleep I'd managed to reach. I spent many half-wakeful hours trying to find a comfortable position.

The earliest study of modern fibromyalgia by Drs. Moldofsky and Smythe explored the complaint of sleep disturbances, documented in 70 percent of patients. Because articles about sleep disturbance were the first to make it into medical journals, physicians are aware that fibromyalgics have problems getting restorative sleep. It's so prevalent that those who don't complain of poor sleep are often told they don't have the disease!

We urge patients to begin with the over-the-counter sleeping aids—diphenhydramine and doxylamine. These old antihistamines made people so drowsy that, when better compounds came along, they were abandoned as allergy treatments and rebranded as sleep aids. They help people reach delta, deep-sleep levels and are even allowed by obstetricians during pregnancy. They are non-habit-forming and safe in small amounts, even for children.

Diphenhydramine and doxylamine are the sleep-inducing ingredients in products such as Tylenol PM, Simply Sleep, Benadryl, Sominex, and Unisom. They're marketed in capsules, liquids, and tablets, and the dosage can be titrated up to 100 mg a night. Many patients don't need as much as the 25 mg basic dose, which leaves them tired the next morning, so we suggest starting at half of that and then moving the dose up or down as needed. Very small amounts can be titrated most easily by using a liquid. About 10 percent of people get adverse effects such as jitters and excitability; for those, obviously these two antihistamines should be avoided.

Melatonin is a hormone released by the pineal gland. It has many effects in the body, where it's eventually converted to serotonin. It's safe and helps reset the sleep clock in the brain. Travelers have used it for years to offset jet lag. Levels of the hormone decline with age, which may explain some of the insomnia of the elderly. Its safety has not been established for children or teenagers because they already produce large amounts. Various papers recommend trying the hormone for at least two months before abandoning it for lack of success. It works best if taken six to eight hours before bedtime since the hormone doesn't often cause daytime drowsiness. Its function is to reset the clock restoring natural sleep, the so-called circadian rhythm. High dosages of melatonin may cause vivid or unpleasant dreaming; if that is the case, a lower dosage can be tried. Depression is a possible side effect if you take higher amounts.

If taken at bedtime, the sublingual form of melatonin provides quicker action and makes for smaller dosages. This introduces it directly into the bloodstream and avoids the digestive tract. The pill dissolves and absorbs within ten minutes under the tongue. With guaifenesin, you'll need to use one that isn't mint-flavored.

We've had some success combining melatonin with diphenhydramine when neither worked as a stand-alone therapy, and there's also evidence that it enhances the action of amitriptyline (Elavil). There are also melatonin-l-theanine combinations available. L-theanine is an amino acid that's been shown to increase relaxation and lower stress. It may help people fall asleep more quickly. Research shows L-theanine can improve the quality of sleep as well—not by acting as a sedative, but by lowering anxiety and promoting relaxation.

Another nonprescription compound is 5-HTP, short for 5-hydroxytryptophan, one of the chemicals in the process leading to the formation of melatonin and serotonin. Doses generally begin at 20 mg before bed, but lower doses are sometimes taken by day to help control pain. Doses as high as 100 mg three times a day have been studied; but as always, the amount should be started very low and moved up slowly. Side effects include dry mouth, daytime fatigue, dizziness, and constipation. Most pharmacies and health food stores carry 5-HTP, which has been used since L-tryptophan was taken off the market when contaminated batches caused some fatalities. This product should not be used within five weeks of treatment with an SSRI antidepressant because of its effects on serotonin.

If patients still can't sleep or don't tolerate the above compounds, they turn to prescription medications. These all have the potential to create dependence, although they vary greatly in this capacity. If our patients must take them, we suggest taking the tiniest effective amount and diligently avoiding nightly use. Sleeping medications are more effective when used sparingly for short-term situations. In as little as three weeks, benzodiazepines can completely lose their effectiveness if used nightly. Using them on alternate nights lowers the probability of habituation and loss of efficacy. Before turning to stronger compounds, first the exact type of sleeping problem should be identified. Do you have a problem falling asleep or remaining asleep? Is early-morning waking the problem? Different medications may work better on these various problems so that solutions can even be addressed on a night-by-night basis. But remember, if your body is accustomed to sleep medications, insomnia will be worse when you don't take them.

Sedatives work by depressing the central nervous system, which in turn leads to a morning hangover. This compounds the problem for fibromyalgics, who already have difficulty functioning at that time of day. Sleeping pills may also cause rebound effects the next afternoon. If patients nap as a result, they may get into a vicious cycle that further intensifies nighttime insomnia. Other side effects are mental confusion, slowed thinking, dry mouth, dizziness, and malaise. The overall quality (not quantity) of sleep is reduced because medications produce less restorative deep sleep and dream sleep. For many prescription sleeping pills, there are serious side effects that include sleepwalking, sleep driving, and other dangerous scenarios to be concerned about. The biggest issue of all is that very few are approved for use beyond a week or two, and fibromyalgia's sleep problems cannot be solved that quickly.

Many medications, such as muscle relaxants, tranquilizers, anti-anxiety drugs, and some antidepressants, are used for sleep due to their side effect of drowsiness. Even over-the-counter anti-inflammatories and analgesics must be viewed in context, since they can cut intracellular energy production. We urge patients with unrelenting fatigue to review their medications. Ever-present exhaustion should not always be blamed on the illness—symptoms of fibromyalgia are usually variable from day to day.

Commonly Prescribed Medications for Sleep Disturbances in Fibromyalgia

The most common group of sleeping pills are known as sedative hypnotics. In general, these medications act by working on receptors in the brain that slow down the central nervous system. Some are used more for inducing sleep, others for staying asleep. Some last longer than others in your system, and some have a higher risk of becoming habit-forming. This is why you should work with your doctor to carefully decide which choice(s) would be best in your particular case.

Benzodiazepines are the oldest class of sleeping pills still in use. (Barbiturates were used up until 1951, but they are now too highly restricted to discuss here.) As a group, they are the most highly addictive. Although primarily used to treat anxiety disorder, they are also approved to treat insomnia. They have longer duration of action than newer medications, which may result in more morning fatigue and even daylong hangovers. They are known for causing falls (mostly in older patients) and problems with memory, and they can impair the formation of new memories. Benzodiazepines make sleep apnea and breathing disorders worse. They can quite quickly lose their effectiveness if used longer than several weeks. The most common of these are diazepam (Valium), lorazepam (Ativan), clonazepam (Klonopin), temazepam (Restoril), and triazolam (Halcion).

These older benzodiazepines are all generic and as such are favored by insurance companies although quantities and strength may be restricted in older patients. These are some of the hardest drugs of any category to quit—they are considered as difficult as heroin. Experts call for a tapering period that can last a year or more, so the decision to use them should not be made lightly. Stopping cold turkey can result in tremors, muscle cramps, and life-threatening seizures. Therefore, it is always important to taper off benzodiazepines slowly with professional help.

The newer drugs designed for insomnia don't have the same chemical structure but act on the same area in the brain (nonbenzodiazepine receptor agonists). They calm the brain and induce sleep by a hypnotic effect. As a class they are commonly known as Z drugs or sedative-hypnotics. These engage a more specific $GABA_A$ receptor and have fewer side effects, along with a lower risk of dependency, although they are still controlled substances and have significant side effects and dependency issues. Ambien (zolpidem) has been on the market the longest of this group. Side effects are headaches, dizziness, nausea, difficulty creating new memories, hallucinations, and unusual nighttime behaviors. Zaleplon (Sonata) has the shortest half-life of all and is used to help patients get to sleep. It's especially effective for those who wake in the early morning and need only a few more hours of sleep. Owing to its shorter half-life, it has less rebound fatigue but is not designed to help patients sleep for a full eight hours. Among its side effects are dizziness, nausea, and a feeling of physical weakness.

In 2004, Lunesta (eszopiclone) was approved by the FDA for difficulty falling asleep as well as staying asleep. Lunesta has an additional side effect of a bitter or bad taste in the mouth the following day. It was initially touted as not causing dependency, but now that's been acknowledged as incorrect. The FDA has also reduced the recommended dose for eszopiclone from 2 mg to 1 mg, following reports that people on higher doses were less alert in the morning and at a higher risk in activities such as driving a car. This followed an earlier FDA adjustment in the recommended dose for zolpidem in women from 10 mg to 5 mg for the same reasons.

Melatonin receptor agonist Rozerem (ramelteon) helps people fall asleep faster but has little effect on the duration of sleep. It is the only sleeping medication that does not carry a warning about dependence and withdrawal symptoms. Headaches and cold symptoms are its most common adverse reactions. Rozerem works by increasing the level of melatonin in the brain by about sixteen times, which could potentially alter testosterone levels. It's possible to experience changes in your sex drive as well as your menstrual cycle when taking Rozerem. It isn't much different than its chemical cousin, plain nonprescription melatonin. But is it worth taking? In a government-sponsored study, patients who took Rozerem fell asleep sixteen minutes faster and slept eleven to nineteen minutes longer than those taking a placebo.

The newest drug is an orexin antagonist—Belsomra (suvorexant). It acts on the brain in a different way and has a somewhat checkered history of approval. It was initially rejected by the FDA at high doses of 30 mg and 40 mg, which they said posed a dangerous risk of next-day drowsiness that could lead to deadly auto crashes. The FDA eventually approved lower doses of the drug—5, 10, and 20 mg. Side effects are confusion, dizziness, impaired coordination (which can lead to falls when added to drowsiness), vision problems, grogginess, depression, and headache. The 5 mg strength was never tested in any studies for efficacy and was a post-study compromise to get on the market.

Another medication used for sleep disorders is Xyrem (sodium oxybate), which is tightly controlled and only approved for a certain symptom of narcolepsy called cataplexy or sudden muscle weakness or paralysis. It's not available in regular pharmacies but is distributed from one central pharmacy. The reason for this is that sodium oxybate is another name for GHB, the so-called date-rape drug. Small studies of fibromyalgics demonstrated some benefit in pain reduction, but the FDA refused to approve it, saying benefits did not outweigh the great potential for abuse. Sodium oxybate can cause serious side effects even when taken as directed. It cannot be taken with antidepressants, alcohol, or benzodiazepines, and withdrawal generally occurs when it is discontinued.

Sodium oxybate must be taken twice a night because it has a short half-life and won't last long enough. The first dose is taken once in bed, as it begins to work very quickly. The second dose must be placed near the bed, and an alarm clock is used to wake the patient for that dose. Users are cautioned about getting out of bed at all during the night, which makes it inappropriate for most fibromyalgics, especially those who are parents and may be called on by their children during the night. Due to difficulty obtaining this drug, it hasn't become very popular.

Getting a good night's sleep may pose dangers for people with mild heartburn and the more than 40 percent of Americans with gastroesophageal reflux disease (GERD). A 2009 study found that people taking Ambien were less than half as likely to wake up during bouts of acid reflux, increasing their exposure to nighttime stomach acid. This backwash can cause damage to the esophagus that may not have occurred had the person woken and swallowed, thereby neutralizing the acid with saliva. This type of damage to the cells lining the throat may increase the risk for esophageal cancer.

All insomnia medications pose a long list of possible side effects, such as daytime sleepiness, dizziness, sleepwalking, sleep-driving, sleep-eating, memory lapses, muscle weakness (sometimes sudden), and hallucinations. The most frequently prescribed one, Ambien, recently prompted the FDA to recommend that doses for women should be cut in half, from 10 mg to 5 mg, for immediate-release products (Ambien, Edluar, and Zolpimist) and from 12.5 mg to 6.25 mg for extended-release products (Ambien CR). Women eliminate zolpidem from their bodies more slowly, for reasons that are unclear. For men, the agency has asked manufacturers to change the labeling to recommend that doctors and other health care professionals consider prescribing lower doses, meaning 5 mg for immediate-release products and 6.25 mg for extended-release products. The longer many of these medications stay on the market, the more issues may be revealed. Taking the smallest dose possible for the fewest days possible is the best advice we can give. None of them will bestow perfect sleep, and the trade-off should be examined carefully.

If you suffer from severe restless leg syndrome that keeps you from sleeping, a dopamine agonist such as ropinirole or pramipexole may be suggested. These two medications were developed for use in treating Parkinson's disease. The most common side effects are nausea and dizziness, but these medications have also been linked to compulsive gambling, eating, and altered sexual habits. This is because dopamine agonists target receptors in the brain associated with motivation and reward; researchers suggest that anyone taking these drugs be screened for compulsive behaviors and then monitored carefully. Another problem with taking these compounds for restless legs is that over time they may lose effectiveness. The problem is intensified because symptoms can return more severely and begin earlier in the night than before.

Be aware that the medications may lose efficacy; patients may need to switch to a different class of drug or take a few weeks off.

Antidepressants for Sleep

Tricyclic and polycyclic antidepressants (the most studied drugs in fibromyalgia) are often prescribed to help patients sleep. Possible weight gain is a side effect, as well as early-morning grogginess, constipation, and dry mouth. Benefits are seen two to four weeks after initiation. If efficacy starts to fade, a monthlong break may be taken every four months. The most common are amitriptyline, doxepin, cyclobenzaprine, nortripyline, and desipramine. Side effects include drowsiness, nausea, headache, and constipation. Trazodone—both a sedative and an antidepressant—is the most commonly used for patients with sleep issues. Small doses should be used in the beginning, and often that's all that is necessary. Other classes of antidepressants such as the SSRIs generally do not help as well with sleep problems.

Muscle Relaxants

Some patients can use muscle relaxants to allow for better sleep with the added benefit of helping with discomfort. This is because their effect is to depress the central nervous system, which has an overall sedating effect on the body. The majority of these drugs do not act directly on the muscles, but on the brain. This same fatigue can make them problematic for daytime use. Tiredness, drowsiness, or sedation effect as well as dizziness, dry mouth, depression, and decreased blood pressure are common side effects. It is hard to think and function normally, even if you take a low dose, so combining them with alcohol can increase your risk of an accident. You shouldn't drive or operate heavy machinery while taking muscle relaxants. Some start working within thirty minutes, and the effects generally last anywhere from four to six hours.

Muscle relaxants can be addictive for some people. Almost all cases of addiction and abuse are due to the drug carisoprodol (Soma), which is a schedule IV controlled substance. That's because when the drug breaks down in your body, it produces a substance called meprobamate that acts like a tranquilizer. People who become addicted abuse the drug because it makes them feel relaxed. Carisoprodol is not recommended for older adults or for those with a history of drug addiction. Cyclobenzaprine is structurally similar to tricyclic antidepressants and has similar anticholinergic side effects such as sedation, dizziness, tachycardia, and arrhythmias; it may worsen heart failure, cardiac conduction abnormalities, and benign prostatic hyperplasia.

Cyclobenzaprine (Flexeril) and carisoprodol (Soma) have been well studied. Comparisons have not shown either of them to be superior to the other. There is very little research regarding which type of muscle relaxant is more effective, so the choice of which medication—or whether to use one at all—is based more on factors such as reaction to the medication, personal preferences, potential for abuse, possible drug interactions, and adverse side effects. Most of the research done on muscle relaxants was done on Flexeril, which has been shown to increase stage 4 sleep. Increasing this sleep stage does help patients feel more refreshed in the mornings. Studies have also demonstrated that this action helps reduce pain in some fibromyalgics. A new timed-release version of cyclobenzaprine called Amrix is also available, but is much more expensive. All other cyclobenzaprine is now generic; there's no brand-name Flexeril available, as such, though the name is in common usage.

Other muscle relaxants are methocarbamol (Robaxin) and metaxalone (Skelaxin). Metaxalone can cause nausea, irritability, nervousness, upset stomach, and anemia. It isn't approved for patients under thirteen or for those with liver or kidney disease. It is the least likely to cause sleepiness of this class.

The last we'll mention is the newer, more potent Zanaflex (tizanidine hydrochloride)—actually marketed to decrease spasticity of muscles in serious spastic conditions. Side effects include mental confusion and hallucinations; this one especially should be used with care. It can also lower blood pressure, causing light-headedness, fainting, and dizziness. Other side effects include dry mouth, blurred vision, constipation, frequent urination or urinary retention, runny nose, speech disorders, and vomiting.

There is a potential for abuse with all the muscle relaxants, and they should not be discontinued abruptly if you've been taking them regularly. Your doctor should prescribe a gradual reduction in dosage. They should not be used with antihistamines, especially in older adults, and never with alcohol at any age.

MARIJUANA

There is much discussion over the use of marijuana for fibromyalgia. Marijuana has been used medicinally for thousands of years. In the United States, doctors could prescribe it until 1942, when it was removed from the US Pharmacopeia. Today more than thirty states have laws legalizing marijuana in some form, and the vast majority of states allow for some medical use. Experts say that one in eight fibromyalgia patients uses medical marijuana, so obviously we get a lot of questions about it. Yet because marijuana is still illegal at the US federal level, very few high-quality studies have been done, and there is still a lot that isn't known.

Medical marijuana is often suggested as a treatment for fibromyalgia because it contains compounds that can offer relief from pain, and help with anxiety and sleep. Two ingredients, called cannabinoids—tetrahydrocannabinol (THC) and cannabidiol (CBD)—are the most common. These are chemical compounds secreted by cannabis flowers. The marijuana plant contains more than a hundred types of cannabinoids, some of which have documented medical value.

Results from certain cannabinoids are so promising that some have been synthesized for legal prescription use, but only one is used for fibromyalgia. Nabilone was approved as an add-on medication for neuropathic pain in 1985. Nabilone is more similar in effect to cannabidiol (CBD) than tetrahydrocannabinol (THC)—it has a therapeutic effect on the body. In two randomized controlled studies, nabilone significantly reduced pain and improved quality of life compared with placebo when taken by fibromyalgics. It was more effective than amitriptyline in improving sleep, and effective in the treatment of inflammatory bowel disease, especially ulcerative colitis. There were significant decreases in anxiety, pain, and functional improvement when taking nabilone. In other countries, such as Canada, it is widely used as an adjunct therapy for chronic pain management. Although considered well tolerated, there were some side effects, including dizziness/vertigo, euphoria, drowsiness, dry mouth, sleep disturbance, headaches, and nausea. Since this is a single chemical, not even plant-derived, it cannot block guaifenesin.

A double-blind controlled study in 2007 demonstrated that smoked cannabis was effective for painful peripheral neuropathy. While noting these results, doctors complained about the method, pointing out that an estimated four hundred chemicals are in marijuana, but the smoke has as many as two thousand. A vape method was developed and a follow-up study demonstrated that smoking and vaporization yielded pretty similar concentrations of THC in the bloodstream but less carbon monoxide—a marker for toxic or noxious gases.

We have seen many patients block by smoking the plant, which burns at a lower temperature than tobacco. Others can puff away safely by using pipes with built-in filters, which trap plant particles, or by vaping. Yet many people still do not like the resulting brain effects. When it comes to marijuana, we just don't know how much salicylate it contains, but it must vary by type and crop. Potential side effects of using marijuana to treat fibromyalgia include euphoria, increased appetite, sleepiness, lowered motivation, and diarrhea.

We have to say, we aren't sure about its ability to block, so use at your own risk and keep track of your symptoms.

Let's also take a moment to explain CBD or cannabidiol, which is another cannabinoid. It is often called hemp oil because it's extracted from that cannabis strain. CBD offers potential medical benefits and doesn't produce the "high" associated with THC. Research has shown that CBD can be an effective treatment for many types of pain, particularly inflammatory pain. Recall that there is no inflammation in fibromyalgia, but many users claim it helps. There is no research yet on CBD's long-term effects or, in fact, on its actual efficacy.

CBD-rich cannabis oil products can be taken sublingually, taken orally, or applied topically. Concentrated cannabis oil extracts can also be heated and inhaled with a vape pen. We have seen references stating that CBD oil contains some methyl salicylate, so we ask patients not to use the oil topically.

You can also find CBD isolate, which is extracted from hemp using CO_2. The resulting CBD hemp oil is purified using a filter to remove all plant material and excess waxes, producing a pure isolate powder with 99 percent CBD. With no measurable amounts of THC or dense plant material, CBD isolate powder has no taste or smell and can be used a number of ways, including vaping or oral consumption. This is the least risky form of CBD when it comes to blocking guaifenesin. If you're using a cartridge, make sure there's no flavor added.

Currently, a transdermal CBD patch is being developed. It would provide a more controlled release of the medication. If this is the pure chemical, it wouldn't block guaifenesin and could even be FDA-approved and -tested.

All the ways of getting cannabis into the body can be separated into two categories. The first group, which is where edibles fall, metabolizes through the liver. The second group, which encompasses everything else (vaporizing, smoking, applying to the skin, dissolving under the tongue), bypasses the liver and heads straight to the bloodstream. We are unsure if edibles will block guaifenesin or even if the answer is the same for all types of them.

CBD can interact with many common pharmaceuticals. At sufficient dosages, CBD will deactivate cytochrome P450 enzymes and have an effect on the absorption of painkillers, statins, blood thinners, insulin, and more. Problems are more likely when consuming high doses of CBD isolate products.

Internet storefronts including Amazon sell unregulated hemp-derived CBD products to all fifty states, despite that fact that cannabidiol is not an FDA-approved dietary supplement. So far, the FDA has sent warning letters to several retailers for mislabeling products and making unproven medical claims. Some products tested by the FDA contained little or no CBD. As with other supplements there's no quality assurance, testing, or oversight, and websites are designed to lure you in with testimonials and a marketing pitch. If you don't know what you're getting, you can't know for sure if you'll block your guaifenesin.

IN CONCLUSION

If there were any drugs that always worked for pain and fatigue, we'd all know about them. The vast amounts of drugs and supplements patients take are ample proof that none is very effective. People who come to us are frequently taking amazing combinations; it's common to see patients on ten or more medications. The saddest part is that even with all those compounds, they are still searching for relief. These days, five brain-altering drug mixtures are almost the norm. Even mathematicians couldn't calculate the possibilities of drug interactions in that interplay. For us, it's mind boggling!

New patients arrive with their drug stockpiles, and in the beginning we don't try to interfere with their products. Once they're doing better, it's time to discuss the notion of purging their list one drug at a time. Luckily, we also see patients who have tried everything and concluded that strong medications are of no real benefit and only result in more symptoms from their side effects.

Polypharmacy, or multiple medications, is a very real problem when suffering has gone on without relief for a number of years. Eventually, medications alone are reason enough for a patient to be disabled. Patients taking heavy narcotics such as methadone, fentanyl, or OxyContin should not drive cars or operate machinery. At work, narcotics certainly make people accident-prone and a possible danger to themselves or others. Some patients may not be able to pass drug screenings because of their medication list.

> More serious is the fact that many of us are taking a lot of drugs at once—often five, maybe ten, or even more. This practice is called polypharmacy and it carries real risks. The problem is that very few drugs have just one effect. In addition to the desired effect, there are others. Some are side effects doctors know about, but there may also be ones we are not aware of. When several drugs are taken at once, those other effects may add up. There may also be drug interactions in which one drug blocks the action of another or delays its metabolism so that its actions and side effects are increased. When the function of an organ, for instance the liver or kidneys, is even slightly impaired, the problem of complications from one or other medication increases. And the more medications taken, the more likely it is that one of them will interfere with the normal function of some organ.
>
>   —*Marcia Angell, MD, former editor in chief,*
>   New England Journal of Medicine

Prescription drugs aren't the only thing commonly used for fibromyalgia.

In response to the lobbying efforts of the multibillion-dollar "dietary supplement" industry, Congress in 1994 exempted their products from FDA regulation. Since then, products of all description—animal, vegetable, and mineral—have flooded the market, subject only to the scruples of their manufacturers, who promise all sorts of miracles in carefully worded infomercials. The so-called scientific facts on labels are often indistinguishable from advertising jargon because they are! Dietary supplements may contain the substances listed on the label in the amounts claimed, but they need not, and there is no one to police them and prevent their sale if they don't. The well-advertised coral calcium products, for example, which claimed to treat everything from cancer to fibromyalgia and arthritis, were found to contain dangerously high levels of lead when finally subjected to independent laboratory testing.

> In an analysis of ginseng products, for example, the amount of active ingredient in each pill varied by as much as a factor of 10 among brands that were labeled as containing the same amount. Some brands contained none at all...The only legal requirement in the sale of such products is that they not be promoted as preventing or treating disease. To comply with that stipulation, their labeling has risen to an art-form of doublespeak.
>
> —*Marcia Angell, MD, and Jerome P. Kassirer, MD,*
> New England Journal of Medicine[3]

According to a recent survey, about 40 percent of Americans use some sort of medical alternative treatment, and most of these are chronic pain patients looking for relief. A new development is that more insurance companies are advertising these services. Only a few actually cover herbs and other dietary supplements because they are of unproven safety and worth. Yet they let sellers advertise their products to members, which can imply benefit. Some HMOs allow doctors to prescribe them although the patient must pay for them out of pocket.

What does this mean? It means that patients who pick these alternatives pay more for health care because they aren't using their drug cards. Every person who uses St.-John's-wort instead of Prozac or red rice yeast instead of a statin pays for it out of pocket and saves the insurance company money. So is it a coincidence that several large insurers are contracted with dietary supplement companies to "deliver discounts" to their members? And the criteria for promoting a product? "If a healthy person can safely take it, we will sell it."

It's not within the scope of this book to agonize over herbal medications, their safety, and their efficacy. Since plant concentrates totally block guaifenesin, it's a moot point for us. We've previously questioned the wisdom of taking tablet concentrates from crushed leaves, roots, or other plant parts that contain at least one hundred thousand various compounds. The dangers of individual idiosyncrasies mount with that volume of chemical contents. While herb users are seeking help from just a couple of these chemicals, they are consuming many more by ingesting the entire extract. The sheer number of components exponentially raises the likelihood of hypersensitivity reactions as well as liver or renal damage. The potential for harm is increased with frequent dosing and questionable purity and potency.

While some herbal formulas with a doctor or health practitioner's guidance can certainly be beneficial, the vast majority of users self-medicate, which can be a recipe for disaster. As these supplements are used more widely, interactions with prescription drugs have been documented as well as side effects—the same as with any medicinal compound, no matter what the origin. Despite what advertising would have you believe, *natural* is not a synonym for *safe*. Medications, quite simply, are poisons judiciously administered. We suggest that any compound that has a medicinal effect on the body should be treated with respect.

There are numerous new warnings about ingesting excess vitamins and minerals. These won't block guaifenesin, but they can interfere with prescription drugs, especially the absorption of thyroid hormone. Very little is known about the effects of consuming large quantities of any substance, and unbalanced components may interfere with the others. Yet vitamins are consistently marketed as life extenders and necessary for good health. Americans take billions of dollars' worth of them a year, and yet not a single one has been actually proven to reduce deaths or illness. Fat-soluble ones such as K and E pose minor risks because overabundance can't be excreted. Vitamin A (beta-carotene) seems downright dangerous in the quantities customarily marketed. Calcium is known to partially block the action of some antibiotics, and magnesium the effects of Neurontin. Very recent studies have cast doubt on the safety of calcium supplementation, showing an increased risk of heart attacks and strokes. Magnesium is often taken for muscle relaxation but can cause diarrhea. Larger amounts of others such as zinc have been questioned for safety by some Alzheimer's disease researchers. Vitamin C in large doses can increase the risk of weight gain when taken with tricyclic antidepressants.

Vitamin D deserves its own paragraph. It's now the darling of the vitamin world. Some well-quoted papers claim that 65 percent of American adults are D-deficient, and nearly every new patient we see is taking or has been told to take large doses of it to help with pain and other complaints.

But is this true? Can it be true? Of course not—how could it be? This conclusion is based on plasma measurements of 25-hydroxy D3 (25-OH D3), which is made in the liver after the sun has radiated certain fatty substances in the skin. The 25-OH D3 undergoes further transition when a kidney enzyme piggybacks another hydroxyl (OH) onto the liver version. This produces

1-25dihyroxy D3 (1-25 OH$_2$), a vitamin–turned–hormone that is four times more potent than the original compound the liver produced. A recent paper in the *Journal of Nutrition* clearly demonstrated that the liver's vitamin D had only a 3 percent benefit to promote intestinal calcium absorption, whereas the more potent form had a 97 percent rate. This clearly shows that the free form of each vitamin (that is not bound to a blood protein) is what matters. It turns out that many tissues, including the bones, seem able to make the more powerful vitamin D form and can meet the body's needs easily.

Parathyroid hormones, estrogens, and certain bone-kidney liaisons do the delicate balancing of the body's vitamin D. The amount you can create from exposure to the sun depends on your skin tone. For lighter skins, fifteen minutes in the sun during the middle of the day provides 4,000 units of D. Think of 1,000 units as a safe number. If you're not sure whether you need supplemental D, make sure your doctor tests for the 1-25 variety. If it's normal, you don't need additional D.

THE HORMONE HOAX

A battery of tests done by a well-meaning physician looking desperately for any abnormality to treat will turn up one or two of these. Patient and doctor often seize upon these as something to "fix." But can you fix fibromyalgia by adding hormones to a system that can't make enough energy? And what happens when you try?

From what we've seen daily in our practice, we think it's necessary to write these pages. It's all too common to see patients taking everything from a single hormone to combinations of many of them. We think as patients it is important for you to understand why this approach could potentially be damaging, and why this approach may in the end actually reduce your energy.

The word *hormone* is of Greek derivation, from the verb meaning "to excite." Simply put, hormones are biochemical products of various glands that are transported to instigate action in a different area of the body. They're messengers! Hormones carry very significant and specific instructions. Once even a small amount enters the system, there's a cascading effect. Unlike some of the other systems we've discussed, this isn't warfare. Quite the contrary—it's total cooperation in the best of biologic sequences. It's skillful diplomacy at its most graceful.

How many hormones are there? Where do their receptors lie? These are mostly unanswerable questions at this stage of technology, which is part of the dilemma we face when we use them. The total number of hormones accrues faster than we ever imagined— new ones are discovered almost annually. In any case, many have not yet been synthesized, so they're unavailable as supplements, making them safe from inappropriate use for the moment. The few we've chosen to discuss are those most frequently prescribed and subject to abuse by both patients and physicians.

Each hormone has a different shape and chemical structure. We bunch them into certain classifications depending on some dominant features. One category whose name you'll recognize immediately is the group known as steroids. Among those are estrogen, progesterone, testosterone, cortisone, and DHEA. Some have an evil connotation earned by abuses by athletes. Others have had reputations because they are believed to have a profound influence on behavior: testosterone and estrogen, for example. Hormones work through receptors much as a diplomat might work through a translator. Without receptors to carry their message into a cell, a hormone cannot work. This is why they only work on certain cells; without the medium, there is no message.

Hormones are produced and designed by the endocrine glands. Once their code is broken by researchers, they can be synthesized or copied in laboratories, and it becomes tempting to use them. Since they are perfect copies of the natural messenger, it is possible now to invade the inner recesses of a cell. Having broken the secret code, we can send orders of our own.

It's the very prowess of hormones that makes them attractive. Both patients and physicians frequently fail to think such potency might serve as a double-edged sword that should be wielded responsibly. Just having massive weapons in our arsenal is not an excuse to use them at every small provocation. We should remember that biological dynamics are never simple; every interjection has the potential for complications. Similar to a law of physics, every action demands a counter-regulation.

The thyroid is a small angel-wing-shaped gland located in the neck above the Adam's apple. It's the body's metabolic thermostat, controlling temperature and energy use. Thyroid hormones have effects on all body processes and on the rate at which organs function. The human thyroid produces a number of hormones, but we're only going to focus on the two of them that are abused. No other hormones are as widely prescribed for such dubious reasons as the thyroid's. Because complaints of fatigue, brain fog, and weight gain are ubiquitous, patients and practitioners zero in on this gland.

The leading output of the human thyroid is hormone comprised 95 percent of the amino acid tyrosine with four attached iodine molecules. This structure is reflected in its medical name, T_4. The remaining 5 percent is the same amino acid, this time carrying three iodine passengers, or T_3. Let's remember this important ratio of 95 to 5, nature's intended ratio for human thyroids.

When the thyroid gland is underproductive, we refer to the condition as hypothyroidism. Since the thyroid controls the metabolism of the body, an underactive gland means that the body becomes sluggish. Low energy and weight gain are the primary symptoms. Thus it's easy to see why many doctors and fibromyalgics think an underactive thyroid might be to blame for at least some of their symptoms.

Luckily, thanks to a superbly accurate test, it is easy to check if you're hypothyroid. A blood test measures the level of the thyroid-stimulating hormone (TSH). This controller is not actually released by the thyroid, but is a messenger sent from the pituitary gland, the so-called master gland of the body. If thyroid hormone levels in the blood fall low, more TSH is released. Test results will reflect this situation, showing an elevated level of TSH. In the reverse situation, if the thyroid hormone levels are high in the blood, the pituitary will cut production of TSH so that the thyroid will curb its output.

Low-thyroid patients may be placed on hormones made from desiccated pig or cow thyroid glands, such as Armour Thyroid (porcine) or Thyro-Gold (bovine). These compounds are held in high esteem by those who provide them, and patients are often told they are "natural"—a term frequently used to inspire confidence that in reality means very little. In this case, especially, it is a dubious claim unless you happen to be a pig or a cow who has an underactive thyroid gland.

A few paragraphs ago we described the mix of T_4 and T_3 produced by human thyroid glands. Animals make a different mix of the two hormones, approximately 15 to 25 percent T_3. Thus it is questionable to tout animal products as natural replacements for humans. More important, the precise human hormones have been expertly synthesized and are readily available in many potencies. Levothyroxine (T_4) and triiodothyronine (T_3) are the true natural hormones, identical to those the human thyroid generates.

In humans we don't normally supplement T_3, because it isn't necessary. Our liver and some other tissues normally convert T_4 to T_3 as needed. For this reason, it's customary to replace deficient thyroid output only by T_4 and allow the system to make its own necessary conversions. There is some debate about adding a small amount of T_3, but the problem with this idea is that it's impossible to discern how much to give. When thyroid hormones are extraneously administered, blood measurements only reflect how much T_4 and T_3 are running loose in the bloodstream. We have no sure way of knowing what all the various tissues might have scooped up for their own use. Only our own internal monitors—the pituitary and the adjacent brain hypothalamus—have the ability to make a precise interpretation of the rapid and minuscule variations on the blood's hormonal combinations.

Each of us has two adrenal glands that sit atop a kidney totally encased in a mound of fat, nature's protection for such important structures. Each gland is made up of two parts, the outer adrenal cortex and the inner medulla. The adrenals release more than forty hormones. Many medications for autoimmune or inflammatory diseases are synthetic models of adrenal steroids.

In this section we'll limit ourselves to hormones produced in the outer cortex, the so-called corticosteroids that so profoundly affect our metabolism and energy production.

These glands are important in their own right but, like the thyroid, take commands emanating from the pituitary and also, in this case, the hypothalamus. This section of the brain sends sequential instructions that result in perfectly timed releases of adrenocorticotropic hormone, ACTH, which enters the bloodstream and then the adrenals via receptors on cell surfaces.

The incoming message delivered by the arrival of ACTH is a report of some kind of disturbing stress, such as infection, trauma, surgery, emotional surges, and even exposure to excessive heat or cold. Upon receipt, the adrenal cortex releases a hormone of its own, a member of the steroid clan. Though you'll recognize it best by the name *cortisone*, it's known in medicine as cortisol or hydrocortisone.

Cortisol is an extremely potent and wide-ranging hormone that has an effect on how the body uses fuel: carbohydrates, fats, and proteins. So we are back in the realm of energy production! In times of duress, the body can release twenty times its basal amount of this hormone. Receptors friendly to cortisol are found in the walls of most bodily structures.

Spurts of cortisol block the effect of insulin and cause the blood sugar to rise. The body's idea here is to give more energy, and it's this action of the hormone that is responsible for the dawn effect where the blood sugar rises to help us wake up and face the day. Cortisol also induces bone surfaces to break down to release calcium into the bloodstream. It steals amino acids from the muscles and promotes their conversion to glucose in the liver. It coaxes fat cells to release their contents, and fatty acids are plucked out for energy needs. These are all controlled responses designed to steal fuel from less essential functions to face an emergency.

Cortisol also impacts the immune system. It depresses the number and activity of immune cells, and various white cells partially disappear from the bloodstream. These are crucial to mounting an attack against infection, bacteria, viruses, and fungi. When cortisol levels are high, the body cannot fend these off and rampant infections are an eminent danger.

There are additional dangers with long-term use of steroids. Cataract formation accelerates, and blood pressure rises, often to dangerous levels. Skin fragility can result in large wounds from minor abrasions because healing is compromised. Internal tissues also become more fragile, making patients poor surgical candidates. Emotions become labile and swing rapidly from depression to paranoia, from excitability to somnolence. There's a gradual progression of arteriosclerosis, and osteoporosis is guaranteed from the hormone's action on bones. Eventually, fatigue replaces the energy that was initially increased. There's more, but this is enough to make our point.

An unfortunate example of hormone misuse has surfaced in recent years—the diagnosis of adrenal fatigue or insufficiency. This is based on ignorance and incorrect or inadequate testing. The rationale seems to be that a little bit of synthetic cortisone shouldn't hurt. Oh, but it does!

Cortisol is particularly dangerous when given for too long and at the wrong time of day, because it has a diurnal variation. It begins to rise in the body and blood in the early hours before you wake, and levels are naturally highest in the morning. Then they drop off a bit before lunch, rise slightly after eating, and drop off again by 4 p.m. Administration needs to be properly timed, or patients will suffer from anxiety, restlessness, and insomnia.

There's naturally perfect harmony in the endocrine system. Pituitary control is very precise. If only a small amount of cortisone-like drugs are ingested, the adrenals may not totally shut down, but they will produce less hormone. Larger or excessive doses put the gland to sleep and completely stop all internal production. No harm is done when the dose exactly equals what the glands normally put out—except that your own glands will stop functioning. Too much will put your own glands into such depression that they won't recover for several months after the outside hormone is stopped. The longer cortisol is taken, the longer the recovery time for your own gland. In the meantime, your energy and stamina will be seriously compromised, and you will have the side effects listed above.

Adrenal fatigue shouldn't be confused with adrenal insufficiency, a legitimate medical condition that can be diagnosed with laboratory tests and has a defined symptomatology. It usually has an autoimmune cause, with symptoms appearing when most of the adrenal cortex has been destroyed, requiring careful dosing of hormones for life. Some liken adrenal fatigue to a milder form of adrenal insufficiency—but there's no underlying pathology that has been associated with adrenal fatigue.

Prior to the adrenal hormones being synthesized, animal glands were used in human beings and administered by injection. The current adrenal supplements you can purchase on the internet are glands of animals like cows and pigs gathered from slaughterhouses and ground up raw. If taken orally, they are digested like any other protein and cannot be absorbed from the gastrointestinal tract, so they are ineffective.

Accurate testing is available for adrenal hormone levels and should not be done by kits purchased over the internet and other unusual ways. This should be done by a medical doctor, because certain medications and supplements can alter the results. It must be done at a precise time of day and can be affected by diet, stress, and physical activity.

Another adrenal hormone, DHEA (dehydroepiandrosterone), is less popular today than it once was when it was touted as a youthing hormone. If you look at the long chemical name you'll see the syllable *andro*, which refers to something masculine. It's there for a good reason.

DHEA and its sulfate companion DHEAS are found in the bloodstream in greater amounts than any other hormone. When such levels circulate, it's a sign of relative impotency, or there wouldn't be a need for so much. Like other "sex" hormones, levels are highest in early adulthood and then slowly fall with age. By age eighty, most people have less than a fifth of what they had in their twenties—hence the notion that taking it might make you feel young again.

DHEA is actually what's called a prohormone, suggesting that it needs to be worked on somewhere in the body to produce a more potent compound. DHEA supplements on the market are a synthetic form. Even after many years of study, the hormone hasn't been tied to any hugely important function. The skin and hair follicles turn it predominantly into testosterone. The liver and other systems have receptors, too, although the reason for them is unknown.

Because it's a precursor of estrogen and testosterone, pumping extra DHEA into an aging system may be fraught with danger. Does it augment the already known increased risk of breast, endometrial, or prostate cancer? Since it is more male than female in nature, women have experienced the same effects from it as from testosterone: excessive darkened hair on the face, breasts, and chest (in a male pattern). Other outward signs of masculine effects are oily skin and acne, sometimes accompanied by detrimental changes in blood lipids.

How much DHEA is converted to estrogen or testosterone seems to be at the whim of the liver. No conversion ratios of either can be predicted. Those who ingest it on a long-term basis should do so recognizing its uncertain peril at the current level of knowledge. In patients whose adrenal glands have been destroyed or surgically removed, only cortisol is routinely provided for replacement therapy. No such attention has been given to DHEA and no negative effects have been evident from this omission.

Research on DHEA to date has uncovered no benefits to improve well-being, cognitive function, or body composition. It possibly could be more effective than placebo in treating depression. DHEA has been studied in osteoporosis, where it had very modest benefits in improving bone density, but was not nearly as effective as drugs approved to treat this condition. These same studies also showed that quality control of the supplements was often low, and there are some known drug interactions. Due to lack of knowledge about long-term effects and little evidence of any benefit, the wisest course is to avoid this hormone.

HUMAN GROWTH HORMONE (HGH)

We've mentioned the mighty pituitary several times—it's usually called the master gland, because it controls endocrine tissue scattered all over the body. Every pituitary is a masterpiece of chemical ingenuity. Most of its many hormones are not yet commercially produced so are unavailable for experimentation or abuse. This is not the case for human growth hormone, or HGH, first synthesized (and thus marketed) in the 1980s. It has widespread effects on the body.

Growth hormone has an obvious function from birth until full maturity. Almost all our bodily structures have receptors that are built to receive and enact its commands. It continues to promote growth during our lives, though in adults its actions are much more subtle—essentially tissue remodeling and repair. Many metabolic functions would slow without it, thus the temptation exists to speed them up by supplementing this hormone to create more energy.

When HGH was first synthesized, the manufacturer subsidized many hundreds of studies looking for uses. You may have seen the studies showing benefit after a certain number of weeks in fibromyalgia. At least for the term of these, a reduction of symptoms was demonstrated in most patients after nine weeks of injections. Whether or not it would benefit symptoms for longer periods or in more patients is unknown. Therapy is enormously expensive, well over a thousand dollars per month. You'll notice that internet searches will turn up these old studies; there have been no follow-ups in recent years.

Like other hormones, HGH should only be carefully used for proper indications. Overproduction from a pituitary tumor is the cause of acromegaly, where all parts of the body enlarge. This thickens facial features as well as enlarging hands, feet, and some internal organs. Hypertension and diabetes develop because of HGH's antagonizing effects on insulin. The heart later succumbs to a general arteriosclerosis. If untreated, sufferers die of heart attacks, stroke, or cancer that originates in the colon. Growth hormone should not be added if pituitary function is normal. Although initially energy may increase, this wanes when these additional diseases strike.

HGH must be prescribed by a doctor and is usually given three or more times per week and only by injection. It cannot be taken orally; any product that states otherwise is a scam, as are extracts extracted from animal tissue. Whatever growth hormone might remain in the desiccated tissue will be digested like any other ingested protein and totally broken down into individual amino acids before being absorbed.

While we're on the topic, we might as well mention the various other organ extracts, secretions, and enzymes. They all suffer the same fate as any other meat in their trip through the digestive system. Erroneously touted for almost any medical condition including some that don't exist, they soak up all too many health dollars better saved for other needs.

The bottom line is that hormones are powerful and not simple solutions. Manufacturing drug and supplement companies strive to make patients and physicians feel there's a need for these products and have made catchy names for conditions that require their use. In the end, it's your body, and you have to think the hardest about what you may be doing to it. Adding the wrong things for you, or some you don't need, threatens that equilibrium and can rob you of the very improvement you were seeking.

To recap, we steadfastly advocate a single, simple medication for the treatment of fibromyalgia—guaifenesin. It's been around for a very long time and is devoid of side effects, so we unhesitatingly prescribe it for persons of all ages. We're especially pleased when new patients come to us with the desire to stick to just one protocol. This way, there is no confusing what gets them well. In time, they'll know that guaifenesin is what got them there and not some complicated combination of things. Although it's tempting to reach for every new golden promise or astounding miracle, it's wise to stick with one modality at a time. Wiser still is to research the proposed treatments thoroughly for safety. When it comes to that issue, guaifenesin wins hands-down.

We hope this chapter has answered some questions but, more important, that it has underscored our basic tenet. First and foremost, we've got to diagnose patients before they are incapacitated, and then fight for treatments that get patients well. Each and every patient should be offered the chance to have the most productive, successful, and complete life possible. Nothing less should be acceptable to us, both as medical professionals and as human beings.

CHAPTER 16

COPING WITH FIBROMYALGIA

*What Will Help While Guaifenesin
Helps Your Body Heal?*

I have been on guai [for fourteen months]—I probably
have another two to three years to clear. These past months
have not been hell at all. They have been the best fourteen
months in a long time for me. I know I am healing. I have
more energy. I have more stamina. I can do more things,
socially, physically, and mentally. So for me, if this is hell—
bring it on!

—*Linda P., Ohio*

In a very real sense, the first day you take guaifenesin is the birth-
day of your new life. You've read the patient stories throughout
this book. They're all true. Yet you must wonder: Authors would
hardly include bad ones, would they? It would be great if we could
all know someone who is on the protocol and is responding well
to guaifenesin. But most people won't be that fortunate. So, if you
aren't that lucky, you'll just have to trust us and our various online
resources. We hope we've given you hope. We hope you'll investigate further and decide to try guaifenesin and reverse your illness.

By now you're also aware there's more to this treatment than just swallowing a pill. We haven't hidden the fact that fibromyalgia reversal is demanding, takes time, and requires both perseverance and dedication. You may encounter people who will tell you this protocol is too restrictive and too complicated. If it's any consolation, we'll tell you straight out: We believe that since you've bought this book and read this far, you've got the guts to persevere!

What's left now is to think about what you can do for yourself while waiting for guaifenesin to do its job. We think it important enough to repeat: If you're taking the correct dosage and you aren't blocking, guaifenesin will work. You don't need to take any other medications. Everything else, as far as we're concerned, is optional and only temporarily useful. But there are certainly things you can do mentally and physically to pave the way toward your new life.

> Patience is my biggest struggle. Over the past month, I've come to a place of accepting that it will take however long it will take. Before that, I was setting specific goals—hoping I could do things I wanted to at six months, a year. This only set me up for frustration. To the best of my knowledge, I developed fibro following a car accident in 1998 (at least that's when I became symptomatic), so I have almost twenty years to reverse. So using the one-month-on-guai-reverses-six-months-of-fibro estimate, I'm probably about a third of the way toward being clear.
>
> —*Marti Thompson, Ohio*

REDUCE STRESS

Don't you want to laugh when you read those words? Poor stress! It's blamed for everything unpleasant that happens to us. For years, it was thought responsible for inducing fibromyalgia, and many doctors still believe that. There's no doubt that chronic pain and fatigue make it a battle even to get up and dress in the morning. Add to this the other things you can't get done, the things you regularly forget to do, and the neglect your illness imposes on your family and relationships. These are all enough to keep you on edge and at fever pitch. Undoubtedly, mental strain intensifies the symptoms of FMS—or for that matter, any chronic illness. That's no surprise, is it? Being sick is stressful. You may have already considered many of the coping strategies we'll suggest, but we think it still helps to see them collected in writing.

One of the first things to do is to get other health worries out of the way. Make sure your doctor has checked carefully for coexisting conditions. Treat anything that overlaps and confounds fibromyalgia. Thyroid function should be checked and treated, but only if it's abnormal. Anemia can make you feel tired and weak, and can greatly inhibit the muscular clearing of fibromyalgia. If you're hypoglycemic or diabetic, don't duck the issue. Start the corrective diet without hesitation. In just a few weeks, you'll have more energy, feel better, think better, and find your irritable bowel gradually improved. Your worries about more serious conditions being the root cause of your many symptoms can be set aside by your doctor—so discuss these underlying fears with him or her. Remember that the internet contains both accurate and not-so-accurate information and must not take the place of a qualified medical practitioner. Don't neglect your health because you have fibromyalgia and you feel lousy anyway.

Review your medications and remember that some of them are certainly compromising how you feel because of side effects. Some depression is normal in chronic illness. Do you really need to take an antidepressant? Sometimes medications are handed out with very little reasoning the minute a doctor suspects fibromyalgia. Read about the effects of the mood-altering drugs and tranquilizers that have stripped your personality of its highs and lows. Understand which ones add to your fatigue. We acknowledge you just need to continue functioning, but it's also logical to question how much a drug is actually helping. It's important to reassess what you are taking periodically. Many medications prescribed for fibromyalgia are documented to decrease in efficacy over time. If you are doubtful about whether something is helping, ask how you should go about reassessing it for both value and side effects. You may wonder what this has to do with stress, but it's pertinent for several reasons. Deep down you're probably worrying about the effects and long-term risks of multiple compounds. Most people really don't like taking drugs. Budgets are strained when paying high pharmacy bills each month, and this doesn't make life any easier. Finally, until you reduce drugs to minimal needs, you can't estimate how this polypharmacy is affecting your mental outlook. Medications used for pain, anxiety, and depression all work directly on the brain.

Besides your prescription drugs, look at the over-the-counter stuff and the supplements you've added over the years. Why did you add them? Because someone told you they helped someone else? Because you read somewhere that they are good for you? These are usually more expensive than prescriptions because insurance doesn't cover them. Wonder more than a bit about side effects and safety, since they aren't often tested for interactions with prescription drugs. This is a new beginning: a good time to repack the baggage you'll carry into the future. We understand the fear of omitting anything on the chance you'll feel worse without it. If you stop something and you realize it was actually necessary, you can always add it back. Your target is to make your regimen as simple as possible. Removing the worry about what medications are doing to your system will lessen that stress.

He suggested Paxil. The effect was slower and more subtle but eventually I had a similar feeling of absence, just emotionally flat. The pain was not touched by either antidepressant. I began to wonder what it was doing to my mind and how dependent my brain was becoming on Paxil. Maybe it wasn't the best mind in town but it was mine and I wanted to be on good terms with it, so I determined to do without Paxil. That was over fifteen years ago and I have not regretted the decision. I look back on those difficult years and am grateful for the lessons learned, for the way that pain pushed me to look for myself and renew my relationship with myself and my faith.

—*Jody D., North Carolina*

STRESS AT HOME

One day I asked my husband what was the hardest part about being married to someone as sick as I was. I expected him to say working all day, then coming home to do the cooking, cleaning, and wait on me. But he didn't, he said it was the loneliness!! I had no idea. At that time I wasn't able to give anything to him, I was a blob. He took care of me and loved me unconditionally. Maybe not perfectly, [but] to the best of his ability. See, I am the luckiest girl in the world!

—*Susie, California*

Next, carefully examine where life is the sweetest—hopefully your home. You should make an effort to share what you are about to begin with those closest to you. If they're interested in reading about your illness and the protocol, you can share parts of this book or materials from our website: www.fibromyalgiatreatment.com. The site also contains a "Love Letter to Normals." Read and adapt it for your own use or use it as an inspiration to talk about what you and they are facing.

Everyone in your household should be given a chance to understand what's happening with your health, possibly especially the children. Reassure them that you're going to get better. The fear of losing a parent is always present, and many children worry more than they let on. So be clear that while there will be things you just can't do right now, it isn't your fault or theirs. If you express yourself simply and clearly and continue to reassure them that all is well, you will diminish their stress and yours. Our time with children and grandchildren is truly the most precious thing that we have to give them. Together think of things that you can do, like bake cookies or decorate cupcakes even if they aren't made from scratch. Board games can substitute for outdoor playing. If your grandchildren or children are old enough, let them read to you out loud. Watch movies with them, or work on simple projects, puzzles. You can color with them, or play with blocks. On better days, as energy permits, short walks together can be marvelously bonding and refreshing. Spending time with children keeps you mindful, in the moment, and releases you from worries and stress. You will be surprised at how much you have to give if you keep it simple and don't burden yourself with ambitious projects and plans. Don't worry if nothing much comes to mind when you read this; Google and other search engines are a fantastic resource for simple things to do with children. For example, there's a Pinterest page called "40 Ways to Entertain Your Kids While Lying Down."

Let family members know what help you need. Be specific and explain why you need it. If they understand that you are beginning a demanding protocol for getting well, it will be hard for them to refuse you. There are three secrets for getting help. First, learn how to ask, and be specific about what you want. Don't expect clairvoyance from your significant other when it's time to mop a dirty floor. Children won't automatically volunteer to haul trash all the way to the curb just because you wish they would. Second, if someone is doing something to help, don't supervise the task. Not only does this expend energy you don't have, it's annoying to those over whom you hover. If it's not the way you would've done it...oh well! There are more ways than one to accomplish things, and perfection in most things is not essential. Third, be absolutely sure to say thank you. Express your appreciation to a child who drew you a picture or played quietly so you could sleep. Be grateful to a spouse or friend who cooked dinner and even cleaned up afterward. Let each know you view their efforts as wonderful. "Do you know what that means to me?" goes a long way as a reward and installs them as participants in your recovery.

"Lower your standards" would make a good motto when you face house and garden chores. This last phrase might contain words of wisdom for us all—even healthy people have too much to do these days. Everyone, not just fibromyalgics, feels stressed out and pressured from all sides. Changes you cultivate during guaifenesin treatment may turn into much healthier habits useful for the rest of your life.

Make simple meals and eat them off paper plates if you don't have a dishwasher. Save some energy by cooking bigger batches of familiar recipes when you feel up to it. Freeze the extra portions for the energy-deprived days that are sure to come. Find easy recipes: This is so easy to do—there are hundreds of websites dedicated to them, even low-carb ones. Women's magazines and cookbooks have plenty of them; some are printed on package labels. Especially in the winter, Crock-Pots can be used for one-dish dinners without supervision, and require less cleaning up. The new electric pressure cookers (Instant Pots) cut cooking time drastically and allow for easier cleanup. There's even a Facebook page called "Dump and Push Start" for Instant Pots.

If your budget allows, there are a huge number of options for meal delivery or services that deliver mostly prepped meals that require only simple cooking to prepare. Many markets will deliver groceries, making online shopping speedy and convenient. You can order bulky things like laundry detergent and heavy items like canned goods and have them delivered at no cost to your home. None of these things were available when we wrote the first edition of this book and seem like answered dreams to us. Don't be afraid to research and try these things—you will be amazed at how much less stressful your life can be without going out, looking for parking, and waiting in line when you don't feel up to it. You can buy salicylate-free products of all kinds and have them delivered, too.

Stop worrying about what's accumulating behind the refrigerator or under the stove. Remind yourself as many times as necessary that there's a time for everything, and this is yours for healing. A spotless house should be low on the list of priorities in life, with health at the very top. When you regain that, you'll have plenty of energy to play catch-up with all of those dusty corners.

Perhaps you can afford to pay someone to help with housework. We're not insensitive to the fact that some budgets won't allow it. However, just having someone come in every couple of weeks or once a month to do the heavy stuff can feel lifesaving. Another possibility is to let your kids or older grandchildren earn extra money by doing housework. It may not be to your satisfaction, but it'll be a learning experience for them. They'll undoubtedly do it in fits and starts, but so what? It's at least a little break when you're about to collapse.

> Even my spouse could see the incredible difference. He now felt guilt-free to serve me with divorce papers. How kind of him. He was going to anyway, he says, but he had been feeling painfully guilty about it. Look how guai even helped his pain!
>
> —*Iris, California*

Nurture your relationships in all the ways that you can. Don't take them for granted or put off doing what you can. If your relationship doesn't survive the symptoms of fibromyalgia, remember that it might have faltered anyway. Some couples get lucky and mend the rifts, but for right now, concentrate on getting yourself well. Don't waste your precious energy being angry or confrontational. Try to be cheerful and be straightforward about your issues. Don't suffer in silence when you are in pain expecting a partner to understand why you are detached or crabby. At the same time, though, it's your responsibility to keep your complaints about others to a minimum. Like you, most people are doing the best they can. Instead, concentrate on yourself and making peace with yourself.

My energy levels are up, the fog lifted almost immediately, and some of my hair is growing back! I am doing things now that I couldn't do a year ago. I wake up in the morning and my legs don't ache. I sleep. FM has taught me to appreciate the little things in life and that in and of itself is a blessing. I also make it a point to live life more fully and to take the time to do things for me. This protocol has worked, and I hope that anyone out there who might be contemplating whether they should do it or not will "Just Do It!" This past week we hosted friends of ours in our home for a week. We were on the go all week long and I managed to get by on just two Aleves, which I took as a precaution since it was that time of the month and I was trying to avoid getting a headache. Yes, I am feeling tired today, but then again, we all are!

—*Susan, California*

STRESS IN THE WORKPLACE

We get a lot of patients who have fibromyalgia. I print the guaifenesin protocol notes for them, along with giving them the name of the book and the website address. I tell them about my progress using the protocol. I'm not at a 100 percent reversal yet, but I am so much better than where I started! I love to read progress reports shared on the support group. I was training for a half marathon back in November 2016 and I was only able to walk about five miles (in three and a half hours). I was a long way behind everyone else. I still feel that failure, but I'm thinking if things continue the way they have I'll start training for another one! I'm also better able to play with my five grandchildren now and go camping with my husband, my kids and grandkids. I no longer think about if I'll have to quit work or find a permanent way out of the pain I was experiencing. I'll be turning fifty-five in December and feel better than I have in a long time. I am so thankful for stumbling onto the blip about the guai protocol! I'm sure God was guiding my computer mouse that day! I pray for all of you out there with this horrible thing called fibromyalgia. May each day be better and each night be more restful!

—*Tammy W., Nebraska*

Job stress and anxiety about it are sure to magnify your symptoms and make your fibromyalgia worse. Stress and anxiety make it harder to eat properly and can exhaust what little energy you have, energy you need for healing. So it's important not to let work situations weigh you down. If it's feasible, schedule a meeting with your supervisor to discuss fibromyalgia and the treatment you're about to start. Keep it simple and honest but be clear that you're going to improve. You can finally promise that in good faith; all you ask is for some tolerance in the weeks that lie ahead.

Quitting is rarely the answer—for several reasons, including adding financial stress to your life—but perhaps a sympathetic boss will let you cut your hours temporarily Before you do this or request any changes, be sure to look at your situation to see what is possible financially. Try to be as thorough and honest as you can, but take into consideration money you might save perhaps by less frequent transportation costs and less need for paid child care.

We should state here that the vast majority of our patients continue to work full-time even during the first months of guaifenesin treatment. Most have already developed coping mechanisms and may require only more rest during cycles. In our office, all of us have fibromyalgia and none of us ever missed work because of our reversals. We know there are stories on the internet about how tough the protocol can be, but we promise we are telling the truth.

You may be able to arrange to do some of your work from

home. Computers have made it easy for employees to telecommute or simply bring chores home, where they can be completed in a comfortable chair and preselected surroundings. While working at home, you can move around, stretch, take breaks as you need them, and work flexible hours. If mornings are very difficult, as they are for most fibromyalgics, you can arrange your time to work later in the evening if you normally feel better at that time. However, be honest with yourself. Working from home is not for everyone; some find it impossible with the distractions and interruptions. When working from home, things like unmade beds, the TV, the internet on your computer, unfinished projects, and a fully stocked kitchen can tempt you away from your work. You should know yourself pretty well. If you are not disciplined enough on your own, you should not jeopardize your job by attempting it. You can read about some of the pitfalls and benefits on…guess what? The internet.

The problem with this simple advice is that by the time many fibromyalgics are diagnosed or begin treatment, they are already having problems at work. Some have taken too many sick days; others have fallen behind and performed badly on days when fibrofog and other symptoms were at full fury. If you've been told that your job is in jeopardy if you call in sick just one more time, you might need to take some proactive steps at the time you start guaifenesin. Your possibilities will be different depending on the size of your company and your benefits package. It's not a bad idea to consider the option of taking time off at the beginning of treatment if you feel it is necessary and you won't be given any help. The Family and Medical Leave Act (FMLA) became law in 1993 and may apply to you if you work for a company that employs more than fifty people. It was enacted to permit up to twelve weeks of unpaid leave for you to reverse a serious health condition. It does require continuing treatment by a licensed health care provider, and that provider must consider fibromyalgia a serious illness that will improve. You'll need to provide documentation from your doctor in a timely fashion and medical records when requested. The law also mandates you'll be restored to the same or an equivalent position with the same pay and benefits unless you are a highly paid worker who is considered indispensable by your employer. You can get better information from your state's board of equalization (by whatever name) or your employer's human resources department, where you can learn about your personal options in detail. The internet is also a source of information about your options, but carefully select what you read—for example, there are many articles posted on the site of a law firm that specializes in disability that may be designed to make you think the process is less complicated than it is.

It's very important not to be too frightened or overreact in advance, especially if your options are limited. We're not all endowed with the same strength, but certainly most of our patients cope with jobs successfully throughout reversal. In fact, despite what you may have heard or read, the vast majority continue working even during the initial days on our protocol. Only a few require a period of absence, and generally not more than a month or two. That's one of the reasons why we've advised you to start on a small amount of guaifenesin and titrate up slowly to find your proper dosage. Taking more medication than you actually need will make you cycle harder. It's far better for you to take the correct amount and sooner experience good days. When these start appearing, it will make it possible for you to catch up with some of your work. You'll be amazed at the energy you have when you start having them. The challenge when that happens is not to attempt to do too much.

Employers are certainly becoming much more sensitive to those with disabilities or limitations. There are many resources available, and often a simple note from your physician will help you make changes. More comfortable chairs, wrist supports for computer work, footstools, and cushions are all things your employer might provide because new laws require reasonable accommodations; a little research on your part can promote coop-eration. We find the best approach is for you to do some research on your own and present options that you believe will help you be more productive. Try to be realistic about what your employer can afford and keep demands at a minimum. Try simple solutions such as a backrest cushion before a five-hundred-dollar chair.

Relationships with co-workers might benefit if you sim-ply tell them that you're beginning a difficult new treatment for your fibromyalgia. Share your hopes and fears and explain that you intend to do your best and continue working as hard as you can. Most people will respond to such a direct approach and will be more inclined to help. Try getting them to understand that a medical problem is the basis of your struggles and that you're doing your best to get it under control. Reassure them that you won't be ill forever.

> Normal are the hours when I forget I am a sick person. Normal is when I keep up with a fit person my age and don't pay for it big time. Normal is when I cry for a normal reason. Normal is when I laugh without being macabre or cynical. Normal is when I don't burn when I think about doctors. Normal is when I want to do something besides watch TV. Normal is not being in pain all the time. I have these normals now and you will, too.
>
> —*Janet, Canada*

THINGS YOU CAN DO FOR YOURSELF

The first thing I did when I prepared to start the protocol was to read everything that came in on the online support group site each day. Every time a progress report or testimonial came in, I cut and pasted it into a document in my computer and saved it. Whenever I was frustrated or thought perhaps that the protocol was not working for me I could then go to all those positive let-ters and read and reread them until I felt better about what I was doing. I wrote my progress reports on a regular basis and saved them as well. That made it easier to realize the progress I was making. I could always go back and look at my own comments so I never lost track of my successes.

—*Bonnie J., Florida*

GET ENOUGH SLEEP—YES, *REALLY*

As we sleep, our bodies all clean out the metabolic debris created by simply existing. That's the time when cells do their housekeeping. Fibromyalgic muscles compile overabundant metabolic leftovers because they're kept constantly contracted, and this prevents the restorative rest needed for a good nighttime cleansing. To a lesser extent, it's the same for the rest of the body, particularly the brain. It follows that a prominent complaint in fibromyalgia is insomnia and the dominant exhaustion this imposes. No matter how tough you are, fitful sleeping makes next-day function impossible. Rest is crucial, so get as much as you can—but realize that it won't entirely solve the problem of fatigue.

When you've had a bad night, occupy the next day with less demanding tasks. Although this is not always possible, choose the simplest ones from your must-do list. On those bad days, enlist others to help by doing what they can. Now is the time for simple meals such as grilled cheese sandwiches, soup, or takeout. If you've frozen a casserole or portions of a larger meal, this is the time to thaw it out. Conserve what strength you have for the most basic and urgent tasks. Recognize that lack of sleep will make your thinking even more cloudy and leave you more vulnerable to mistakes and accidents. Exhausted as you are, you'll need to be somewhat proactive.

A good general rule is to grab what rest the disease allows whenever you can. Snatch naps when you have to when it's possible. Keep them brief and find a way to wake yourself before you lapse into a prolonged coma. You've got to remain tired enough to sleep that night. When you start yawning in the evening, forget the next TV show and go to bed earlier than usual. Sometimes it requires a Herculean effort to propel yourself from your chair into the bedroom, but do it. Dozing in your chair or on the couch is not as restorative as sleeping in a quiet room. Your spouse isn't enjoying your company, especially if you're snoring. Your workplace may have a back room or a private area where you can rest at lunchtime or during breaks. A small, inexpensive futon can be stashed on a shelf along with a small pillow. Even half an hour can make a difference if it's spent stretched out with your eyes closed.

Schedule sufficient bed hours; it's counterproductive to aim for seven hours when you know you need nine. Set your alarm half an hour earlier than usual if you really must finish some task from the night before. You'll complete it much more rapidly when you're rested. It may also help to set the alarm earlier, take your morning dose of pain medication, and then press the snooze button while waiting for it to take effect. In this way, you'll feel better when you get up and start moving. Starting your day with a shower even if you don't feel like it can loosen your muscles and at the same time wake you up.

If you're a light sleeper, relaxation tapes, quiet fans, and white-noise machines can make it easier to stay asleep. Make sure your bedroom is dark and your mattress comfortable. When purchasing a new mattress, ask for a trial period and a money-back guarantee—there's no one kind that helps everyone with FM. On painful nights, little adhesive heat pads for muscle pain may be used, or apply a simple old-fashioned hot water bottle. Don't risk electric heating pads when you sleep because of the danger of burning yourself. If you use one, be sure to get one that has an auto turn-off feature. Don't overlook simple aids such as earplugs or sleep masks if your room has features that keep you from fully relaxing. Exercise in the afternoon will also help, as will gentle stretching after a shower or a bath before bed.

Do we even need to mention here that electronics disrupt sleep and make it even more difficult for fibromyalgics? You may be tempted to ignore the many good studies that show that blue light emitted from iPads, smartphones, tablets, laptops, and other electronic devices profoundly mess up sleep patterns even in normal people, but you shouldn't. Well-designed investigations have documented that the blue light they emit reduces levels of melatonin, our natural sleep hormone. This results in it taking longer to fall asleep but also in less restorative REM (rapid eye movement) sleep once you do drift off. Double-blind studies have also shown that people using electronics before sleep are less alert the next day even after a full eight hours, and that they have delayed circadian rhythms.

If you must work in the evenings on electronic devices, download a filter to cut their blue light emissions. Without a filtering app, users are exposed to an alarming amount of blue light, especially if you are lying in bed and have your screen just a few inches from your face. Apple electronics come with an app called Night Shift. For Android users, there are a number of free downloadable fixes such as Night Filter or f.lux. Actual blue-blocking filters can be applied to screens. It will also help to turn brightness down and hold the screen farther from your face. Experts say that without a blue-blocking program you should stop using electronics two hours before you plan to fall asleep. Also limit the amount of time you spend using devices in the evening. One study showed that an hour of use had no significant impact on melatonin suppression, but after two hours the suppression level was significant.

Car lights and streetlights can also suppress melatonin. If you must drive at night before bed, you can purchase amber goggles. These can also be used in your home or while watching TV if you do that before bedtime. LED lighting is another culprit, although proximity to the eye is a large factor so small screens are usually singled out.

Chronic suppression of melatonin could have other health consequences, and these are amplified in patients with fibromyalgia who have other reasons for poor sleep including stiffness and pain. Reading printed material or using an e-reader that does not emit light such as certain Kindles is certainly a better solution. Tempting as it is to ignore these paragraphs, we advise that you do pay heed.

Self-treatment with over-the-counter medications should be used only for a short period of time. It's important to make sure that nothing you take will interact with any other medications you take. The over-the-counter sleep compounds are low doses of older antihistamines of which drowsiness was a side effect. They can cause things such as dry mouth, blurred vision, and weakness. Magnesium often helps with muscle relaxation but may cause diarrhea and nausea. It is often suggested that calcium be added to magnesium at bedtime to counteract the diarrhea. You will find more about medications for sleep in chapter 15.

Without medical reversal of fibromyalgia, everything gets even worse, including insomnia, and nocturnal tissue cleansing remains incomplete. During guaifenesin reversal, you'll still have to temporarily make do with whatever downtime you can muster. Making rest a priority and finding workable solutions to avoid unwanted wake cycles are essential for restoring your ability to cope on a daily basis. (See chapter 15 for guidance on getting better sleep.)

My insomnia started when I was a teenager. It got progressively worse over the years, particularly after an extreme reaction coming out of surgery. I almost lost my job. I had to take Remeron for four years to help me sleep, but later was able to wean myself off and start sleeping somewhat normally again. I did notice that during times of stress, I would hardly sleep at all. Not even strong sleep medications could put me to sleep. I thought I must be just plain crazy, as I had never had such bad anxiety along with the severe insomnia I was experiencing. I thought about suicide, but was always too scared to go through with it. A friend who was on the guaifenesin protocol convinced me to try it. I had heard of it, but didn't believe fibromyalgia was real or, if it was, that the solution could be so simple. I was wrong. Within two weeks on the protocol, my anxiety completely disappeared, and my insomnia began to improve. Sleeping medications began to work. After a year, I was down to 1 mg of Ativan, and now after two and a half years on the protocol, I only need Benadryl to help me sleep. I take 600 mg guaifenesin twice daily, and have been amazed at how much better I feel. Now I react to stress in a "normal" way, and a "bad night" of sleep is getting only six hours! I can honestly say that learning the TRUTH about fibromyalgia has both physically and mentally healed me. I realize my story is a bit more extreme than others, but please don't take the chance of getting to where I was before you believe in this protocol.

—*Christie B., Clovis, California*

TAKE WARM BATHS

I recently spent a week at my mother-in-law's apartment in New York City. Because the shower had variable temperatures in the space of a few minutes, I couldn't deal with it, so I took a bath. I was immediately sold on the idea because it made me stop and relax and also made my muscles feel much better. I vowed to make the time for at least one bath a week, and I do. Bubbles in the bath help me relax more because I can't see my body and it's like being in a cloud.

—*Valerie, Nevada*

Hot or warm baths will soothe sore muscles or joints and ease the aching pains of the FMS day. They're relaxing and may help you fall asleep—though not in the tub, please! Epsom salts, powdered milk, cornstarch, or mineral or emu oil can be added to the water. Do not use the oils if your skin doesn't need them, but buttermilk and powdered goat's or cow's milk contain a gentle exfoliator called lactic acid. It can also help to soothe irritation, and is a mild, nongreasy moisturizer. Oatmeal can be added if you suffer from itchy skin. If you have dry, itchy, or irritated skin, remember to use warm water rather than hot. Turn off or dim as many lights as possible to set a pleasant atmosphere in the bathroom or bedroom.

Heavy fragrances should always be avoided, especially in bath products. Even if you can tolerate the smell, the added chemicals can irritate the skin and even make it difficult to relax. Some patients report that a mildly scented candle is a wonderful addition to this quiet time, although others find any amount of scent annoying. If you have noisy children or a spouse who enjoys loud TV, play a relaxation tape or quiet relaxing music to make your bath more soothing.

Warm showers work best in the morning. That's when you must loosen muscles that stiffened during the night, yet not get so relaxed that you want to go back to bed. Baths do their best work at night, showers in the morning. Body lotions designed for use in the shower can do double duty in the bath and will soften and moisturize your skin for the entire day. They also help calm the itchy skin so common in fibromyalgia—but be sure to avoid products with fragrances, which can be irritating.

If you have long hair, wear a shower cap. It will keep you from having to wash and style your hair each day. Many (in fact most) dry shampoos on the market are salicylate-free. This alone can save a lot of energy. Holding up your arms to style your hair— well, you know that some days you just can't manage it.

UNDERSTAND YOUR DEPRESSION

The fact is that FMS is a potentially debilitating inherited illness that not only affects our entire bodies but is progressive. It is nothing to take lightly and nothing that can be fixed with an antidepressant. I just had one of the best years of my life, am very active, very happy even with this illness, and yet my physician wanted to put me on an antidepressant to ward off hot flashes. Ridiculous. No way will I subject my brain to a mind-altering substance when I am very happy with my brain. I have had to take charge of my own health when it comes to fibromyalgia.

It's my body and my decision.

—*Jody D., North Carolina*

A certain amount of depression and frustration is considered normal with chronic illness. Most patients instinctively understand and don't want to take medication for it. Antidepressants certainly have a place in serious depression, but as we've seen, they have effects on the body that are less than desirable if there are other choices. Depression is one of the most common complications of chronic illness, and about a third of people with medications struggle with symptoms.

Try a few tricks to coax your brain out of a funk while you're waiting for guaifenesin's benefits. Easier said than done, but you can trick the brain to fend off some of the facets of your depressing thoughts. It's perfectly normal to chafe against your limitations, mourn losses, and feel sad at being deprived of the stamina to do what you used to do. Yet you can find new activities to replace some lost ones and, in less demanding ways, spend time with those you love. Overcoming such obstacles to enjoy quality of life will certainly contribute to your well-being. You can regain your self-confidence, and guaifenesin can give you a sense of hope for the future that you've been missing.

Depression in fibromyalgia may stem from feeling defeated in trying to meet some unrealistic standards, self-imposed at home or work. It is often the result of feelings of inadequacy and helplessness. You may miss the social interactions and spontaneity of your pre-sickness life. It is easy to fall into a rut where depression becomes chronic and takes over your life.

Recognizing your limitations is a good place to start and might help you cope as you are able to examine and erase self-inflicted rules. Concentrating energy on doing what you do best helps immensely and should be a goal. To do this, you must often find ways to unburden yourself from tasks you dislike, such as housework. But even then, there are often parts of work you do around your home that give you satisfaction and a sense of accomplishment that you can still do and do better if you are able to let other things go.

When it comes to housework, you're not alone: Women and often men say that looking around their unkempt homes puts them into an immediate tantrum. If the deplorable state of your house is a major cause of your anguish, put changing this at the top of your priority list. Lower your standards, and remember that most people with children and busy lives don't themselves live in magazine-picture-perfect rooms. We've addressed this, but get outside help if you can afford it. If being in an imperfect home is that depressing to you, paying for a little help should take precedence over less important things.

Worth thinking about if you need extra income to pay for help doing routine tasks that weigh you down is using your talents to supplement your income. For most people, doing things they are good at is a depression fighter. For example, if you're adept at sewing, you might earn extra money to help pay for a cleaning helper. Embroidering school and club uniforms or costumes might be right up your alley. Holiday tablecloths or place mats might be sold at craft fairs or online, or be accepted for sale by small boutique stores. You can save money if you make presents of your wares. Besides just earning compliments for your skills, some recipients and their friends might offer to pay you for similar productions. You don't know until you put it out there.

Exercise is a fantastic way of fighting depression and feeling blah. Simply getting out for a walk can really make a difference. Walking to or sitting outside in a park, weather permitting, is a great change of pace. If you live in an area where year-round out-door exercise isn't a good option, check with local indoor shopping centers to see if they have a mall-walking program. Joining an exercise class at the YMCA or a local recreation department (many have programs tailored for arthritis) can get you out of the house, and you may even make some new friends. Curves is a franchise popular with women who have fibromyalgia because the workout can be adapted to the day's stamina. It's also inexpensive, and if you have Medicare and supplementary insurance, it may well be free. Other insurances and Medicare Advantage plans offer other options.

Search the internet for what's available near you. Many neighborhoods have small gyms that may not have the latest fanciest equipment you'll never use but do have quiet hours that make them appealing to us.

Water exercise classes are helpful, especially for patients who are overweight and may have joint issues. Here, too, you will find many classes for seniors or patients with chronic pain. Remember that any kind of exercise will trigger your feel-good endorphins, and don't forget to check with your insurance to see if they will cover costs. Many offer programs for patients with pain, stiffness, or arthritis, especially with a letter from your physician.

Obviously, these are suggestions for the depression that arises from living with a chronic pain condition. If you struggle with serious, clinical depression, be sure to work with your doctor. But if you're stuck in a rut and blue—we hope these ideas will start you thinking.

JOIN A SUPPORT GROUP OR START YOUR OWN

Be careful. There are some groups claiming to be support groups that are actually venting grounds. That is, the people in the group do little more than moan and groan about what a lousy hand life has dealt them. A little venting is good for the soul and the health of everyone. But if the entire discussion is centered on moaning and groaning, it will drag you down into the depths of negativity. Avoid negative groups.

—*Devin J. Starlanyl,* The Fibromyalgia Advocate[1]

Communicating with other fibromyalgics is very comforting. It hauls you out of isolation, and quite likely, you may help others in the process. If you're looking for an in-person group, that's a bit tricky because face-to-face support groups are giving way to online groups, including many on Facebook. These work well for patients with fibromyalgia because they often don't feel well enough to get dressed or drive across town. There's an online group available for the guaifenesin protocol, which you can access from www.fibromyalgiatreatment.com. There are other groups on the internet that feature the guaifenesin protocol, but not all promulgate accurate information. Though they may offer friendships and support, be sure to check any information they disseminate with what is on our website and in this book. We are not affiliated with any other groups despite the fact that some do use our names and information.

If you live in a large city, you may find more than one fibromyalgia support group. If you live in a smaller area, you should search for chronic pain or arthritis groups if you don't find something specific for fibromyalgia. Local newspapers publish calendars with schedules of groups dedicated to helping various medical conditions. Health care providers who deal with fibromyalgia may know of a group. Local hospitals are another resource; they often have meeting rooms used by local support groups.

Visit each and select the one that gives you positive feelings. Ideally, a group serves two functions. First, it should afford members a venue for expressing feelings and releasing frustrations. Unfortunately, this is where too many of them stop. Meetings are full of sad stories strongly accentuated with moans and groans, week after week. Tales of pains, failed therapies, and poor spousal and family support are part of each person's litany. It sounds like a competition for who's the worst off! These are negative organizations. Forget them! You're already low enough emotionally. The second thing you want from a support group is dedication to improving the quality of its members' lives. It should be a forum for suggestions that help you cope with daily functions. Members can share resources and information about fibromyalgia, good care providers, and ways to make day-to-day life easier. Some even organize car pools, shared child care, or potluck meals. They do just what the name implies—offer support for members. When one individual isn't feeling well, others will come to the rescue. Helping with household chores, doing a little shopping for you while doing their own—just a few practical things that an understanding friend can provide. Loneliness is terrible, but your life brightens when you call a buddy and speak to an empathetic ear.

> I call people by the wrong name. I called my new daughter-in-law by her sister's name and then a few weeks later I called her by my own sister-in-law's name. It's embarrassing. I must come across as a total idiot to a lot of people in those situations when I can't recall the simplest things; fumble, drop, and spill things; and ricochet off walls and doorways.
>
> But I've learned that when I'm in a group of people who share my experiences, that all falls away. It is so wonderful to know that everyone there understands exactly what I'm talking about and why I can't remember my own name or what day it is, and there is so much warmth and acceptance that I can soak it up and coast on it for a long time afterwards.
>
> —*Anne Louise, Minnesota*

If no acceptable support group exists in your area, consider starting one of your own. We must stress *acceptable*. Many of our patients have gone to more than a few and left disenchanted. Discussions too often center on a new pain pill, sleeping potion, antidepressant, "my doctor said," and the hot new herbal concoction of the day. You're far better off with a guaifenesin support group devoted to a single protocol designed to heal you, not simply applying patches to your symptoms.

Starting an organization is not an enormous task, so don't be frightened at this thought. As with everything else, simplicity is the notion of the day. You can start by getting together regularly with a fibromyalgic friend or two. You'll be amazed how quickly that sprouts into a sizable group, although there are benefits to keeping your group small. Once under way, work on constructive things: Discuss the protocol and where to find good salicylate-free products; collect simple recipes and helpful tips for improving the quality of your lives. We've included it a number of times in these pages, but once more, here's the website: fibromyalgiatreatment.com. Claudia and the administrative team are dyed-in-the-wool guaifenesin protocol supporters and totally knowledgeable about the disease and our treatment. The same website will keep you up to date on any new research and information that will help you.

I have been on guai for about seven years. I am so much better. I remember when I first started cycling; the depression hit me so hard. I was in a craft store with my mother and I just started bawling. That was about a month into the protocol. I just felt so much sadness for no reason. I felt overwhelmed with sad emotions and I couldn't explain them.

Things are so much better now—but I still cycle my brain. It's my worst symptom and sometimes it's hard to realize that's what's going on. Keep on keeping on and you will see the light!

—*Pam S., Pennsylvania*

GET SOME EXERCISE

After months of being bedridden and unable to leave my house, the very thought of standing up and stretching or going for a walk was painful. But I had to do it. I started slowly. I began with gentle stretches while lying down. Then I was ready to start walking. My house made a small circle inside, and I decided that I would start there. The best part about it was that I didn't even need to change into exercise clothing. I could wear my jammies. Each day, I made moving my goal. Get up. Stretch. Walk. Repeat. Get up. Stretch. Walk. Repeat. I celebrated the small victories with each minute I added. Eventually, my routine included sneakers, workout gear, and a pedometer that would track my minutes to miles. Walking in circles is my daily norm. Find your daily norm and embrace it. Gentle exercise is the key. The more you move, the better your muscles will feel and the more energy you will have.

—*Chantal H., Michigan*

We've already beat this into the ground, but it's important to remember that only one thing has been proved over and over in countless studies to help control the symptoms of fibromyalgia. Not reverse the disease like your guaifenesin will do, but rather lead to feeling better in the short term, with long term benefits, too. As your fibromyalgia improves, you'll want to be in the best physical shape you can be to enjoy it. If you put off exercising until you are well, you'll have to tackle getting back into shape then. So why not start by taking small steps now? And you can. No matter how daunting it sounds, you absolutely can. There's no doubt even modest exercising will make you feel better. We discussed this fairly extensively in the previous section. Besides improving pain thresholds, releasing endorphins, and rebuilding mitochondria, exercise has a positive effect in relieving depression.

In this high-tech age, we often forget how simple things can be. Exercise doesn't require fancy-colored tight-fitting designer togs, shiny equipment, hundred-dollar shoes, or a racing bike. You don't need to join a gym or even buy weights that match your leotards and sweatbands. The sight of well-toned athletes working out with huge resistance equipment is intimidating and looks too hard to try. The reality is that very few people look that good. Most of us don't have those perfect bodies or the money to buy fashionable outfits just for exercise. Many more people stay healthy by taking long, peaceful walks, especially with a companion, human or canine.

You can begin early in the treatment, but go easy and start out moderately. Ambitious jump starts are predictors of certain defeat. You can begin by walking around the block or gently stretching on your living room floor with a computer program, DVD, or book to guide you. Some of these are designed particularly for fibromyalgics, and you can find them on the internet. You'll appreciate hints that help you recognize and abide by your own limits of tolerance.

Exercise should never be done when your muscles are cold or tired. Do some mild stretching, or take a warm-up walk, even a warm shower before you begin. In her book *The Fibromyalgia Advocate*, Devin Starlanyl offers an excellent rule of thumb for evaluating an exercise program: "If mild soreness disappears after the first day, you can repeat it on the second day. If it persists to the second day, postpone any exercise until the third day. If soreness persists on the third day, your exercise routine must be changed. This rule of thumb is true for any treatment, such as massage or electrical stimulation."

I started slow, walking around the block. One day I walked five blocks to buy a lottery ticket (hope blooms eternal) and five blocks back. It almost did me in, but I survived. Now I can walk to the grocery store, and if I am too fatigued, I take the bus partway to save a few blocks. It's like Claudia once said—you will be in pain whether you are home or not. You will be worn out at home or you can get out and be just as tired. Sometimes it is like I am moving in a fog but at least I am moving. A few times I've called my friend in San Diego on my cell phone and the walk doesn't seem as long because we are talking the whole time.

—Janice, Minnesota

For those who prefer structured programs, an internet search or an organization such as the Arthritis Foundation will direct you to those that meet your needs. If available, an aquatic program is often the easiest and has been shown in studies to be as beneficial as walking. It's designed for those with limited mobility and empowered by enlisting the soothing buoyancy of warm water. There are beginner group workouts that offer exercise in class-like settings. They're not hard to find. One secret is to join a class designed for senior citizens; the pace is usually slower. However, if getting out of the house, driving to a local pool, changing into a suit (and getting there on time and with regularity) sounds like more than you can do now, save it for when you start to feel better. Getting out of the house and exercising in the group are beneficial when you are ready to do them.

The key is to make it as easy as possible for yourself. The value of any exercise is determined by the number of people who stick with that particular modality. We encourage patients to keep searching until they find a regimen they can enjoy and tolerate that fits into their schedule and routine. Yoga, Pilates, tai chi, and other disciplines all have advocates. The consensus is: Carefully graduated workouts that avoid overdoing things progressively promote energy and a wonderful sense of well-being. You should plan to do more as you feel better—you have no idea how good this will feel!

After about three months on the guai, I decided to try exercising on my stationary bike again...I have found that when I am really hurting, if I ride the bike for at least fifteen minutes, the pain begins to ease up. It is really hard to convince myself to get started when it hurts to even walk, let alone really exercise. But the benefits are worth it. Evenings are my worst times, and I find that if I ride my bike for about thirty minutes just before bedtime, I get rid of a lot of my pain and become very relaxed. This promotes a good sleep that often leads to a better day afterward.

—*Marilyn J., North Carolina*

TRY MASSAGE AND MANUAL THERAPIES

I have had pain all my life but was told it was growing pains. I have chronic back pain at times so severe I can't function. The muscle spasms are so bad it feels like I have ropes in my back. This was much worse during pregnancy. I discovered then that if I roll on a tennis ball in the areas where it felt just like knots, it would make the pain radiate somewhere else or it hurt right where it was, but either way it always felt better. What I have read tells me I am actually rubbing on trigger points.

—*Liz, Kentucky*

Bodywork and *manual therapy* are general terms that refer to manipulation of the body (by a licensed practitioner) to aid in relaxation and to relieve pain. Massage is the most common form of manual therapy. Manual therapy is a little different. It uses teaching and techniques to help patients who position their bodies unnaturally because of pain and stiffness. The aim of all the different forms of therapy is to reposition the body and allow for pain relief by more natural movement and posture. This reduces stress on the body and, in turn, eases pain.

When it comes to massage, practically no one discounts the soothing power of human hands. Yet there are hypersensitive people who cannot tolerate being touched. If you're one of these, you know it and can skip this section until you feel it becomes applicable to you. For most people, trained therapists who understand fibromyalgia and use gentle massage can temporarily ease muscular pains and pacify jangled nerves. As long as you both bear in mind that the benefits are transient, you'll do fine.

Carefully avoid deep tissue work and stay away from deep tissue massage—these techniques will increase pain. Rolfing in particular is a form of deep tissue massage that applies a great deal of pressure to muscles and can even leave bruising. The wrong kind of massage can bring immediate pain that may last for days. While it is occurring, you won't realize until much later how badly you've been hurt. Make sure that any practitioner you visit understands fibromyalgia. Read printed material about the proposed treatment before you submit to it and be sure it's appropriate for your condition. Do not be afraid to speak up if something is painful or doesn't feel right. Bear in mind that the lumps and bumps of fibromyalgia can't be jackhammered out by using bare-knuckled attacks. That can cause tissue damage and greatly disturb already distressed structures.

Some patients get relief from acupuncture, and many medical researchers support its benefits. As with chiropractic approaches, investigators have found little lasting benefit. Feeling better for a few better hours or days is wonderful and should not be discounted, but will not improve your fibromyalgia. Ask your doctor and support group for recommendations if you don't know where to start.

Chiropractors treat the body as a connected system and strive to adjust your skeletal structure back into balance through adjustments, manipulations, and stretches to relieve pain. Many are very adept at diagnosing fibromyalgia, especially when they discover that their adjustments don't hold for as long as expected. Several studies have shown chiropractic care to be helpful to relieve some pain and discomfort. Discuss with your doctor about whether you might be helped by this. Then be sure to search out a doctor of chiropractic who understands the unique symptoms your body presents.

When using chiropractic services or acupuncture, make it absolutely clear that you cannot use herbal products offered as medications or on the skin. Even though you think you've explained this thoroughly, be vigilant to make sure that you were understood and that your practitioners comply. Ask to personally see the list of the ingredients of any product used on your body. Do not take a practitioner's word for something being "salicylate-free."

Highly endorsed by fibromyalgics is the Feldenkrais Method. In a series of lessons, patients are taught how to integrate their body movements so they can function with less effort and pain. Instructions are individually structured as a series of altogether smooth and gentle activities. Similar disciplines such as the Alexander Technique, Trager approach, and Bowen Therapy also have staunch supporters, but our experience with these is minimal. To be honest, any type of stretching and movement done regularly will help your body. You will have additional benefits from some training that will show you better and less stressful ways to move and position your body.

YOGA AND PILATES

We all know by now that exercise is a crucial component to health and to managing fibromyalgia symptoms. But for people who are very deconditioned and ill, exercise as we commonly think of it—gyms, biking, and running—is impossible, and if it is attempted, results in a flare of more pain, fatigue, and even worse sleep. But two very popular forms of therapy can be very helpful and quite often are taught together: yoga and Pilates.

Pilates was developed as a means of rehabilitation and strengthening by developing a strong "core." Fibromyalgia exercises can be performed sitting in a chair, standing, or lying on a mat.

Yoga teaches mind and body awareness, including both muscle stretching and strengthening and meditation as well as breathing exercises that will help with relaxation. You can find many resources on the internet for patients with chronic pain and even specifically with fibromyalgia. Practicing gentle stretching, strengthening, and relaxation helps improve your ability to move throughout the day with less pain and fatigue. Once your body is strengthened and helped by these non-aerobic exercises, you can move on to what's described in the section on exercise in this book.

After any kind of treatment, except massage, plan on resting. Your body has just had a significant workout. If your muscles are already getting tight, take a warm shower to relax them.

Unfortunately, the above therapeutic approaches can be expensive. Not every patient has insurance coverage, and even sound, hands-on treatment is often rejected as unnecessary. Medical insurance carriers usually regard massage as a luxury except following an accident, and not for extended periods. However frustrating this is, it will help to accept when you understand that these modalities will, at best, provide only brief comfort, and that none of these disciplines is required for healing. Yoga and Pilates may be taught at local recreation centers, libraries, and other places. You can also purchase DVDs for use at home, some even tailored for patients with fibromyalgia.

There are colleges of massage therapy that charge much smaller fees than do the professionals. I had my second visit at my local school and I am still sold on the idea. I even took my sisters-in-law and the four of us got in on a two-for-one special: $10 a person! They are now sold on the idea, too. One important note: Although there may be one main address for the school, there are often additional locations of that school in different cities in your state. Take Utah, for example—there is one school, but it has three different locations throughout the state. Contact the schools in your state for more information on additional locations.

—*Sharon H., Utah*

DO SOMETHING YOU LOVE EVERY DAY

I used to put "baking cookies with my son" on my list almost every week because we would talk while we were cooking, and he loved that. I would tell him about when I was a little girl and how I used to watch my mother bake, and it made me happy to remember good things. If I did nothing else at all that day, at least I did that. I made a vow not to flog myself for what I could not do—not to sit and watch other mothers running after their kids and beat myself up anymore. Instead I focused on the tasks I had made for myself…and counted myself lucky when I could do them.

—*Cathy, California*

Most detrimental of all to your emotional health is to stop doing things that are important to you. You must somehow keep in touch with yourself and the person you were before fibromyalgia took over your entire being. That's hard to do when you feel so rotten—very hard. As the disease progresses, many people retract into some inner sanctuary that conserves strength only for essential activities that can't be shoved aside. Such a move is logical but ultimately counterproductive. Far better to streamline unavoidable chores by trimming wasted effort while still retaining everything that lends charm to life.

I found that there were activities I had stopped doing long ago, such as playing the piano and sewing, that really make me feel good…If I am sad or stressed, perhaps experiencing early warning signs of an approaching flare, I make sure to spend some time involved in such an activity. It makes me feel better and my life feels enriched.

—*Mary Ellen Copeland, coauthor,*
Fibromyalgia and Chronic Myofascial
Pain Syndrome[2]

Start by deciding what you really enjoy doing and what makes you feel good. You have to provide some time for your partner and children, but of similar importance, what do you particularly love to do? What makes you feel better? Possibly it's gardening, painting, reading, or solving crossword puzzles. Do you like strolling in the evening or just sitting quietly in the morning sun sipping a cup of coffee? Choose something so wonderful that it usually makes you lose track of time.

Make a list of all the things that were important to you when you still felt well enough to do them. If you love watching your son play soccer, jot it down. Logging on to a Facebook group that serves the needs of others may be to your liking; that's a major joy to include. Going to the library, art museums, concerts in the park...which of these pastimes do you miss? Many music schools and colleges provide plays and entertainment at reasonable prices in a less rigid setting. Maybe you haven't considered these lately. Maybe you don't recall the importance of just getting out of the house and out of yourself, even if it is just to sit on your deck in the sunshine.

Finish the list and get a calendar with unusually big spaces. For each day, make a simple entry. Write in what you plan to do for yourself. It might be working in the garden for whatever time you can safely expend, or going in the afternoon to watch your daughter practice softball. It could be a morning trip to a farmers market or making time to watch a movie you've been meaning to see. If it's an outdoor activity, have something you want to read or download a favorite movie or television show that always makes you laugh.

It's true that life isn't just made up of fun time. So you'll have to add a chore or two to the daily schedule. At least they also give the satisfaction of a mandatory job completed. Pick a single item for each day from your list: changing bedsheets, cleaning out the car, or organizing the refrigerator. Marketing and errands could be necessities for another day. Con yourself into thinking that vacuuming is part of your exercise program—which, by the way, new studies have determined that it is!

Every day, try with all your might to satisfy your plan. If you can muster the discipline, you'll start getting in touch with the wonderful person you were and still are. Even if no one else praises your effort, pat yourself on the back for the strides you've made. Life will be enriched and more meaningful to you. You'll subdue some of your recent demons and gain respect for your steadfast resolve. You're now a doer, not just a viewer. Mounting confidence will smooth your interactions with friends, family, and even doctors. Your new focus is on the road ahead, and you're now unstoppable on your drive to health.

Before I became symptomatic with fibro, I loved to dance. Ballroom, folk dance, belly dance, turning on the stereo and boogieing in the living room. Gradually, that became harder and harder (my pain is largely concentrated in my legs and hips). My goal is to be able to return to dancing, and the stories I read on this board give me hope that this will happen. I am working on strengthening my lower body muscles so that I can ease back into dancing again.

I hope my story will help any fibro sufferers who are struggling with the decision of beginning the protocol. What held me back was that it wasn't a quick fix; it could take years. But I read posts that showed me that there were benefits to be had along the way, that even a longtime sufferer could experience good days after a few months. That helped me get started. I have been extremely grateful for the stories others have shared here; at times they were an absolute lifeline.

—*Marti T., Ohio*

CONCLUSION

R. Paul St. Amand, MD
Associate Professor of Medicine
Endocrinology—Harbor/UCLA

Very many years ago I never thought there would be a "now." There was no sigh of relief when Claudia and I stuck a final period onto the first edition in 1999: The end was not in sight. Yet clairvoyance was confident that I would summate my doctoring life far earlier than this. Twenty years have elapsed between that then and this now. I might even reach my ninety-second year before this volume is published.

Please tolerate my having appended my academic title to this closing letter. It was earned over a sixty-two-year career on staff at my postgraduate alma mater, UCLA. I would like to think I merited it and that it was not gifted that simply. It did take a lot of continuing study and lots of polishing by my peer professors, chiefs, and research associates. Cumulative years have provided me ample moments to reflect on the huge corps of silent teachers I've needed to get this far. They will never be known to you. In their ranks are the countless authors who penned the overwhelming number of papers I've read in my cherished journals. Add erudite lecturers braving critical audiences at ever so many conferences. It's from no lapse of memory that I do not remember their names, but they all taught me.

Deeply embossed in my aged brain are shared discussions or

fleeting phrases I snatched in passing from my savant professor-colleagues. Patiently they shared their superior knowledge and allocated me time under their tutelage while we worked our clinics. Them I know well. Pensive faces of those living and dead are mine to keep, and they flash before me right now as I type. They buried me in great debt, one I know I shan't repay. It would be considered gauche if I dared whisper how much I've loved them all.

Unrewarded are the readers among you who might barely remember some unique contribution you made to what I presume to know. Far more of you who've been my patients have no idea how much you taught me. You complained, recited symptoms, jabbed me with questions even though too often I lacked answers. Could you possibly know you were teaching this sometimes insecure, would-be healer? I address these words to each of you because you too are among my revered, though unlisted, coauthors. I've happily accepted you into my collective teacher staff. I readily acknowledge how little could I have written in these pages without you and the professionals. But you were in the special group that gifted me with thanks and hugs. You even dared show me love.

I'm sure you guessed there would be words of accolade for my co-workers Claudia and Gloria. I seriously doubt they themselves long dwell on their impact in our mutual, professional lives. My teary nostalgia surfaces when, alone, I charm myself reminiscing about these unlicensed and unwitting practitioners of medicine. They've served alongside me for over thirty years. I smile whimsically when I think about their sometimes subtle, other times blatant lectures that sought to teach their subservient "boss." I ponder over so many dedicated years; so many calming words; so many admonishments to prod this reluctant internet-learner; so many times the need to flip him a life preserver and always just in time. There are countless among you who've profited from the advice and moments of conversation they've given you. You do see their respective roles on my teaching staff, don't you?

So why am I expending many words just to confirm how many skillful people and fellow sufferers it has taken to get you to this end dialogue? In gratitude, I belatedly offer praise and thanks to my aggregate teachers. Simultaneously, I'm trying to impress you, the reader, with how much we had to mine from collective skills to create these pages.

You, the new folks, have just labored through much print doing your best to decipher alien words. Did we possibly instruct you sufficiently to let you master fibromyalgia, hypoglycemia, and their fellow-traveler conditions? Have you mastered enough from these chapters to capture the protocol to your benefit? We'll continue in direct contact with many of you; others grace our unrelenting schedule. Remember that your failures would be ours. We pride ourselves you will get well. But our reserved concern is for those whom we cannot touch, actually or figuratively. Book in hand and internet in sight, they will be winging it alone.

Those of you who have not become hooked on narcotics are in luck. Adverse publicity and governmental edicts against promiscuous abuse of those drugs have greatly benefited you because of physician reluctance to prescribe such. That's a big plus, since you'll avoid the torture of future weaning.

Throughout this book, we've been writing about metabolism and how it has gone awry. By now you well realize that it can be perturbed from many directions. We've harped on fatigue from sickened mitochondria—very basic chemistry. You've learned about the microbiome and its jolly or punitive bacteria. You've word-skirmished with the metabolic syndrome. You've endured facts that made you wince a bit: Fats are friends—carbs are curses. We relented a bit by saying, *Don't die of frustration, nibble on one occasionally, but don't let those tasty morsels become part of your regular diet ever again.* You've been told that your chow does greatly affect you, and that salicylates are ubiquitous. It has taken far more than just a few short sentences to tie all of this mishmash together. We trust we've succeeded.

As of this writing, we're still hopeful there will arise a prominent spokesperson for fibromyalgia. Such a champion would need the ability to rouse and motivate enough individuals to action. From their followers would come funds necessary to finish current genetic work. Gene miscreants need to be exposed. Their effect on aberrant biochemistry would lead to the elusive blood test to facilitate diagnosis and serial follow-up of patients.

Quoting myself from our third edition: "Each of us who has conquered the disease owes something to those still sick. As wonderful as it is to get a person well, we remain saddened for those who will never learn about our protocol. As long as we receive emails and letters detailing lifelong struggles with pain, fatigue, and relationships, our victory is not complete and our job is not yet done. We hope this book will provide the initiating impetus for human chain letters. As you get well, you progressively incur a debt, and you should plan how to repay it. You can only do that by helping others who are still searching for the path you've already walked. Please, reach out and take someone by the hand."

Since I am unlikely to write a fifth edition, permit me to make a last request. Bring the others along, since there will be no Claudia, Gloria, or Paul St. Amand to drive the team. Do as Facebook and other internet aficionados are doing. Tell people to send pictures of products showing lists of ingredients that initially stump protocol newbies. Please take the lead until such time when versatile physicians can do so with a blood test.

Repeated waves of our virtual magic wand brought some wishes to fruition. Countless individuals are now bouncing sound advice off the cloud, helping to salvage the ailing. Progressively more people in foreign lands are doing the same using their internet highways. Funds permitting, several of the newly informed make the trek to us. They return home better equipped to rescue not only themselves, but also fellow citizens. We're aware of their successes as confirmed by others they refer to us. Our teaching army will surely cultivate ever more of the human crop that's thirsting for help. From those rehabilitated cripples will come new enlistees to grow the force. There are ongoing favorable reverberations; new get-well treaties to be signed, more non-alienated people who will learn what should be our motto: "Happiness is freedom from pain."

Those who say something can't be done should not interfere with those who are doing it.

Gratefully yours,
R. Paul St. Amand, MD

NOTES

Chapter 1. An Invitation to Join Us and Find Your Way Back to Health

1. Frederick Wolfe, "The Fibromyalgia Problem," *Journal of Rheumatology* 24, no. 7 (1997): 1247–49.
2. W. R. Gowers, "A Lecture on Lumbago: Its Lessons and Analogues," *British Medical Journal* 1 (1904): 117–21.
3. F. Wolfe, H. A. Smythe, and M. B. Yunus, "Criteria for the Classification of Fibromyalgia," *American College of Rheumatology* 33 (1990): 160–72.
4. F. Behm, I. Gavin, O. Karpenko, V. Lindgren, S. Gaitonde, P. Gashkoff and B. Gillis, "Unique Immunologic Patterns in Fibromyalgia," *BMC Clinical Pathology* 2012: 12–25.

Chapter 2. The Fibromyalgia Syndrome: An Overview of Symptoms and Causes

1. A. Bengtsson and K. G. Henriksson, "The Muscle in Fibromyalgia: A Review of Swedish Studies," *Journal of Rheumatology* 16, supplement 19 (November 1989): 144–49.

Chapter 3. Guaifenesin: How and Why It Works

1. *Physicians' Desk Reference* (Montvale, NJ: Medical Economics, 1999). Entry for Humibid, 1698.

2. C. M. Ramsdell, A. E. Postlewaite, and W. Kelley, "Uricosuric Effect of Glyceryl Guaiacolate," *Journal of Rheumatology* 1, no. 1 (1974): 114–16.

3. Julia Lawless, *The Encyclopedia of Essential Oils* (Lanham, MD: Barnes & Noble, 1992), 106.

4. *Physicians' Desk Reference for Herbal Medicines* (Montvale, NJ: Medical Economics, 1998).

5. *Physicians' Desk Reference* (Montvale, NJ: Medical Economics, 1999). Entry for Humibid, 1698.

Chapter 4. The Fly in the Ointment: Aspirin and Other Salicylates

1. *Science*, November 18, 1984.

2. A. R. Swain, S. P. Dutton, and A. S. Truswell, "Salicylates in Foods," *Journal of the American Dietetic Association* 85 (August 1998): 950–59.

Chapter 5. Patient Vindication

1. J. Feng, Z. Zhang, W. Li, X. Shen, W. Song, C. Yang, F. Chang, J. Longmate, C. Marek, R. P. St. Amand, T. G. Krontiris, J. E. Shively, and S. S. Sommer, "Missense Mutations in the MEFV Gene Are Associated with Fibromyalgia Syndrome and Correlate with Elevated IL-1 beta Plasma Levels," *PloS One* 4, no. 12 (December 30, 2009): e8480. doi: 10.1371/journal.pone.0008480.

Chapter 6. Hypoglycemia, Fibroglycemia, and Carbohydrate Intolerance

1. P. Genter and E. Ipp, "Plasma Glucose Thresholds for Counterregulation After an Oral Glucose Load," *Metabolism* 43, no. 1 (January 1994): 98–103.

Chapter 8. The Brain Symptoms: Chronic Fatigue and Fibrofog

1. Harvey Moldofsky, "Nonrestorative Sleep and Symptoms After a Febrile Illness in Patients with Fibrositis and Chronic Fatigue

Syndromes," *Journal of Rheumatology* 16, supplement 19 (1989): 150–53.

Chapter 11. Genitourinary Syndromes

1. J. J. Yount and J. J. Willems, "New Direction in Medical Management of Vulvar Vestibulitis," *Vulvar Pain Newsletter* (Fall 1994): 5–7.

Chapter 15. Medical Band-Aids: Currently Promoted Treatments for Fibromyalgia—What You Don't Know Can Hurt You

1. Frederick Wolfe, "The Fibromyalgia Problem," *Journal of Rheumatology* 24, no. 7 (1997): 1247–49.
2. Don L. Goldenberg, "A Review of the Role of Tricyclic Medications in the Treatment of Fibromyalgia Syndrome," *Journal of Rheumatology* 16, supplement 19 (1989): 137–40.
3. Marcia Angell and Jerome P. Kassirer, "Alternative Medicine: The Risks of Untested and Unregulated Remedies," *New England Journal of Medicine* 339, no. 12 (September 17, 1998): 839–41.

Chapter 16. Coping with Fibromyalgia: What Will Help While Guaifenesin Helps Your Body Heal?

1. Devin J. Starlanyl, *The Fibromyalgia Advocate* (Oakland, CA: New Harbinger Publications, 1998), 227.
2. Devin J. Starlanyl and Mary Ellen Copeland, *Fibromyalgia and Cronic Myofascial Pain Syndrome: A Survival Manual* (Oakland, CA: New Harbinger Publications, 1996), 161.

INDEX